ALIVE
AND
WELL

ALIVE
AND
WELL

YOUR SURVIVAL GUIDE
FOR THE HEALTH CARE APOCALYPSE

Martha Howard, M.D.

of Wellness Associates of Chicago

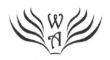

Produced by
www.alvinwriter.com

Cover & Interior Design and Layout
Jiyas Suministrado-Morales

Editing
Frances Ibañez
Alvin Ramirez

This book is dedicated to my husband, children, grandchildren, parents, and grandparents.

ADVANCE PRAISE

At last, a readable, informative and practical guide to help you through the maze of questions and options concerning healthy life choices. Dr. Howard explains historically how we have come to our current medical crossroads and presents a more natural approach to improved health and well-being for body, mind and spirit, rather than the health industry's obsession with pills as the "final answer." I especially love Part 2—a "dictionary" of chronic illnesses with natural solutions, followed by preventive measures to maintain a healthy lifestyle. This is a medical guidebook that should be in everyone's personal medical reference library.

— **Alice Nixon**, L.C.S.W., CEO, Brain Breakthrough www.brainbreakthrough.com

Dr. Howard makes feeling better, feel oh so good. If it wasn't for Dr. Howard diagnosing my dairy allergy, I might still be suffering from migraine headaches and dry eyes. Traditional doctors couldn't find a solution except to prescribe heavy duty drugs. And they said I might have a very complex "autoimmune disease" called mixed connective tissue disease. Why didn't they suggest a simple IgG test which tests for 90 foods like Dr. Howard did? What a relief to find out that it was food allergies and not a mysterious autoimmune disease or incurable migraines. Shortly after Dr. Howard diagnosed me correctly, I felt so good that I decided to learn to ride a motorcycle and went on a motorcycle trip through Morocco. Can you imagine someone with migraines and dry eyes doing that? The combination of eliminating dairy from my diet (and later gluten) plus acupuncture treatment and Chinese Herbs has worked wonders. Thanks to Dr. Howard, I've been headache-free for 24 years and my general health and wellness continues to be great.

— Deborah Chapman

Dr. Martha Howard has put together an informative, persuasive guide that empowers us to take control of our own health. *Alive and Well: Your Survival Guide for the Health Care Apocalypse* lifts the veil on what Dr. Howard calls the "Five Horsemen of the Apocalypse"—the major players in our nation's health care system. Not only does her book reveal the systems and policies that are making us sick, it is filled with scientific evidence and clinical examples about effective strategies for making ourselves well. This book could impact generations to come.

— Ruth Buczynski, PhD, licensed psychologist, president of The National Institute for the Clinical Application of Behavioral Medicine

Maybe like you, I was "fairly" healthy and didn't really pay much attention to any of that... I was very busy! Then, I noticed I didn't feel very well, didn't have much energy and was in pain all the time. They called my disease fibromyalgia; it had no cure. Luckily, I was referred to Dr. Howard. Not only did she cure the "incurable" with protocols like she provides in her book, she also gave me information about making healthier choices: her DOs. I absolutely know her experience (it's in the book!) has added many quality years to my life.

The book teaches self-care, making wise choices, gives information to assist in finding appropriate (reliable and knowledgeable) care and provides great options for making healthy changes all on your own. Without the information provided, I would never, either have understood the huge impact environmental sensitivities and food additives were having on my well-being. They were really dragging me down. After I got Dr. Howard's input, made some changes, that's all better, too!

Spending time with the book is just like having time with an exceptional friend, it is always about becoming more; it is focused, very clear, straightforward and often humorous. Every time I read it, there's always something new: I learn more about the systems in which we are so enmeshed, the diseases so many have (they believe with no cure), and other ways, perspectives and points of view to help my life be healthier and more sustainable.

Doctor Howard's practice has been a perfect proving ground for the invaluable information in her book. With her skills of observation, true care for her thousands of patients, coupled with her open-minded dedication to science and discovery, the information she offers is not only deep, it is also proven and, most of all, it is practical.

To sum it all up: I enjoy and use Dr. Howard's valuable information. I count on it. It works! I cannot recommend her book more highly... it is a treasure to use and a joy to give to others.

— Jan Cross

I have known Dr. Howard for 30 years. She is an excellent doctor who has helped many thousands of patients. Dr. Howard is a very keen observer of the medical-industrial complex and understands its strengths and weaknesses. She knows when the medical system can help, and when it can't. This book outlines a path to get healthier and stay healthy. It is also a guide for improving or reversing chronic illness while avoiding the toxicities of current allopathic remedies. Her advice is practical, affordable, and not influenced by the profit machines of either the pharmaceutical or supplement industries. There is much wisdom in these pages, and very helpful suggestions for a better, healthier life.

— Chris O. Costas, M.D., F.A.C.P
Chairman, Department of Infectious Diseases
Presence St. Francis Hospital, Evanston, IL

I love this book! Here's a doctor who is a wellness wonder-worker rather than a pill pusher. *Alive and Well, Your Survival Guide for the Health Care Apocalypse* tells you exactly how the food, health, pharmaceutical, and agricultural industries are making you sick, aided expertly by the political "industry." Even better, this book gives you a blueprint of what you need to do to stay well. And it's not about just diet and exercise—it has much more about the true foundations of good health: stress-busting methods, resilience-building, community connection, and spiritual support. Of course, my favorite stress reliever is laughter. You will want to know what Dr. Howard's book says about laughter and your health, and to put it into action immediately!

— Loretta LaRoche
Internationally Acclaimed Stress Expert, Humorist, Author, Speaker and TV personality

FOREWORD

I am a veteran investigative reporter and medical reporter. My stories in the Chicago Sun-Times led to the American Medical Association selling off tobacco stocks held by its Physicians Retirement Fund and the AMA president selling his tobacco farm in Georgia. Other stories on ethical and financial breaches led to the AMA firing two CEOs and seven other top executives. The fox is guarding the henhouse.

But you don't need to be an investigative reporter to know our medical and food industries are a mess, and neither one puts patient interests first. As a patient, a parent and a citizen, I can see firsthand that we are in trouble. Our collective and individual health is in jeopardy.

Martha Howard, MD, the author of "Alive and Well: Your Survival Guide for the Health Care Apocalypse," and an old friend of mine, points out in her book that we are in the middle of a healthcare apocalypse. She explains what has gone wrong and why. She helps you understand the system, which will help you navigate your way through this maze.

But Dr. Howard also addresses the common ailments that affect us. She does not take a pill-for-every-ill approach. Rather, she is among the pioneers who take an ecological approach to healthcare, considering the inflammatory effects of disease—often impacted by the foods that we eat and the air that we breathe. She tells us how diet, exercise, environmental clean-up in our homes, stress reduction and a few (not too many!) nutritional supplements can help us control and potentially reverse what ails us.

Martha took a personal interest when I was diagnosed with type 2 diabetes in summer 2017. She sent me the chapter on diabetes that you are about to read. It was clear, easy-to-read and informative—just what I needed when I was so vulnerable as a new diabetic.

She offered me advice and support. It helped tremendously. Within six months, I had reversed the course of diabetes. I saw an endocrinologist who said I should frame my glucose readings—the best he'd seen in years—and put them on my refrigerator (an apt place). He told me I likely could "cure" my disease and get off the diabetes med I was taking.

Dr. Howard offers similar support and advice in her book to readers coping with many common diseases, such as heart disease, arthritis, depression, irritable bowel syndrome, insomnia, and many other illnesses. I can't promise you a "cure" with this book and neither does she. Be cautious of anyone who ever does. But read Dr. Howard's science-based advice with an open mind. Know that help is on the way.

Dr. Howard's ecological approach takes into consideration not only food but exercise, stress reduction and the development of resilience and community ties. She follows traditional Chinese medical practice of "treating the root of disease," not just the symptoms. She aims to protect not only the patient but also the planet. That's holistic medicine to the nth degree.

Get ready. This book could alter your health and life—for the better.

— **Howard Wolinsky**
Flossmoor, Illinois
January 2018

Howard Wolinsky is co-author with Tom Brune of "The Serpent onthe Staff: The Unhealthy Politics of the American Medical Association." He also is co-author with his wife Judi Wolinsky of the best-selling "Healthcare Online for Dummies."

DISCLAIMER

This book is intended as a reference only. It is not a medical manual. It is not intended as a substitute for any diagnoses or treatments that may have been prescribed by your doctor. If you suspect that you have a medical problem, we urge you to seek competent medical help.

Mention of specific companies, organizations, or authorities in this book does not imply endorsement by the author or publisher, nor does mention of specific companies, organizations, or authorities imply that they endorse the book, its author, or the publisher. The author has no financial connection with any products mentioned. Internet addresses and telephone numbers given in this book were accurate at the time it went to press.

Copyright 2018 by Martha H. Howard, M.D.

TABLE OF CONTENTS

Part II: Chronic Illness—What's Making You Sick and What You Can Do About It

Part III: Preventive Health Care Strategies

Recipes

INTRODUCTION

Ever wonder why you're suddenly sneezing when it's not "allergy season"? Having stomach cramps after guzzling milk? Waking at 3 o'clock every morning, mind racing with worries, pulse heightened, and can't get back to sleep? Not sleeping because your partner is snoring? Feeling heavy, exhausted, uninspired before you've even begun your day, so you reach for a 5-hour energy shot before downing your usual pot of coffee with vanilla-flavored creamer? Popping B12 vitamins like mad? Discovering your socks have left indentations around your ankles after sitting at your desk all day and realizing you neglected to take a walk during your lunch break because you were wolfing down your ham-and-cheese on rye with extra mayo while continuing to work because you're a multitasker and that report was due at 1:00 p.m., the conference call was at 1:15, and now you've got your volunteer gig after work and the grocery shopping and then your two kids have soccer games simultaneously at opposite ends of the city?

If any of the above sounds familiar, or if your version of these struggles differs, let's admit it. We're human beings, and one of our best defenses is denial. In the rush of life, it's a lot easier to ignore what's going on with our health and just keep "dancing as fast as we can."

Here's the thing. Have we come to accept this rush through life in a not-so-healthy state as the norm? While all of this is going on—people not sleeping; people crouched over desks in cubes with flickering fluorescent lights buzzing overhead, wolfing down soggy lunches because of deadlines; people coughing and sneezing, feeling tired all the time, or trying to ignore that stomach pain. Are we settling for "this is as good as it gets"?

And even when we don't settle for the "background fog of ill health" as the norm, and try to do something about it, are we being ignored or dismissed?

Let's say you're feeling sick again, but you just saw your doctor and you were told it was your "usual" irritable bowel syndrome? Or they might have said that it was probably just "inflammation" and you might want to take an anti-inflammatory drug for a few days.

Is it possible that what your doctor may be dismissing as "inflammation," "irritable bowel syndrome," "acid reflux," or "chronic sinusitis" could be your body's reaction to a common food sitting in your fridge or pantry—something you eat daily without a second thought? Or a common indoor air pollutant like your fabric softener, your plug-in air "freshener" or the fire- retardant chemicals riding on your household dust? It's just not enough to give your set of symptoms a label and write a prescription.

The purpose of this book is to help you dig yourself out of the piles of confusion and disinformation that surround the effects that your food, activity, environment, and your mental and emotional states can have on your well-being and move forward to a healthier life.

I almost chose to write under a pen name, because this book is not about me. It is about you—staying alive and well despite the many hidden (and some not-so-hidden) factors that are affecting your health. I have always told the people who come to see me that, above all, I am a source of information. What they do with the information is their decision. I believe that health care providers need to stop trying to "fix" people and instead form a partnership, giving them what they need to know to help themselves. And I believe in working with information from reliable, scientific sources. Recently, more of these sources are scientific studies from countries like Denmark or Sweden who still have health care research establishments that are not compromised by profit-driven politics. But there is still good research being done in this country as well. That said, if you are someone who regards only double-blind studies as evidence—no matter how compromised by financial conflicts of interest they may be and dismisses all clinical evidence as "anecdotal"—no matter how compelling it may be, then this book may not be for you.

I recognize that staying alive and well is increasingly difficult here in the United States because of the past 60 years of food industry and health care industry history. There are limits to individual solutions because of the institutional nature of the problems. More than a half century of chickens raised with antibiotics, fed with pesticide-laden grains, and penned in chicken prisons have come home to roost. We have food deserts, and a junk food epidemic.

On the up side, some of those roosting chickens are becoming healthier. There has already been some change in the way many chickens are raised because of the demand for antibiotic- and hormone-free organic chickens. There are at least a few food trucks in the city food deserts and an urban farming movement. There is an increasing move toward organic whole food, rather than junk. Large grocery store chains have had to begin offering organic foods to be competitive in the market. One state, Vermont, has even reorganized its whole agricultural and food marketing system with a farm-to-table initiative that began in 2011.

However, our own creative solutions are being opposed by food industry hucksterism. And there have been deliberate, repeated political attempts to destroy health care and health insurance in the United States. We have seen a rise of what I call neo-feudal leadership in the health care industry, food industry, and political industry (yes, industry—politics for the sole reason of individual and corporate profit). These so-called leaders have become all too focused on putting more money into their own offshore bank accounts and appear to have forgotten completely that they are supposed to serve the population at large. There are still dedicated people in all these industries, but as of 2018, they are being shouted down. At this moment, the average person in our country must plow through a blizzard of lying, cheating, and stealing just to buy decent food and get health care. And more and more people can't afford food or health care at all.

Will the resourcefulness and dedication of people who support health and well-being for everyone in this country (rather than just the privileged few) prevail? Only if we all work for it. In 2018, we have different and discriminatory health care systems for members of the government and for people in the general population. I recognize that people with more money have always had better access to health care, but I don't believe that dual systems of care, one for members of the government, and one for the general population, have ever been legislated in any other country, much less one that is supposed to be a democracy.

What to do? You may start by realizing that staying busy and putting your health on the back burner or listening to health care providers who aren't listening to you isn't working. You may also become aware of your own "health environment"—the snack in your hand or the spray in your home that may be affecting your health. Once you get started, you will also find additional responsible people and information to help you.

Of course, making different health care decisions can require big changes—and you need to learn how to make them. But you already know this. What you may not know is that big forces operating behind the scenes are affecting your individual health and the health of everyone in this country in a major way.

Initial Survival Tips for the Health Care Apocalypse

It could be that the health care apocalypse has escaped your notice, or that you are quite understandably hoping that if you ignore it, it just might go away. Maybe you are one of the shrinking number of Americans who still has decent health insurance. Maybe you are part of the 40% of Americans who *don't* have at least one chronic illness. Or maybe the news has been so depressing lately that you just can't bring yourself to watch it—to find out what is making us all so sick. Or maybe some of the major players are almost too big to notice. They are so much a part of our "atmosphere" that we don't know how their actions affect our health. So, here are your first three important survival tips, and an introduction to some of the major players.

1. Watch out for the health care. It could kill you.
2. Watch out for the food. It could kill you.
3. This Apocalypse has Five Horsemen, not four.

Big Med: Disease manager and not-so-silent killer
Big Pharm: Robber baron
Big Food: Sugarholic, additive-obsessed huckster
Big Ag: Master of chemical attack strategies
Big Pol: Profit-mad healthcare demolition expert

This last player is being paid by the other four horsemen to make laws that protect their profits, not our health.

These five often work in pairs, threesomes, foursomes, or all together. The pain-killer (opioid) epidemic is a perfect example. As recently as fall 2017, an ex-DEA agent said that both Big Pharm and Big Pol were fueling the epidemic (meanwhile, we thought they were supposed to be helping to stop it!)

"In the midst of the worst drug epidemic in American history, the U.S. Drug Enforcement Administration's ability to keep addictive opioids off U.S. streets was derailed – that, according to Joe Rannazzisi, one of the most important whistleblowers ever interviewed by 60 Minutes. Rannazzisi ran the DEA's Office of Diversion Control, the division that regulates and investigates the pharmaceutical industry.

"In a joint investigation by 60 Minutes and *The Washington Post*, Rannazzisi tells the inside story of how, he says, the opioid crisis was allowed to spread—aided by Congress, lobbyists, and a drug distribution industry that shipped, almost unchecked, hundreds of millions of pills to rogue pharmacies and pain clinics providing the rocket fuel for a crisis that, over the last two decades, has claimed 200,000 lives." [1]

But don't take the word of just one whistleblower. A Harvard study says the same thing, and their report, "Fixing a Broken Pharmaceutical Market" stated: "In this article, we argue that non-rigorous patenting standards and ineffectual policing of both fraudulent marketing and anticompetitive actions played an important role in launching and prolonging the opioid epidemic." [2]

This is just one example of the behind-the-scenes actions of the Five Horsemen of the Healthcare Apocalypse. But even this one act of health sabotage for profit has had a huge effect on our health as a nation, and it illustrates a big point: All the Five Horsemen represent groups that are supposed to support healthcare. After all, groups are comprised of people and people have families and families often have kids, and in community groups, aren't we supposed to be looking out for one another? Well, when it comes to health care, that's not happening. What's worse, these so-called supporters have mounted a constant attack on our personal health, our health as a group, and our whole healthcare system. We are on our own in a health care war zone.

Before we officially talk about the anatomy of the health care apocalypse, and how to survive and even thrive in it, let's put up some warning flags, so that the five horsemen don't continue to operate behind the scenes. Simple awareness can be your first survival move.

I have characterized these entities as the Five Horsemen but make no mistake. These symbols are not cartoons, and they are not funny. They represent what I believe to be major forces in our country that have turned a nation of healthy, energetic people—the adults I saw around me in the 50s—into a nation of the chronically ill.

Big Med—Red Warning Flags

Red Flag 1: _In America, medical errors are the third leading cause of death!_

When I warned you to look out for Big Med, and said health care could kill you, I wasn't joking. According to a study by Johns Hopkins University researchers, published in _The British Medical Journal_, and reported by _The Washington Post_, this is what death in the U.S. looks like under Big Med. Big Med is doing a disastrous job of management, and is often behaving just like an abusive parent or spouse—who lures you with promises and then locks you in the closet, hurts you, or even kills you.

When the very institution that is supposed to take care of our health becomes the third leading cause of death, something is terribly wrong, and needs to be changed.

This chart from Johns Hopkins University, has the apocalyptic title: Death in the United States. Medical error is the third

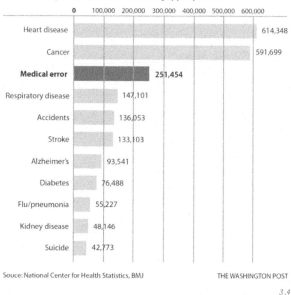

Death in the United States

Johns Hopkins University researchers estimate that medical error is now the third leading cause of death. Here's a ranking by yearly deaths.

Heart disease	614,348
Cancer	591,699
Medical error	251,454
Respiratory disease	147,101
Accidents	136,053
Stroke	133,103
Alzheimer's	93,541
Diabetes	76,488
Flu/pneumonia	55,227
Kidney disease	48,146
Suicide	42,773

Souce: National Center for Health Statistics, BMJ   THE WASHINGTON POST

3,4

leading cause of death, topped only by heart disease and cancer. According to the researchers, 251,454 people die from medical error every year. That's 688 people a day, 28 people an hour, nearly 1 every two minutes!

Red Flag 2: _Among developed nations, American health care is dead (pun intended) last._

The American health care industry is last among developed nations in health care outcomes—the results people get from health care. It is also last in access to health care—too many people in this country do not have access to health care nor can they afford it. Our health care industry has only one "first"—it is the most expensive! This is not happening in other developed countries. According to the 10th Annual Global Prosperity Index, released in November 2016 by the London-based Legatum Institute, and reported by _Business Insider_, here are the countries (in two cases, city-states) that have the top sixteen health care systems in the world. The USA is _not_ on the list.

1. Luxembourg
2. Singapore
3. Japan
4. Netherlands
5. Sweden
6. Hong Kong
7. Australia
8. Israel
9. Germany
10. Belgium
11. New Zealand
12. Norway
13. France
14. Qatar
15. Canada [5]

Red Flag 3: _Chronic illness is the new normal. More than half of American adults—60%—have at least one chronic illness._

Chronic illness can be defined as a disease or condition that lasts longer than 3 months. According to a Rand Corporation research done in 2017, 60% of Americans have at least one chronic illness, and 42% have multiple chronic illnesses. Here is what they say about these apocalyptic chronic illness statistics:

> "This... updates previous versions with more recent data on the prevalence of multiple chronic conditions (2008–2014) and associated health care utilization and spending. It also analyzes functional and other limitations for those with multiple chronic conditions. In 2014, 60 percent of Americans had at least one chronic condition, and 42 percent had multiple chronic conditions. These proportions have held steady since 2008. Americans with chronic conditions utilize more—and spend more on—health care services and may have reduced physical and social functioning." [6]

Big Pharm—Red Warning Flags

Red Flag 1: Big Pharm can act like a robber baron.

> "I don't mean to be presumptuous, but I liken myself to the robber barons," said Martin Shkreli, who acquired U.S. rights to Daraprim, a drug that treats toxoplasmosis—a parasite that is dangerous to pregnant women, the elderly, and people with compromised immune systems. It can cause seizures, blindness, and birth defects in babies of infected mothers. At the end of 2015, Shkreli jacked up the price of a single pill more than 5000%, from $13.50 to $750. Shkreli refused to apologize, and compared himself to John D. Rockefeller, saying he would never apologize as long as what he was doing was legal."

NOTE: As of this writing, Martin Shkreli is awaiting sentencing on a fraud conviction, and his bail is being revoked because he offered someone $5000 for a hair from Hillary Clinton's head. [7]

Red Flag 2: Watch the needless markups by Big Pharm.

Shkreli is a terrible example of a drug price gouger. But he's not the only one. Drugs cost excessively more in the USA than in other countries. Here's a price comparison chart from 2016.

Medication	U.S. Avg Price	Canada Avg Price	U.K. Avg Price	Spain Avg Price
Celebrex[8]	$330	$51	$121	$164
Copaxone (MS)	$3,900	$1,400	$862	$1,191
Cymbalta (depression)	$240	$110	$46	$71
Enbrel (auto immune)	$3,000	$1,646	$1,117	$1,386
Gleevec (leukemia)	$8,500	$1,141	$2,697	$3,348
Humira (arthritis)	$3049	$1,950	$1,102	$1,498

9

Red Flag 3: Big Pharm can act as a deadly addiction machine.

One of the most widely used and deadly pain killers is OxyContin. It was aggressively marketed, and the marketing contained a dangerous lie—that it was the only pain killer that would last for 12 hours. But it didn't work that way for many people. Instead, it would wear off sooner, leaving withdrawal symptoms and terrible pain in its wake. The company knew this, but did they have their reps tell doctors to prescribe it more often? No, they advised the doctors to tell the reps to keep up the 12-hour dosing schedule, but to give stronger doses. What happened? More people got addicted! In 2007, the company was taken to court, pleaded guilty to misleading doctors and patients, and was fined 600 million dollars—a mere wrist slap. How could that much money be just a drop in the bucket to this company? It's simple: from 1995 to 2015, they made 35 billion dollars on the drug. OxyContin is just one of the pain killers in a flood of opioids on the market, causing an epidemic of addiction and death. Here's what the CDC 10 has to say about opioid overdose: "Opioids, (including prescription opioids, heroin, and fentanyl) killed more than 33,000 people in 2015, more than any year on record. Nearly half of all opioid overdose deaths involved a prescription opioid." [11-13]

Big Food—Red Warning Flags

Red Flag 1: Big Food is a sugarholic, and sugar is one of the main foods that is making you sick.

The prestigious medical journal _JAMA_ published an article in its September 12, 2016 online issue with documentary proof that in the 1960s an industry group called the Sugar Research Foundation, knowing that sugar was a principal cause of coronary heart disease, paid scientists to point the blame at fat. This deliberate disinformation generated decades of "low fat" manufactured foods that were advertised as healthy but were loaded with health-destroying sugar, starch, and trans-fats.

In my opinion, this criminal cover-up was one of the biggest factors in ruining the health of the last three or four generations of Americans. [14]

Thanks to the sugar industry's big lie about sugar and heart disease, we are in the eye of a huge disease storm—the heart disease, diabetes, and obesity epidemics. As I have already said, 60% of adults currently battle at least one chronic illness, and 42% have more than one. And it is even more disheartening that children are developing middle-aged diseases—Type 2 diabetes, high cholesterol, and high blood pressure.

Red Flag 2: Big Food can be a con artist, a hustler, a tease, and a pusher.

When you deal with Big Food, be prepared for disinformation, deliberate exploitation of the addictive qualities of food, junk science, and downright falsehoods. Here's a telling fact about Big Food from Michael Moss, author of the must-read book, *Salt Sugar Fat: How the Food Giants Hooked Us.* A man who recently retired from Big Food had invented a very popular line of pre-packaged kids' lunches. His daughter will not let his grandchildren eat them! And he doesn't eat them either. He has become wise to the harmful nature of junk foods and has become part of the movement for healthy school lunches. [15]

Red Flag 3: Big Food is obsessed with chemical additives—artificial preservatives, sugars, flavor and texture enhancers, and dyes.

If you eat processed foods, there is almost no way to escape at least one of these chemicals in your food—and many processed foods have all of them. These additives have been studied extensively and most of them have been proven to be harmful, causing everything from skin rashes to strokes. The EU and the UK have banned many of them. And it's not just additives—food-processing chemicals such as n-hexane or methylene chloride can leave residues that end up in your food. It is well worth your time to learn more about these additives and chemicals and stay away from them. See the Allergy section in Part II and the Food section in Part III for more information.

Big Ag—Red Warning Flags

Red Flag 1: Like Big Food, Big Ag is chemically obsessed. But they don't mix them in food, they spray them on it.

The bottom line is, pesticides that have been shown to be harmful to humans are routinely sprayed on crops and end up in your food. One of the chemicals Big Ag has been spraying on your food is chlorpyrifos, a chemical of a class that was originally developed as a nerve gas. It has been so widely used by Big Ag that a 2012 study found chlorpyrifos in the umbilical cord blood of 87% of the newborns tested in an agricultural community. Why is that so bad? Chlorpyrifos has been proven to cause brain damage in children. (Big surprise—a nerve gas chemical causes brain damage!) Despite a June 27, 2017 protest from The American Academy of Pediatrics, a recent proposed ban on chlorpyrifos was rejected by Big Pol, so that Big Ag can continue to spray it on your food. [16, 17]

Another popular Big Ag pesticide used widely in the United States is glyphosate. Here is a list of other countries that have proposed bans or have imposed restrictions on its use because of concern for risks to human health:

Argentina, Australia, Belgium, Bermuda, Brazil, Canada, Colombia, Denmark, El Salvador, England, France, Germany, Italy, Luxembourg, Malta, Netherlands, New Zealand, Portugal, Scotland, Spain, Sri Lanka, Sweden, Switzerland.

As of September 2017, four countries have completely banned the use of glyphosate: Belgium, Malta, The Netherlands and Sri Lanka. In Argentina, nearly 30,000 doctors demanded that glyphosate be banned because of reports of its association with cancer, spontaneous abortions, birth defects, skin diseases, respiratory illness, and neurological disease. [18]

Red Flag 2: _Big Ag disrupts hormones and creates superbugs._

Some of the most dangerous "additives" to food are the antibiotics and hormones fed to animals in the process of trying to produce more meat faster. Eating chicken, beef, pork, or other meats from animals fed with hormones can disrupt your own hormones. One of the best examples of this is bovine growth hormone in milk. Feeding antibiotics to animals to keep them from getting sick even when they are being raised in horrible environments creates superbugs that become resistant to all antibiotics. Antibiotic-resistant superbugs have already become a global threat. Here are a few of the latest CDC statistics from their online infographic "Antibiotic Resistance, The Global Threat":

<u>Annual deaths, illnesses and extra hospital days in four countries</u>

- EU: 25,000 deaths per year with 2.5 million extra hospital days
- India: 50,000 babies died in one year with resistant infections, usually passed on from their mothers
- Thailand: More than 38,000 deaths per year, with 3.2 million extra hospital days
- USA: More than 23,000 deaths and more than 2 million illnesses.[19]

Big Pol—Big Red Warning Flag
Health care demolition alert!

Big Pol has been witnessed repeatedly trying to destroy health care coverage for at least 23,000,000 people. I am not going into detail about the health horrors of Big Pol. I'm just saying that instead of doing their job, which is to help to provide health care so that our country stays vital and strong, Big Pol is doing just the opposite and trying to dismantle health care in this country! And as always, there's a money angle—it has been estimated that 40% of the money from cutting health care coverage for that many would go to the top 1% of the people with the highest incomes in this country.

For now, that's it for the basic warnings about the Five Horsemen. It is important to keep in mind, from the beginning, that they are not invincible, and the apocalypse is not inevitable. Conditions can change in a short time, depending on our actions. Of course, we are not going to engage the Five Horsemen in a full frontal old-school battle, nor are we going to ignore them. Maybe we will see them immobilized in the same way that hundreds of tiny Lilliputians tied down Gulliver. Who knows? For now, our challenge is to create and organize our way out of the health care apocalypse and live to see the Five Horsemen riding away into the distance.

Alive and Well, Your Survival Guide for the Health Care Apocalypse—Outline

A man I once worked for did a lot of speaking and teaching. He always said that to be understood fully, first tell people what you are going to tell them, then tell them, and finally tell them what you just told them. So here is what I am going to tell you.

Part I: The Anatomy of the Health Care Apocalypse

Part 1 is about the forces that have created the apocalypse: disinformation that is making us sicker, not healthier; the normalization of chronic illness, a broken diagnostic system, and out-of-date methods, and a possible solution to these problems. Here are the topics:

1. The Five Horsemen of the Apocalypse have misled us for decades—led us to believe that we have the best medical system in the world, that drugs will cure all our ills, that we have the best food, that agricultural chemicals, hormones and antibiotics are not harmful, and that our politicians are operating democratically to regulate foods, drugs and chemicals for our benefit.
2. Chronic illness is the new normal and pills are not the answer.
3. Big Med has a broken diagnostic system that hides threats to your health. It is content with label-only diagnoses that give a name to groups of symptoms, rather than looking for causes.
4. Big Med is out of date. It is too much like a high-tech dinosaur from the old barber-surgeon era. The old doctors had knives, leeches, and laudanum. The new ones have scalpels, scopes, gamma knives, blood thinners, and an epidemic supply of opioid drugs.

5. Possible solution—a new ecologically-oriented health care model

Part II: Chronic Illness—What's Making You Sick and What You Can Do About It

The usual health industry routine is to give your illness a dysfunctional diagnostic label and then throw a pill at it! These labels fail to get to the root of the causes of the diseases and make it too easy to keep you coming back for more pills. Part II is about a whole different way of looking at common chronic illnesses and their diagnoses. You will learn preventive, scientifically studied, alternative ways to approach them. The supplements and methods you will find here have decades of clinical success and scientific studies to back them up.

Here's a list of the chronic illnesses in Part 2:

Common illnesses: Allergies; Alzheimer's; Arthritis; Cardiovascular Disease; Chronic Fatigue and Fibromyalgia; Anxiety, Depression, and Post Traumatic Stress; Diabetes, Eczema and Psoriasis; Migraines and other Headaches; GERD and IBS; Insomnia; Menopause; Obesity; and Sinusitis.

Every one of these illnesses has inflammation as a component. One of the main contributors to these inflammatory illnesses—delayed-type allergies to foods—is still generally ignored by the American healthcare industry. The industry is content with a broken diagnostic system that usually doesn't consider causes of illness. Even the newest buzzword in the medical industry, "inflammation," doesn't help. Your practitioner may tell you that part of your disease is "inflammation," but most providers are still not looking for the causes of the inflammation. This aspect of the broken system can keep you in a cycle of inadequate diagnoses and prescriptions for drugs that don't really help you. You will learn ways to escape from that cycle.

The suggested alternatives can be simple or complicated—as simple as getting rid of your old feather pillow and down comforter, or as complicated and detailed as learning to supply yourself with food free from agricultural chemicals, chemical additives, hormones and allergenic foods. Either way, comprehensive management that considers your whole system and everything in your environment can change your health for the better.

Part III—Preventive Health Care Strategies

In Part III, I will give you specific plans for diet, exercise, and stress reduction, and resources for the development of emotional intelligence, resilience and community support. You will learn how all these methods can be used to prevent illness, move toward a much better state of well-being, and replace "disease management" with true health care. You will discover that this preventive type of care is based on a new ecological, environmental model of health and illness. I will talk about options for recovery from chronic illness, so that you can begin to see your way out of the default idea that with chronic disease, the only way to go is down.

Now that you have been introduced to all the players, and you have some idea of what you are about to read, here is Part I.

PART I:
Anatomy of the Health Care Apocalypse

Problem 1: The Five Horsemen of the Apocalypse Have Been Conning Us for Decades

I am going to repeat what I just said in the Red Flags section of the introduction about disinformation from the sugar industry because this point is so important, and in my opinion, so central to the steep decline of public health in the United States in the last 50 years.

The prestigious medical journal *JAMA* published an article in its September 12, 2016 online issue with documentary proof that in the 1960s, an industry group called the Sugar Research Foundation—knowing that sugar was a principal cause of coronary heart disease—paid scientists to point the blame at fat. In my opinion, this cover-up has been one of the biggest factors in ruining the health of the last four or five generations of Americans. [14]

Thanks to this deliberate, dishonest scheme, we are in the middle of heart disease, diabetes, and obesity epidemics. Children are developing middle-aged diseases—Type 2 diabetes, high cholesterol, and high blood pressure.

From the 60s on, the entire manufactured food industry fell right in behind the sugar industry and used every marketing trick in the book to convince everyone that "low fat" snacks loaded with sugar and trans fats would be "healthy." In my lifetime, cola drinks, once sold in 6-ounce glass bottles, are now in giant plastic 32- or even 64-ounce bottles. Foods with a "healthy profile" like yogurt and oatmeal have been hijacked and marketed with sugar loads higher than sugary cereals or sodas.

Our diet of sugary, salty, fatty, processed foods laced with additives and pesticides has pushed American health off the edge.

Sugar, salt, processed fats, preservatives, additives, dyes and agricultural chemicals have all helped turn food into a monster: a source of disease instead of health.

And what about the medical industry? How is it working for us? Not at all. A June 2014 Commonwealth Fund study says this:

> "The United States health care system is the most expensive in the world, but this report and prior editions consistently show the U.S. underperforms relative to other countries on most dimensions of performance. Among the 11 nations studied in this report—Australia, Canada, France, Germany, the Netherlands, New Zealand, Norway, Sweden, Switzerland, the United Kingdom, and the United States—the U.S. ranks last, as it did in the 2010, 2007, 2006, and 2004." [20]

The report evaluated these areas for each country:

Quality, Access, Efficiency, Equity, and Healthy Lives. Here are the U.S. rankings:

Quality	Number 5 of 11
Access	Number 9 of 11
Efficiency Number	11 of 11
Equity	Number 11 of 11
Healthy Lives	Number 11 of 11

That's a terrible report card for the most expensive health care system in the world: C for quality, D for access, and F for Efficiency, Equity, and Healthy Lives, with an overall average of F— and a dead-last ranking among all the countries surveyed. And I mean *dead* last. Those bad rankings translate into illness and death for Americans. Worst of all, the area that is most directly related to health outcomes for people in the U.S.—Healthy Lives—is one of the worst.

As I have said, 6 out of every 10 adults in this country have at least one chronic illness. Emory University published a chronic illness study in 2016 in *Psychology, Health & Medicine.* The medical illnesses considered included asthma, cirrhosis of the liver, diabetes, heart disease, AIDS, lung cancer, pancreatitis, and stroke. Mental illness and substance abuse were also included. [21]

What is the result of all this for the average person? Poor care at high cost, and an industry that is basically using your sick body as a cash cow. Medical "business as usual" is big business. Huge profits are being made from the disaster that is our current state of public health in this country—profits from health insurance premiums, office visit fees, outpatient procedure fees, hospital fees, and ridiculously overpriced drugs.

Are food, exercise, stress reduction, or resilience building the usual first-line remedies for illness? Unfortunately, no. The go-to remedy is prescription drugs, and their prices have gone completely out of control. You have already read about a drug pricing scandal and have seen some drug price comparisons in the introduction. Here is another drug scandal. In 2016, the cost of a two-pack of EpiPen—the lifeline for many severely allergic children and adults—skyrocketed from $461.00 to $608.61. This was not the first price increase. In 2007, the cost of a two-pack was $93.88. By 2015, it had already increased to $317.82. Overall, the price increase since 2007 is more than 500%. There has been massive public pressure, and a response by the company: they will sell a generic two-pack for $600, but the brand name version will still cost $1000. But there is hope. As of January 12, 2017, one of the drugstore chains has already produced an alternative two-pack that will cost $109.99.

The EpiPen prices aren't the end of it.

There are countless more abuses in both the medical and food industries. The whole idea that drugs should be marketed aggressively to the public is such a common practice now that people have forgotten that it is wrong to do it at all. Marketing food as an addictive substance instead of a support for health is equally common, and equally wrong. Many books have been written about the hype in both industries. I would encourage you to read at least these two: *The Truth About the Drug Companies: How They Deceive Us and What to Do About it* by Marcia Angell, M.D., published by Random House in 2004; also, mentioned earlier, *Salt Sugar Fat: How the Food Giants Hooked Us* by Michael Moss, published by Random House Publishing Group in 2013.

Problem 2: Chronic Disease is the "New Normal," and Drugs Are Not the Answer

Here are a few more facts and figures about chronic illness in the USA.

- As of 2012, one in four American adults had two or more chronic conditions; 50 percent had one or more; 13 percent had at least three. And you have already read that those numbers have gone up in 2017. *In only five years, the percentage of Americans with at least one chronic illness has increased from 50% to 60%*, and the percentage with at least two chronic illnesses is 42%.

- Seven of the top 10 causes of death in 2010 were chronic diseases. Of these, heart disease and cancer accounted for nearly half of all deaths.

- One out of three American adults is obese.

- 45.3 percent of people age 65 or older have two or more chronic health problems.

- Nearly 70 percent of Americans take at least one prescription drug, and more than half take two, according to researchers at the Mayo Clinic and Olmsted Medical Center. The most commonly prescribed were antibiotics (17%), antidepressants (13%), and opioids (13%). [22]

- According to a 2015 study published in *JAMA*, between 1999 and 2012, antidepressant use by Americans nearly doubled, increasing from 6.8% to 13%. [23]

- In 2011, 52 percent of American adults didn't get enough aerobic exercise or physical activity.

- Thirty-eight percent of Americans say they eat fruit less than once a day, and 23 percent say they eat vegetables less than once a day. [23]

On a positive note, the October 25, 2016 issue of *JAMA* published a "Viewpoint" article entitled "Chronic Disease Prevention: Tobacco Avoidance, Physical Activity, and Nutrition for a Healthy Start." The article stated that an hour a day of moderate to vigorous physical activity for children is the standard, and less than half the children in the United States meet it. The authors also point out that the Healthy Hunger-Free Kids Act (HHFKA) passed in 2010 has provisions that would improve quality of foods and drinks available in schools. They say that if its standards were applied to all schools, it would be number one in reducing childhood obesity, in a group of 40 different interventions.

It is incredibly heartening to read even a short "opinion piece" article from a major medical journal calling for prevention of chronic illness and naming physical activity and nutrition as two of the three most important preventive methods. Clearly, these people know that when it comes to chronic illness, drugs are not the answer.

What happens when we make drugs the answer? Antibiotics are a perfect example of the "pill as magic bullet" idea gone horribly wrong. I have already talked about deaths, extra hospital days, and the number of illnesses caused by antibiotic-resistant superbugs. The overuse of antibiotics in the agricultural, food, and medical industries has created monster germs that are resistant to all known antibiotics. The most recent of these is pan-resistant Klebsiella, already responsible for one death in the United States. In addition to the threat of an antibiotic Armageddon, all drugs have at least two problems: they have side effects, and they are overpriced.

It could be a wise move to ask what else you might be able to do before you begin taking a drug. Make no mistake—the purpose of this book is to tell you how to prevent illness and stay healthy. Saying that all prescription drugs are bad is just as bad as saying that they are always the best, and first-line solution to chronic illness. Instead, what I'm hoping you will learn is how to use nutrition, hydration, activity, sleep, stress reduction, resilience, emotional intelligence, and other drug-free methods to help release you from chronic illness and lessen your dependence on prescription drugs.

Why not "just take the pills"? Prescription drugs are expensive, have many side effects, nearly all of them suppress symptoms rather than addressing underlying problems. They are often the "go-to" fix when there are other equally good or better solutions.

Worse yet, drugs can be a direct cause of illness, ER visits, and hospitalizations. *According to a 2013 CDC report, 79.3% of all visits to a hospital ER were linked to reactions caused by drug therapy.* Nearly half of all Americans (48.5%) said they had used at least one prescription drug in the 30 days before they were surveyed, 21.7 % said they had used three or more prescription drugs, and 10.6% had used five or more prescription drugs.

Even drugs traditionally thought to be "safe" can cause problems. In my 35 years of practice, I've seen a lot of people taking pills for arthritis, cholesterol, diabetes, reflux, (GERD) and more.

Their doctors had not tried to tell them about better quality food and water, more activity, better sleep, and stress reduction.

Four chronic illnesses top the list for being treated with so-called "safe" pills that are not so safe.

1	High Cholesterol
Causes	Diet, obesity, heredity, age, gender
Drug problems	Statin drugs prescribed to lower cholesterol can cause muscle pain, and more rarely and seriously, rhabdomyolysis, which is a breakdown of muscle tissue. Statins have also recently been linked to causing increased blood sugar, leading to diabetes. [24]
2	Diabetes
Causes	Excessive weight, high glycemic diet, inactivity, heredity, diseases that cause insulin resistance
Drug problems	Metformin is just one of the many drugs prescribed for diabetes. It is currently considered by many to be a benign "starter" drug for almost everyone first diagnosed with type 2 diabetes. Recently, however, we are learning that metformin may be associated with memory loss. Other commonly mentioned side effects include taste problems, headaches, nausea, vomiting, diarrhea, cramps, bloating, and lowering vitamin B12 to inadequate levels. [25]

3	High Blood Pressure
Main causes	High salt diet, obesity, inactivity, chronic kidney disease, smoking, drinking, heredity
Drug problems	Hydrochlorothiazide, again thought to be a benign "starter drug" raises blood glucose, contributing to diabetes, and may cause dizziness, nausea, vomiting, diarrhea, and other problems. [26]
4	GERD (Gastroesophageal Reflux Disease)
Main causes	Formerly called heartburn, this is now a common chronic illness. It is also one of my least favorite dysfunctional "label-only" diagnoses. In my clinical experience, I have seen that in most cases, GERD is caused by adverse reactions to foods. Remove the foods and you remove the GERD. It is rare for most doctors to look for food reactions, and common for them to prescribe proton pump inhibitors—(PPIs).
Drug problems	Recently, experts have raised concerns over these drugs, which were once considered quite safe. They now have been found to affect vitamin and mineral absorption and may lead to iron deficiency anemia as well as deficiencies in B12, calcium, and magnesium. Emerging evidence also shows that people in the early stages of PPI therapy may also be at higher risk for pneumonia and other infections. [27]

The top ten drugs between April 2014 and March 2015, ranked by number of prescriptions, were as follows:

Drug	Number of Prescriptions
Synthroid	21,561,481
Crestor	21,478,776
HFA	18,203,939
Ventolin	15,298,228
Nexium	13,776,325
Advair Diskus	21,561,461
Lantus Solostar	9,635,935
Vyvanse	10,413,999
Lyrica	10,022,365
Spiriva Handihaler	9,635,935

28

2015's Number 1 Drug, Synthroid

It is surprising that thyroid disease is so common in America that Synthroid was the most commonly prescribed drug for at least a year. Here is one possible explanation.

In 2006, the National Research Council (NRC) issued a report, which stated that the Environmental Protection Agency's safe drinking water standard of 4 parts per million of fluoride puts people at risk for increased damage to teeth! And it also increases the risk of bone damage. What about the thyroid disease/fluoride connection? According to that same NRC report, there is evidence to show that fluoride adversely effects thyroid function; it is linked to elevated levels of thyroid stimulating hormone (TSH). And when TSH is elevated it means that the thyroid is not producing enough thyroid hormone. If you have this condition, you are then given Synthroid, or some other form of thyroid hormone.

The thyroid/fluoride connection is pretty much universally denied in the American health care industry. However, Western European countries do not add fluoride to their water, yet tooth decay has dropped as sharply there as it has here in the United States. This suggests to me that fluoride has very little, if anything, to do with our improved dental health. And in Japan, fluoride is actively banned. Officials there have stated that "fluoride may cause health problems." [29]

Bottom line? Our overzealous water fluoridation problem may have had the unintended consequence of exposing millions of Americans to thyroid problems. [30, 31]

2015's number 2 drug: Statins

Once you are diagnosed with high cholesterol, the "standard of care" is to give you a statin—the drug that made number 2 on the list of most prescribed drugs and is thought to be close to stealing Synthroid's number 1 spot.

Statins have many known side effects, including memory loss, elevated blood sugar, muscle pain, muscle and liver damage, as well as digestive discomfort. However, the side effect that completely took me by surprise is this: *statins can cause you to eat even more foods that are bad for you, at the very time when you need to be changing your diet to healthier foods.*

A new UCLA Health Sciences study confirms that statins give people a false sense of security that encourages them to eat too many calories and fatty foods. The researchers compared people who took statin drugs from 2009–2014 to people who took them 10 years earlier. They discovered that a decade ago, people taking statins consumed fewer calories and less fat, but today they consume more. Today's statin-takers also have a higher body mass index than those who took statins 10 years ago. [32]

"We believe this is the first major study to show that people on statins eat more calories and fat than people on those medications did a decade earlier," said the study's primary investigator, Takehiro Sugiyama, MD, who at the time of the study was a visiting scholar at the David Geffen School of Medicine at UCLA. The 2014 study, "Gluttony in the Time of Statins," was published in *JAMA*. "We believe that when physicians prescribe statins, the goal is to decrease patients' cardiovascular risks that cannot be achieved without medications—not to empower them to put butter on steaks," said Dr. Sugiyama. [32]

I couldn't agree with him more. It is a sad day when a medication encourages a diet that is less healthy. The first steps toward wellness will always be the ones I have already mentioned—eating and drinking healthfully, exercising, sleeping well, reducing stress, and increasing positive connections with friends, family, and community. Yes, some people who are dedicated to living well may still have to take medications, but drugs should rarely be our first-line treatment.

"Inactive Ingredients" in Drugs—A Hidden Hazard

Another poorly-recognized hazard of pills is that most of them contain known allergens—dyes, cornstarch, cane sugar, and the milk sugar lactose. I had a patient who was diagnosed with a "lupus-like syndrome"—an "autoimmune disease" of unknown origin. I suspected an allergic response, tested her, and it turned out that her illness was caused by a systemic allergic response to the FD & C Blue 2 dye in her blood pressure medication. When she changed to a dye-free medication, the illness resolved. Many of the so-called "inactive ingredients" in medications can be the source of delayed-type allergic reactions—which do not cause hives or an immediately swollen throat, or swollen lips, but instead bring about generalized inflammation. If you have delayed-type reactions to foods, additives, or dyes, you may react to drugs that contain these as "inactive ingredients." After all, inactive does not translate to "harmless" or "hypoallergenic!" A good example is asthma inhalers that contain lactose.

I have had many patients who were reactive to dairy (both the milk protein, casein and the milk sugar, lactose) react to asthma inhalers that contained lactose. Imagine this—these people were allergic to dairy. Their lungs were already irritated to the point that they had asthma, and they were given a medication that contained one of their major allergens, lactose. The doctors who prescribed the inhaler had no idea, and neither did the patients.

Here is the story of Ann C., whose lung congestion was caused by food allergies, who was diagnosed with "asthma" without checking for allergies. She had an underlying, undiagnosed allergy to dairy that was the actual cause of her lung congestion yet was given a dairy (lactose)-containing spray to use—for 6 years!! I happened to see this on social media in the month before publishing this book and received her permission to use it. Here is what she said:

> "Check any meds you are on too. I was on Advair for 'asthma' for about 6 years. My asthma kept getting worse in the winter, to the point they were going to start adding other asthma meds (at this point, I was 40 and on 10-12 RX for various things). I got horribly sick. Crashed. Dr. kicked me out of the clinic. Went alternative. First thing Integrative Dr. did was test me for IgA and IgG food allergies and intolerances. I had IgA allergies to soy, gliadin, and casein. I was allergic to cow milk. I never had asthma--it was a milk allergy. That Advair asthma inhaler I was using 2x/day for 6 years? FIRST contraindication states: Do NOT use if severe allergy to milk proteins (casein, whey).
>
> Do they test you first for milk allergy—IgE and IgA— before putting you on asthma meds? No."

So that was 6 years of a misdiagnosis and a medication that made her lung congestion worse instead of better for Ann C—all because of failure to consider and test for delayed type allergies to foods.

In addition to the many incidents of "inactive ingredient" reactions that I have observed in my own practice, there is a report from several years ago in the *New England Journal of Medicine* regarding two women, ages 58 and 81, who experienced dangerously low blood pressure after taking a generic version of the popular anti-GERD medicine Prilosec. It turned out that the drug contained soybean oil. Both women were allergic. [33]

Drugs—both their active and "inactive" ingredients—are clearly a big player in the Health Care Apocalypse! So is our broken diagnostic system. Ann C. suffered needlessly for 6 years because of a combination of two of these players. Here is more about our current diagnostic system.

Problem 3: Big Med Has a Broken Diagnostic System that Hides Threats to Your Health

Our current system, based on disease management rather than health care or prevention, increases the likelihood of giving you a "diagnosis" that too often parrots what you just told the doctor. Some common label-only diagnoses are "Irritable Bowel Syndrome" or "Gastro-esophageal Reflux Disease" or "Chronic Sinusitis." These say nothing about the cause of your illness. You are put in your diagnostic category. You are given the pills or procedures that match that category. It is a closed loop.

This is a good example of the way "label-only, diagnostic category diagnosis" scores an epic fail:

You: "Doc, my bowel is irritated."
Doc: "You have 'Irritable Bowel Syndrome.' Here--take this
    pill." (Meanwhile Doc doesn't bother to try to find out

that you might be reacting to a common food, like dairy or wheat.)

You: "Doc, I have chronic sinus problems."

Doc: "You Have 'Chronic Sinusitis,' here, take this pill." Meanwhile Doc fails to ask you about allergies. You are allergic to feathers, and Doc sends you back home to sleep on your feather pillow, snuggled up with your down comforter right by your nose. All night. For 8 hours.

If this is happening at your doctor's office, you may suffer from months or years more of diarrhea, headaches, nausea, and stomach pain before you find out that you are reacting to a common food that you are eating every day. Or, you may have more years of sinus infections before you find out about the feathers and get rid of that pillow and comforter. Meanwhile, your dysfunctional diagnosis and the drugs that go with it can "paper over" your problem, while the hidden causes steal away your health.

There are many well-disguised health bandits out there. The air, the air is everywhere, and it's full of allergens. There are common allergens like dust and mold, and those that are often not well recognized—volatile organic chemicals from paints, wallboard, carpet, or air "fresheners" that can cause sinus problems, asthma, and even neurological problems. Water can be a major hazard, as we have recently learned with the lead-contaminated water in Flint, Michigan. Poor sleep, constant stress, and lack of exercise take their toll.

As you have already seen with the case of Ann C.'s "asthma", in my experience, the number one candidate for the "diagnosis that never gets made" is delayed-type reaction to foods. These delayed-type allergies can cause inflammatory reactions in your body and brain, and result in many symptoms—arthritis, eczema, "GERD" (acid reflux), "irritable bowel," migraines, psoriasis, sinusitis, and more. It's not enough to call these "inflammation" and give you an anti-inflammatory, a migraine drug, topical steroid creams, or repeated rounds of antibiotics.

Let's talk more about the common, overlooked, contributory cause of all the illnesses I just mentioned: delayed-type allergy to one or more foods. These reactions are not found by skin testing because they are not an immediate type reaction like a peanut-type allergy. They do not cause hives, or make your lips swell, or your throat close. And they do not show up on skin tests. Most doctors are still ignoring this type of food reaction completely or brushing it off as "just an intolerance," while they focus on allergies that cause the immediate-type response.

These delayed-type reactions are far from "just an intolerance." Medically, there are four types of allergic response, all classified as "hypersensitivities," and further divided into four types: Type I, Immediate type; Type II, Cytotoxic; Type III, Serum sickness or immune complex disease; and Type IV Cell mediated. These are all brought about by different types of immune response. We will consider only Type I and Type III here because they are the responses most often related to foods.

Immediate-type reactions are the ones that our current medical system tends to call "real allergies." They are a histamine response, mediated by the immune globulin IgE, the mast cells, and histamines. They cause you to get hives, immediate swelling, and can bring about the deadly and dangerous anaphylactic response, which makes your lips and tongue swell, your throat close, and takes you immediately to the ER. Obviously, it is important to pay attention to this deadly type of allergic response.

However, even though delayed type responses are slower, that doesn't mean they should be ignored, or dismissed as "just intolerances." These reactions are mediated by the immune globulins IgG and less often, IgA or IgM. These antibodies attack the food proteins and create "antigen-antibody complexes," (the food protein and the attacking antibody, stuck together) which cause inflammation in many organs and tissues—the linings of the sinuses, esophagus, stomach, small and large intestines, the linings of the blood vessels, the joints, the connective tissues, and even the brain.

In current practice, Type III delayed-type responses are generally thought to be caused only by injected foreign proteins or drugs, not food proteins. The resulting illness is called "serum sickness" or "immune complex disease." In my clinical experience, this lack of recognition of food proteins as a possible cause of Type III allergic response has been the source of many wrong diagnoses and the cause of many years of suffering for people with delayed-type reactions to foods.

Here's one of the problems. These illnesses involve food, and that's one of the last places Big Med is likely to look. When it comes to food, Big Med has an attitude: "Just don't go there." Of the more than 140 medical schools in this country, only 32 have nutrition courses. Of the 32 schools that do teach any nutrition, the average total time scheduled for the classes is 24 hours. To be fair, many dedicated health care practitioners do their best to encourage their patients to eat better, but saying, "you need to eat better" just may not be enough.

As I have said, delayed-type reactions to food proteins are often the source of illnesses that get label-only diagnoses: "Irritable Bowel Syndrome," "GERD," "Fibromyalgia," "Chronic Sinusitis," "Eczema," "Psoriasis," Atopic Dermatitis," "Mixed Connective Tissue Disease," and even "ADD," and "Generalized Anxiety Disorder." (Yes, there is a food-mood connection, which I will explain later.)

I have been aware of Type III reaction to foods since 1982 and have seen 35 years of often dramatic clinical results from checking for this problem, testing for delayed-type reaction to foods, and removing the allergenic foods from my patients' diets.

I was taught about the delayed-type reaction to foods by two different MDs—John Robinson, M.D. professor of Immunology at

Loyola-Stritch School of Medicine, and Francis Murphy, M.D., my supervisor and mentor at St. Joseph Hospital. Neither one of these doctors had any difficulty explaining the immunological process behind delayed-type reactions to foods, and both were very sure about it as a clinical entity and medical problem. I am surprised by the level of denial and controversy around it that exist today. I can still hear Dr. Murphy talking about it. He used to say, "I call it the Irish catarrh—it can give you everything from migraines to hemorrhoids! If I could just stop the parents from giving bread and milk to the kids who have it, it would be great, but that's the first thing they always want to give them."

In those days, Dr. Murphy told me that he had observed that the tendency to react to foods, (especially wheat and other gluten grains and/or dairy) ran in families. My immunology professor told me that it was a genetic trait, which is "variably expressive." It can be expressed at birth, and then you have an allergic infant who gets eczema, or ear infections, or diarrhea if they are given a dairy based formula. Or they begin to get symptoms after they are started on solid food and given crackers or toast. These reactions can also come about later in life. The genetic trait can get "turned on" with a pregnancy, a viral illness, surgery, or repeated antibiotics. Wheat and dairy are not the only sources of these reactions. Corn, oats, eggs, soy, and other foods can cause them.

Problem 4: Our Medical System Needs an Update

The current medical system has many faces. At best, there are still dedicated doctors who take good medical histories, listen to their patients, and do their best to practice preventive medicine. They do this despite losing precious time entering endless data into electronic health record systems and battling insurance companies to pay for services that they have already completed. There are good and useful prescription drugs. Emergency room doctors and procedures still save lives. For example, one of my patients, a woman in her 40s with two young children, had a stroke. They extracted the clot and restored her to perfect health. In the old days, having the stroke would have condemned her to months in rehab, trying to learn to talk all over again, and trying to learn to walk, with almost a guarantee that she would never walk or talk again the way she did before the stroke. That didn't happen to her! She ran a marathon in October.

But the "dark side" of modern medicine is creeping up to overtake many of the gains that we have made. I believe this has happened for two reasons:

1) In the last 35 years, we have transitioned from a nation of individual practitioners doing their best to restore their patients' health, to a corporatized, profit-driven, profit-motivated medical industry.

2) Allopathic medicine has always been focused on disease management rather than prevention. "Modern medicine" is not so modern. It is high tech, but the ideas behind it have failed to catch up with advances in science and are more related to the old-school model of the "clockwork universe."

The outdated "clockwork" model is not really working for anyone but the few who make big profits from it. Why? Because it is so far behind the real science of the way our cells, bodies, minds, and environment work. At its worst, our current medical industry reminds me of an old, out of control wind-up clock. How can we work with an old clock in this era where the correct time is instantly in front of us on our cell phones? The answer is that we can't. And for those who believe that our current level of medical technology is progressive, it could be said that allopathic medicine is still pretty much at the level of being like the old barber surgeons, but with more high-tech tools. Unfortunately, our current medical system is all about disease rather than health, and the methods are still cut, burn, and poison.

The old surgeons had leeches, knives, cautery, arsenic, and opium. We have blood thinners, knives, cautery, chemo. And we have opioid-based pain killers. In 2000, 4400 people died from overdose of these drugs. In 2014, the number had skyrocketed to 18,893. By the time of this writing, 2017, the epidemic has shown no sign of slowing down. We need a new model, one that translates scientific discoveries in fields like cellular biology and epigenetics into clinical medicine.

At my alma mater, Loyola Stritch School of Medicine—the school that admitted me as an older woman who openly said that she wanted to do acupuncture, this problem was pointed out to me in an unforgettable way. Who did it? Of all things, a professor in the Department of Surgery. (Sorry, but I'm not going to reveal his name.) This professor was feared by all the medical students and known for rapping us on the knuckles if we started to make a wrong move in surgery. Everyone in my class and all the professors knew that I had learned acupuncture, and I had already helped some of my classmates with it. One fateful day, the professor's secretary contacted me, and issued a summons. I was to come over to an area in the hospital the next afternoon and bring my needles. The professor wanted me to demonstrate an acupuncture treatment on one of his patients who had intractable abdominal pain. I was quaking in my shoes. I was sure he had called me over there to tell me how ridiculous it was that I had learned acupuncture, and even more ridiculous that I intended to use my precious medical degree to practice it.

I marched bravely over with my needles and managed to stop shaking long enough to put them into the patient, in the right places. As soon as they were in, he said he had called me over to talk to me, and I thought "here it comes." Here's what he said, "You know, in 100 years when we look back on the medical methods we are using now, we will see that they are so barbaric, if we don't laugh, we'll cry. I brought you here to encourage you to keep on with your acupuncture. It is one of the medicines of the future. Don't let anybody pull you off into another field. Keep on doing your acupuncture." I was practically in shock, but I recognized great advice when I heard it, and I thank him for it to this day. And that brings us to the next category, medicine of the future.

Possible Solutions: Working Toward a New Health Care Model

There is a better health care model than the one we are currently stuck in. This model focuses on preventive health care rather than disease management, and on the foundations of good health rather than on symptom suppression. When your health gets out of balance and illness happens, the preventive medical model looks for the real causes of your problem, rather than giving you a label-only diagnosis. It draws from a wide range of alternatives in treating your illness—all those areas I have already mentioned like food, water, environment, exercise, sleep, stress reduction and the building of resilience.

The preventive medical model puts an end to dismissing you with a pill.

With the new model, solutions are beyond biomechanical. This new approach to health care breaks out of the world of compartmentalized specialists who look at one part of your body and do not consider the other parts, much less the environment you are living in. The preventive model of health care is based on the understanding that every human being is an ecosystem, operating within a larger ecosystem.

The goal of the new model? To generate the best state of health for the greatest number of people! This is a giant contrast to what appears to be one of the main goals of the current medical industry—the profiteering and price gouging I wrote about at the very beginning of this section. We are in desperate need of a medical system with a view of health that matches advancements in science, the complexity and demands of our lives, understands that a healthy population benefits everyone, and recognizes that we are interactive systems, with multiple factors that contribute to our health.

Here is a perfect example of a budding branch of medical practice that needs to be part of the new model—Deprescribing! Deprescribing is in its infancy. There is still no universal definition of the process. A study in the *British Journal of Clinical Pharmacology* has proposed a definition. "Deprescribing is the process of withdrawal of an inappropriate medication, supervised by a health care professional with the goal of managing polypharmacy and improving outcomes." [34]

The deprescribing process consists of doing a systematic review of medications, identifying inappropriate medications, and designing and monitoring a withdrawal plan. In one small randomized, controlled Australian study of deprescribing for elderly patients with a mean age of 84, an intervention group of 47 and a control group of 48, the preliminary results were astonishing.

Twelve intervention participants and 19 control participants died within 12 months of randomization—that's 26% mortality in the group that received the deprescribing, versus 40% mortality in the control group. There were no adverse outcomes for any patients who had the deprescribing done. Of 348 medicines targeted for deprescribing in the group, 209 were successfully discontinued. The people who did the study are quick to point out that it was small. However, it is very hopeful, and indicates the need for more research. [35]

In Part I of *Alive and Well: Your Survival Guide for the Health Care Apocalypse* you have learned about the ways the Five Horsemen of our medical system can affect your health. Parts II and III are about addressing chronic illness and practicing prevention—so that you come out healthier instead of sicker. You will learn how to:

- Discover hidden threats to your health: learn what is in in your food, water, and environment, so that they are a support to your health, not a threat.

- Eat and drink in a healthy way

- Do exercise that you enjoy and have time for.

- Sleep well

- Lower stress, build resilience and emotional intelligence, and have more positive experiences with family, friends and community.

While we work toward the new medical model (and notice, I said work, not wait) it can be life-saving to get more information, and to find practitioners who can help you with more advanced approaches to your health. This book is intended to be one of your guides.

PART II:
Chronic Illness—What's Making You Sick and What You Can Do About It

The purpose of this section is to show you a different way to think about chronic illness. A kind of fatalistic attitude toward chronic disease seems to prevail in the medical industry. It's as if the only way to go is down—as you live on, you gradually get sicker and sicker, and take more and more pills. However, I believe that many common chronic illnesses can be reversed, or possibly even resolved. Why? Because I have seen it happen thousands of times over the past 35 years. All the "disease entities" you will read about here in Part II have a few important characteristics in common:

1. One of their major causes is inflammation, and it is important to find its sources.
2. Some of the principal sources of inflammation are allergenic foods, airborne allergens, chemical contaminants, and undiagnosed chronic infections—including dental infections.
3. There may be deficiency in one or more basic vitamins or minerals.
4. There are lifestyle issues—stress (including post-traumatic stress and adverse childhood experience), lack of exercise, poor diet, poor sleep, or lack of emotional support.
5. There may be issues at a cellular level, such as pregnancy loss because an inadequate supply of omega 3 fatty acids can cause neural tube defects in a fetus.
6. There may be "epigenetic" factors—conditions handed down over the years that are not genetic but are a hidden influence on your health. These can involve anything from a famine among your ancestors, to ways of looking at the world and operating in it that you have "inherited" and have become so much a part of your internal environment that you don't even notice them. Bringing these hidden health hazards to

light, and addressing them, is a major step in reversing and preventing chronic illness.

Part II is far from a complete list of all the things you need to do to address chronic illness. It is a set of suggestions—knowledge that comes years of clinical experience and observation, and methods that have worked repeatedly over time for my patients and for me. These "clinical pearls" are intended to get you started in the right direction, so that you can navigate (and often avoid) the world of the health care apocalypse.

All the illnesses listed here are likely to have delayed-type reactions to common foods as an inflammatory component. Removing inflammatory foods from your diet is therefore a major part of improving or reversing these illnesses and may even put them into remission. Diet, exercise, reducing stress, increasing resilience, and building family and community connections are all basic foundations of good health, so you will find repeated information about them here. I have included material on all these basics for each chronic illness. This is for the convenience of readers who want to use this book by reading Parts I and III, and then consulting the segments in Part II that are related to their own illnesses. There is another thing to keep in mind here. Paying attention to these basics of good health is not a cure-all for all chronic illness. For genetic illnesses, long-term degenerative illnesses like Parkinson's or ALS, or advanced stages of the illnesses listed here, although you will not get regression or remission from these lifestyle changes, it is still possible to improve your general state of well-being with the methods described in Part II and Part III.

ALLERGIES—THINKING OUTSIDE THE "ALLERGY BOX"

The way the medical industry treats allergies is one of the top candidates for a major update. The purpose of this part of the book is to help you address your allergies by making your own changes now, because it may be a long wait for any change in the medical industry. Remember Ann C. and her 6-year misdiagnosis? And her lactose-containing asthma inhaler that made her worse, not better?

You don't have to do this alone. Again, remember Ann C. She found an integrative doctor who tested her for delayed type food allergies. There are many dedicated allergists, internists, family practitioners, pediatricians, and integrative practitioners out there who are taking good medical histories, trying to find out the source of your allergies, and working to help you deal with them. They would be first to say that the medical industry's "name a symptom, prescribe a pill" approach needs a change.

I have already discussed the difference between immediate and delayed-type allergic responses. I have said that immediate-type responses are the kind that usually go into the standard "allergy box." I have talked about the kinds of illnesses that can result from delayed-type allergic responses and pointed out that these responses can even cross into the brain and cause inflammation there. This inflammation, which can show up as mental symptoms like ADD, anxiety, depression, or insomnia can be persistent, and pervasive. For more about the neurological effects of reactions to foods, see David Perlmutter, M.D.'s excellent book, *Grain Brain*.

If you suspect you might have delayed-type allergic response, you and your practitioner are going to need to think outside the "allergy box." Your symptoms will be very different than the Type 1 response. They will be inflammatory and may happen hours or more after you eat the offending food. Your symptoms will usually be grouped together and placed in a diagnostic category like "GERD" or "irritable bowel syndrome" or "chronic sinusitis" or "migraine" or "fibromyalgia." If you suspect that you have delayed-type allergies to foods, make sure you find a practitioner who is knowledgeable about this type of allergy, and is able to test you for it. One reliable lab that does this type of testing is Meridian Valley Lab in Tukwila, Washington.

Here is a checklist of symptoms that may be associated with delayed-type reactions to foods:

o   Abdominal pain
o   Abdominal bloating or swelling after meals
o   Belching or passing gas after eating
o   Bowel movements after eating
o   Feeling tired or falling asleep after eating
o   Nausea, vomiting
o   Constipation or diarrhea
o   Acid reflux ("heartburn")
o   Nasal congestion or discharge
o   Frequent sinus congestion or infections
o   Asthma, wheezing, shortness of breath
o   Irritability
o   Difficulty concentrating, "brain fog"
o   Memory loss
o   ADD, ADHD
o   Anxiety or Depression
o   Migraines or other headaches
o   Insomnia
o   Dizziness, loss of balance
o   Muscle or joint pain and/or swelling
o   Skin rashes, eczema, psoriasis

Might you have food allergies? On a scale of 0 to 5 (with 5 being the most), rate how much these symptoms bother you.

	Symptoms	Scale of 1-5				
1	Abdominal pain	1	2	3	4	5
2	Bloating or swelling (after meals or in the evening)	1	2	3	4	5
3	Belching or passing gas after eating	1	2	3	4	5
4	Frequent bowel movements after eating	1	2	3	4	5

5	Tiredness or falling asleep after eating	1	2	3	4	5
6	Nausea, vomiting	1	2	3	4	5
7	Constipation	1	2	3	4	5
8	Diarrhea	1	2	3	4	5
9	Acid reflux, burning stomach or esophagus	1	2	3	4	5
10	Nasal congestion or discharge	1	2	3	4	5
11	Frequent sinus congestion or infections	1	2	3	4	5
12	Asthma, wheezing, shortness of breath	1	2	3	4	5
13	Frequent mood swings, irritability	1	2	3	4	5
14	Difficulty concentrating, "brain fog"	1	2	3	4	5
15	Hyperactivity, ADD, ADHD	1	2	3	4	5
16	Anxiety	1	2	3	4	5
17	Depression	1	2	3	4	5
18	Memory loss	1	2	3	4	5
19	Headaches	1	2	3	4	5
20	Migraines	1	2	3	4	5
21	Dizziness, loss of balance	1	2	3	4	5
22	Insomnia	1	2	3	4	5
23	Muscular pain	1	2	3	4	5
24	Joint pain or swelling	1	2	3	4	5
25	Skin rash/eczema/psoriasis	1	2	3	4	5

Look at your numbers, and then check the guide below, to learn how likely it is that you might have food allergies.

If you have no symptoms over a 1 or 2 level, and a total of eight or fewer symptoms, then you're probably not allergic to foods.

If you have four, five, or more of these symptoms, even at a 2 or 3 level, you might have food allergies. Try a paleo-type elimination diet to see if most or all your symptoms go away.

If you have levels of 4 or 5 on two or three of the symptoms listed, consider looking for a qualified practitioner to test for delayed-type food allergies.

If you have levels of 4 or 5 on three, four, or especially on five or more of the symptoms listed, consider getting tested as soon as possible.

One of the best examples of the problems that can happen because of failure to consider or check for delayed-type responses to foods comes from the early days of my practice, in 1988. A man in his mid-40s came to my office because he was told he had "chronic sinusitis." [36]

This had been going on for at least 10 years, and he had had many rounds of antibiotics. He had also lost about 50% of his hearing. I sent him to an allergist, whose report showed that he was allergic to feathers, dust, and mold. He had been sleeping on a down pillow, with a down comforter, and he did not have dust barrier covers on his pillows and mattress. He got new "down alternative" pillows and comforter, put dust barrier covers on his new pillows and his mattress, and cleaned up any mold that was in his house. But clearing up his environment didn't completely clear up his sinuses! So, I sent a blood sample to Meridian Valley Labs to check for IgG (delayed-type) reactions to foods. The report showed delayed-type allergies to gluten grains (wheat, rye, barley, spelt, kamut, triticale, and farro) and dairy. It turned out that foods were just as big a cause of his congestion as the feathers, dust, and molds. He was surprised when his "chronic sinusitis" went away. His hearing improved a little—about 4%, but the damage had been done by years of chronic inflammation. I have seen him periodically over the years, his hearing has stayed stable and his sinuses have stayed clear. I was very upset at the time that all the doctors he had seen had been content to put him in the diagnostic category "chronic sinusitis" and had given him round after round of antibiotics, without even considering allergies. I decided at the time that I would make sure that did not happen to any of my patients.

In addition to delayed-type food allergies, environmental chemicals are another item that generally tends to fall outside the "allergy box." Think of your indoor and outdoor environment as an ecosystem that has a constant impact on your health. And find a health care practitioner who thinks that way too! One reason your pills might not be working is that no antihistamines or other medications will suppress your allergy symptoms if you are breathing, eating, and drinking allergens that fall "under the radar." Make sure that your practitioner is not 50 years behind the times— looking for the common indoor and outdoor allergens—dust, mold, cats, dogs, pollens—while you may be reacting to one or more of the following:

- scented dryer "sheets" or liquid fabric softener (currently the number one cause of indoor air pollution)
- formaldehyde in your clothing, carpeting, paints, and furniture
- artificial scents in plug-in or spray air "fresheners," and scented candles
- cleaning chemicals
- chemicals and dyes in cosmetics and other body products
- fire-retardant chemicals on furniture, carpeting, clothing, and even computers
- "health" drinks that have artificial sugars and dyes

- chemical preservatives, artificial sugars and dyes in junk foods and so-called "healthy" manufactured foods
- pesticide residues on fresh fruits and vegetables
- pesticides in wheat products made from wheat sprayed with agricultural chemicals to make it "wilt" for easier harvesting

For lists of safe and contaminated foods, body products, and household products, your best resource is www.ewg.org. You can find "Dirty Dozen" and Clean 15" lists of foods, detailed lists of safe cosmetics, including sunscreen, and even lists of computer companies that have pledged to stop using fire retardant chemicals—PDBEs—in their computers. And before you shake your head, saying to yourself "this is impossible, allergens are lurking everywhere," remember that it is possible to filter your water and air, clean your place, and to buy and eat whole unprocessed foods, organic as much as possible.

Even if your allergies are strictly airborne, better food can help you. The wrong foods can add fuel to the inflammatory fire. Inflammatory foods can worsen pollen and other airborne allergies for some people. These foods are: dairy, wheat, corn, processed foods, food additives and dyes, trans fats, and refined sugars.

On the other hand, eating foods rich in anti-inflammatory compounds can make things better. Researchers proved this in a 2007 study conducted with 690 children, 7 to 18 years old, on the island of Crete.

The research team discovered that 80 percent of the children they surveyed ate fresh fruit and 68 percent ate fresh vegetables, at least twice a day. These were primarily Crete's local produce: grapes, oranges, apples, and fresh tomatoes. The study showed that eating those foods helped to protect the children against wheezing, sneezing, and runny noses. Eating nuts was also linked to less wheezing. On the negative side, eating margarine, a processed food containing trans fats, increased the children's allergy symptoms. [37]

So, if you have allergies, eat from this list more often:

- Dark green, leafy vegetables
- Deep yellow and orange vegetables
- Onions, garlic, ginger, cayenne, and horseradish
- Wild and organic fish

Avoid these totally:
- Dairy
- Wheat
- Corn
- Processed foods
- Food additives and dyes

And drink plenty of water, about two quarts—6 to 8 glasses—a day.

The common airborne allergens are in the "allergy box" so I will not address that subject in detail here. That said, if you suspect you have airborne allergies, I recommend that you get tested to find out what they are, and how to avoid them. Many health care practitioners still tend to say that you can't avoid airbornes and will tell you to just take antihistamines. However, you may be able to do a cleanup of your indoor environment and keep outdoor air and pollens out of your indoor air. Here is a beginning guide to cleaning up "in the box" allergens. For more detailed instructions, I recommend *Prevention* magazine's September 12, 2017 article, "19 Ways to Allergy Proof Your Home" by Jonathan Psenza, N.M.D. He has a good list in his book, *Dr. Psenka's Seasonal Allergy Solution*. I agree with him that indoor air pollution is one of the top five threats to human health! Here's his list, with my additions and edits:

- Use an air filter. Consumer Report's November 2017 top recommendation for a reasonably priced filter is Blueair Blue Pure 211, which costs $250.00. Another, less expensive but very good filter is the SurroundAir filter, which has a combination of HEPA and charcoal/zeolite filters, and a UV light. If you have central heat, you can use a highly rated system air filter and change it according to instructions.

- Use dust mite barrier covers on pillows, mattress and box spring. And minimize dust by getting rid of heavy drapes, blinds and other window treatments, and carpets. If you can't get rid of your carpet, use Capture carpet cleaner on it every six months. Use down alternative pillows, or if you are not allergic to down, get hypoallergenic down pillows and cover them immediately with a dust barrier cover so that they will not become "dust buckets." As much as 1/3 of the weight of old, uncovered pillows may be dust mites!

- Clean every week with non-scented eco-friendly cleaning products, and vacuum frequently with a HEPA vacuum.

- If you have pets, make sure you are not allergic to them. If you find that you are reacting to them, you can use Earth Bath Wipes (nontoxic) every two weeks on your cat or dog, vacuum up pet hair at least twice a week with a HEPA vacuum, use a lint roller on your couch and chairs, and find an extra comfy spot, out of your bedroom, for your pet to sleep.

- Get an inexpensive humidity gauge to measure your humidity and keep it around 40%.

- Check for mold and get rid of it. You may have to get a professional to do this.

- Pay special attention to bedrooms and keep them dust and chemical free. Cleaning chemicals coming into bedroom air from the closets can be a problem. I had one patient who developed cedar fever from a bedroom sauna. Another patient became very allergic to many chemicals after being exposed over time to mothballs in the chests of drawers in her bedroom. Do not use mothballs. They are extremely toxic.

- Avoid using "air freshener" plug-ins, diffusers, wicks or sprays anywhere in your home, and freshen your air naturally with essential oils, if you are not allergic to them.

- Avoid scented candles.

- Change clothes after work, and shower before bed. Take your shoes off at the door and wear slippers that you do not wear outdoors. Give guests washable slippers or shoe covers.

- If you have grass, tree, or pollen allergies, keep outdoor pollens out of your indoor air by using your air conditioner, and be sure it has a clean filter.

- Grow your own air filters (get plants that help clean the air— areca palm, lady palm, bamboo palm, rubber plant, dracaena, English ivy, pygmy date palm, banana leaf ficus, Boston fern, peace lily). And remember, spider plants went with the astronauts to the moon because of they are such great air-cleaners!

- Use eco-friendly non-scented cleaning products and body products, without VOCs—volatile organic compounds, dyes, milk wheat or oat proteins, or parabens.

- Make sure your plastic products are BPA free.

- Make sure your non-stick pans are PFOA free.

- Make sure your furniture, computers and TV are free of fire retardant chemicals.

- Use non-VOC interior paints and varnishes.

- Dry your laundry the old-fashioned way—fragrance-free detergent, no fabric softener or dryer sheets. Dryer sheets are currently the number one cause of indoor pollution.

- Avoid smoking, and do not let guests smoke in your house.

- Frequently vacuum (with a HEPA-filter machine) and shampoo carpets.

- Remove your shoes at the door and slip into house slippers once you're inside.

- Clean your home furnace vents regularly and use a high-quality furnace filter. Clean air conditioner filters regularly.

Your home should be a safe sanctuary—not a place that makes your allergies even worse than they already are. Remember, no air filter will overcome a bedroom carpet full of 10-year-old dust and dust mites, dusty bedroom curtains and blinds, or a mattress and pillow full of dust, so be sure to do the basic dust cleanup in addition to using the filter. No filter will work for mold if there are high levels of toxic mold in your indoor air. If that is the case, your living space will need professional mold remediation.

Allergy Supplements and Medications

Instead of antihistamines, I recommend at least a trial of the herb butterbur. Butterbur has a scientific record of allergy relief. In a 2002 *British Medical Journal* study done in four Swiss and German clinics, 125 hay fever sufferers were split into two groups. One took the prescription antihistamine Zyrtec, and the other took Butterbur extract. After two weeks, they were both equally effective in relieving allergy symptoms.

Another study was done using Allegra in 2005. The butterbur and Allegra both relieved allergy symptoms equally, and both were superior to the placebo. [38]

You also may get help from bioflavonoids. In general, bioflavonoids, (including quercetin, catechin, and hesperidin) are antioxidants that are also natural antihistamines and strongly anti-allergenic. Quercetin comes from apples, onions, and tea (among other foods). Catechins are found in green tea, and hesperidin is found in citrus fruit. You can find combination bioflavonoid supplements; one that has helped many of my patients is D-Hist. [39]

Probiotics also lower allergic reactivity by balancing the gut ecosystem and helping to lower inflammation. My favorite is Renew Life Ultimate Flora, which comes in several strengths and is widely available. I take a 50 billion capsule every day, and I've been using it with all my patients for more than seven years now, with great results. It has a good spectrum of beneficial bacteria, and it's convenient to travel with because it doesn't need to be refrigerated. (Of course, you don't want to keep it in your hot car, but room temperature is fine.)

Vitamin E has some possibility of calming your immune system's reaction to allergens and lessen your symptoms, though the evidence isn't overwhelming. In one 2004 study, 112 people with hay fever were given either 800 IU of vitamin E or a placebo for 10 weeks. They also continued to take their anti-allergy medications during the study, and researchers recorded the amounts of pills they took. Those in the vitamin E group reported having significantly fewer nasal symptoms—particularly stuffiness—than people in the control group. [40]

Side Effects of Antihistamines

One compelling reason for trying an allergy clean-up, changing your diet, and taking supplements is this: antihistamines and other allergy medicines have side effects. Common antihistamine side effects include blurred vision, confusion, difficulty urinating, dry mouth, drowsiness, dizziness, nausea, and vomiting. Restlessness or moodiness also can occur in some children. Older antihistamines, such as diphenhydramine (Benadryl), for example, can make you drowsy—so drowsy that driving or doing anything else that requires your complete attention may be impaired. Newer drugs, such as fexofenadine (Allegra), may cause side effects that include coughs or stomach upsets. [41]

Even more alarming, antihistamines are strong anticholinergic drugs. This means that they oppose the effects of choline, a nutrient needed to keep your brain healthy. A study published in *JAMA* in 2015 found that higher cumulative use (long term, regular use) of strong anticholinergics increases the risk of dementia by as much as 50%. [42]

Side Effects of Other Allergy Medications

Pseudoephedrine (Sudafed), the popular decongestant, also has negative side effects. Though you can buy it over the counter in any drugstore, it's a stimulant that can raise your blood pressure and cause a variety of cardiac side effects. And if you're a *Breaking Bad* fan, you'll remember that pseudoephedrine is one of the ingredients used to concoct homemade methamphetamine—that's why most drugstores have it under lock and key these days. Interestingly, when herbal supplements (often, a weight loss product) make headlines for causing fatal or serious side effects, it turns out that most of those supplements contain the herb ephedra, or the ephedra compound ephedrine. This compound is nearly identical to pseudoephedrine (the word means "fake ephedrine") in Sudafed.

I tell my patients to avoid Sudafed and supplements with ephedra in them, and to use a simple saline nasal spray instead, or a nasal wash such as NeilMed Sinus Rinse. If you use the nasal wash you must be very careful to clean the bottle thoroughly and use sterile water and the sterile packets included in the kit. If you don't think you can do this, don't use it!! Use the saline spray instead.

Other allergy medications with known side effects are corticosteroid inhalers. These have been linked to osteoporosis. They can also lower your immunity and increase the risk of nasal and sinus infections. [43]

Not many practitioners advise allergy sufferers to move, but some still do. You don't have to!

At one time, physicians treating people with severe allergies or asthma might have given their patients the conventional wisdom of the day, which was to suggest they move to a dry, desert-type environment like Arizona, where they'd supposedly be less likely to encounter pollen and other allergens. But now we know that moving might not be so helpful after all. The largest, most comprehensive study ever conducted on the prevalence of allergies from early childhood to old age was published in 2014 in the *Journal of Clinical Immunology*. It analyzed data compiled from blood tests of some 10,000 Americans who were part of the National Health and Nutrition Examination Study (NHANES) in 2005 to 2006. The researchers concluded that people who are prone to developing allergies are likely to develop an allergy to whatever is in their environment —no matter where they live, says Darryl Zeldin, M.D., scientific director of the National Institute of Environmental Health Sciences. [44, 45]

So, allergy sufferers, you can rest easy and stay put, unless, of course, you live close to a coal-fired power plant, for example, or some other obvious source of pollution.

Clinical Pearls for Allergy

1. Make sure your diagnosis is correct and complete. Find a practitioner who knows how to "think outside the allergy box" and will test for both immediate and delayed-type allergic responses to foods. Ask whether your practitioner will also consider chemical allergens like fabric softener, fire retardant chemicals on clothing or furniture, air "fresheners," moth balls, scented candles, and fragrances and dyes in cosmetics and body products, as well as food, pollens, dust, and molds. And find out if your practitioner is open to the use of supplements and does not insist on exclusive use of pharmaceuticals to address allergies.

2. Start using chemical, dye, and fragrance-free body and cleaning products as soon as possible.

3. Do a complete allergy assessment and clean-up in your home.

ALZHEIMER'S DISEASE

There is a groundbreaking study about reversing Alzheimer's Disease that was published in fall 2014. I would think that by know, practitioners would at least be trying it with some of their Alzheimer's patients, but this is not yet happening. Most doctors simply prescribe Aricept.

Part of this may be that although the results of the study were remarkable, the study is small, and the program involves supplements and activities, not drugs.

The pilot study, "Reversal of Cognitive Decline: A Novel Therapeutic Program," was published in the journal *Aging* by Dale E.

Bredesen, M.D., director of the Alzheimer's disease program at UCLA's David Geffen School of Medicine. [46]

Dr. Bredesen and his team created a personalized, therapeutic approach that combined diet, exercise, and specific supplements. The therapy was designed to improve the mental deterioration associated with Alzheimer's disease and other dementia-related conditions.

Each of the 10 participants had aspects of the program tailored specifically to them, but some elements were common to all. Here's a snapshot of Dr. Bredesen's treatment approach:

- Eliminating all simple carbohydrates, (gluten grains and all other grains, starches and sugars) and processed foods from the diet.
- Increasing consumption of fruits, vegetables, and nonfarmed fish.
- Following a strict eating pattern with a minimum of 12 hours fasting between dinner and breakfast, and a minimum of 3 hours fasting between dinner and bedtime.
- Improving oral hygiene using an electric flosser and electric toothbrush.
- Sleeping for at least 7 to 8 hours per night.
- Exercising for a minimum of 30 minutes, four to six days per week.
- Decreasing stress by meditating twice a day and doing yoga.
- Where appropriate, female participants resumed taking previously discontinued hormone replacement therapy.
- Taking supplements, including melatonin, methylcobalamin (B12), vitamin D3, fish oil, and coenzyme Q10 each day.

The dosages for the supplements listed in #9 above that I use for my patients are as follows. The brands are all free of major allergens.

Melatonin—3 mg before bedtime.

Methylcobalamin (B12)—this must be a type that is meant to be taken sublingually (under the tongue) because often older adults lack the "intrinsic factor" in the gut that makes the body able to absorb B12. Kal makes a spray methylcobalamin that works well.

Vitamin D3—this should be tested and the dosage should be individualized. More than half of older adults in the U.S. need at least 2000 IU a day.

Fish oil—this is a must! A safe and inexpensive brand is made by NOW foods called Ultra Omega 3. I like it because it is steam distilled, and carefully quality controlled to eliminate any mercury. It is also concentrated, resulting in 2½ times the essential fatty acids contained in most fish oil supplements (750 mg vs. 300 mg). The dose for almost everyone is one gel daily.

Co-Q10—this supplement increases energy at a cellular level. My usual recommended dose is 300 mg. 300 mg gels can be purchased inexpensively at Costco (Kirkland brand).

Here's the amazing outcome: At the time of this writing, 10 people had been studied. Prior to beginning the program, six of them had to quit working or were struggling at their jobs; after completing the program, all were able to return to work or continue working—with improved performance.

The great news is that these people have continued to show improvements as long as 2 ½ years after their initial treatment. No pill exists that can even come close to results like this. Why? Because a "one-trick pony" pill designed to suppress symptoms simply does not have the power to change the basics of your mind and body. Only a multifaceted program that addresses all your physical and mental processes can do that!

According to Dr. Bredesen, "What this program says is that we are all contributing to our own Alzheimer's disease by the diet we choose to eat, by the way we sleep, by the stress we have in our lives, and of course by our genetics." Bredesen then went on to say that we can alter our cognitive decline by changing those factors in our lives. [46]

I am happy to say that virtually every aspect of the UCLA program matches what we do in our recommended prevention plans.

Clinical Pearls for Alzheimer's Disease

- Make sure you or your family member's diagnosis is correct.

- Try the Bredesen plan.

ARTHRITIS

The experts at the Arthritis Foundation list 21 different diseases on the Foundation's A-Z arthritis web page. But by far the most common form of this "wear-and-tear" disease is osteoarthritis (OA), which affects some 27 million Americans. That's because this painful condition occurs when the cartilage that cushions your joints begins to wear out and tear down, and as a result, your bones start rubbing against each other. Just thinking about that scenario is enough to make your joints ache. [47]

There is no known cure for osteoarthritis. Its symptoms develop slowly, over time. In the beginning, you might think of your newly discovered aches and pains as something that's not such a big deal—until a few years or more later, when they really start getting your attention. The all-too-familiar symptoms can include:

- Sore, stiff joints, especially after inactivity
- Stiffness after resting that disappears with movement
- Pain that worsens after activity or at day's end

You can experience arthritic pain in any joint, but arthritis most commonly targets the hips, knees, and neck. You can also experience arthritic pain in your hands. X-ray evidence shows that the finger joints (the distal and proximal interphalangeal joints of the hand) are most often affected by osteoarthritis, but they don't generally cause a lot of pain.

As the months and years pass, especially under certain circumstances, the aches and pains can limit your activity. That's when you start thinking twice about engaging in treasured activities, such as playing tennis or hiking.

Fortunately, unless you already have an advanced case of arthritis, you can generally lessen your arthritis pain. Starting an anti-inflammatory diet, doing the right kinds of exercise at the earliest twinges of arthritis, or even before that, and reducing your stress give you your best shot at slowing the disease's progression and keeping your joints as pain-free as possible [47].

Age Is Just One Osteoarthritis Factor

We used to think of osteoarthritis (derived from two Greek words meaning "bone" and "joint") as a condition that naturally comes with the territory of aging, one that few people are lucky enough to sidestep as they get older. But now we know better. At a major Arthritis Foundation workshop held in Chicago in 2012, participants agreed that osteoarthritis is an umbrella term for several different subtypes of the disease based on different causes. [48]

Let's look at the triggers they've identified so far.

Genes. Researchers are particularly keen on unraveling the connection between genes and osteoarthritis. Their work has led so far to the discovery of three genes linked to a higher predisposition for acquiring the disease, and they continue to seek others. But, caution the experts, we're far from being able to say that certain genes lead *directly* to the disease—and even farther away from being able to offer treatments. "The hope is, as we identify more osteoarthritis susceptibility genes, we'll be able to offer new treatments," says John Loughlin, Ph.D., professor of musculoskeletal research at Newcastle University Musculoskeletal Group in England. In an interview with *Arthritis Today,* Dr. Loughlin, who is also secretary of the Osteoarthritis Research Society International, additionally noted that one day, we might be able to help people predict their osteoarthritis risk based on their genetic profile. [49]

Injury. One arthritis subtype, called post-traumatic osteoarthritis, is caused by traumatic injuries to the hip, knee, or ankle. In fact, some 12 percent of the worst arthritis cases are triggered by an injury. Research now shows that 10 to 20 years after a traumatic knee injury, such as an ACL or meniscus tear, 50 percent of the injured people will develop post-traumatic osteoarthritis.

Obesity. Being overweight can also lead to osteoarthritis, and you don't need to be a physiologist to understand why. When you put more pressure on joints than they're designed to handle, it stresses and compacts the cartilage cushion, causing it to degrade. But wait, there's more. Researchers now understand that fat tissue releases chemicals that increase inflammation—and that can wreak havoc on cartilage. Researchers have put one such chemical, the hormone leptin, under study. They've learned that higher leptin levels in fat tissue are directly related to the narrowing of joint space in the hip (an arthritis sign). In other studies, high blood levels of leptin paralleled high pain scores in people with osteoarthritis.

Aging. Obesity, genetics, and injury all play a role in causing the disease, says Richard Loeser, Jr., M.D. Dr. Loeser is a distinguished professor of medicine in the division of rheumatology, allergy, and immunology and director of basic and translational research at the Thurston Arthritis Research Center at the University of North Carolina at Chapel Hill. "The age-related changes in the joint contribute to its [osteoarthritis'] development," he says. Which begs the question, so why don't we all have osteoarthritis after a certain age? In a Dutch study of more than 80 people ages 89 to 91, 63 percent had arthritis-free hips, 51 percent didn't have arthritis in their knees, and 29 percent didn't have arthritis in their hands. So, who makes it to their golden years free of arthritis? People who tend to escape its clutches even into their 8th or 9th decades share these factors:

- They've maintained a normal weight.
- There's no family history of nodal arthritis of the hands (a type that tends to run in families).
- They produce low levels of inflammatory compounds called interleukin proteins.
- They've performed heavy physical labor throughout much of their lives.

As Dr. Loeser explained to *Arthritis Today,* "The message we're trying to get out is that OA is not simply a degenerative disease of aging. It's an active, inflammatory disease. Your joints aren't like automobiles that wear out over time," he noted. [49]

Conventional medicine has very little to offer people with osteoarthritis except pills (nonsteroidal anti-inflammatory drugs, known as NSAIDs) with their worrisome side effects, injections of steroids or joint-cushioning gels whose effects "wear off" over time, and surgery—which often can have limited effectiveness. That said, I have seen many cases of successful arthroscopic surgery and joint replacement. Sometimes it is the only way.

An anti-inflammatory diet, strategic supplement use, stress-relief techniques, and gentle movement to help you ease pain and loosen joints can help you. Let's start with diet.

An anti-inflammatory food plan benefits many of the chronic illnesses we are discussing here. Why is this? Because so much disease has underlying "inflammation," and so much of that inflammation, in my opinion, is caused by inflammatory reactions to common foods. It is very important to find out whether you have delayed-type allergic responses to the common food allergens.

And in addition to avoiding certain foods, there are foods you should eat more of—foods that can be helpful when it comes to easing the pain and stiffness that having osteoarthritis imposes. I ask my patients to add extra daily servings of these foods, and to be careful about avoiding certain foods that are especially inflammatory. If you are in the early stages of osteoarthritis, you'll probably see that within a month or two your pain will begin to ease, and your joints will be moving smoothly and more comfortably. These foods will work better if you are in the early stages. If your knees or hips are already "bone on bone" you may have to find a surgical solution.

Eat these foods more often:

- Wild Alaskan salmon and other cold-water fish, especially sardines
- Freshly ground flaxseed (add to smoothies and salads)
- Organic, omega-3-fortified eggs
- Avocados
- Walnuts
- Tart cherries, blueberries, and other low-sugar berries (off season, you can often find frozen organic berries at your supermarket)
- Garlic, onions, and scallions

Stop All Dairy

Arthritis is a perfect example of the reasons we've crossed dairy foods off our food plan. Over the years, I've observed that when osteoarthritis supposedly "runs in the family," reactivity to dairy also "runs in the family." I've had many patients whose arthritic pain literally disappeared when they got off dairy, so in my experience, it's well worth a trial if you have arthritic pain. And I would add gluten grains to that as well, but more about that later.

I remember clearly, even though it was years ago, a patient whom I will call Tricia C., who came to see me in the late '80s for acupuncture for her arthritis. Tricia was in her mid-50s and had arthritic pain in her hands. She even had some swelling in her finger joints that looked like the kind that doesn't go away. I suspected that she was reactive to dairy, and suggested she stop eating it as part of our treatment.

She went on a dairy-free diet and came weekly for a series of 10 acupuncture treatments. Her hand pain completely disappeared, and what was even more amazing to me (and to her) was that the swelling in her joints near the ends of her fingers reduced. I had learned in medical school that this kind of arthritic swelling was progressive and not reversible, but I saw something different in this case, and I began to treat people in my practice with the understanding that it might be possible to reverse their arthritis.

At around the same time, my dad started to complain that he was having trouble with his fingers, too. He had pain and swelling, including little hard bony nodules on top of the joint called Heberden's nodes. These were thought to be irreversible, and if they caused him trouble, the only known option was to have them surgically removed. He lived 3 hours away, so it was impossible for me to give him weekly acupuncture treatments. But he was someone who would follow my instructions to a T and was willing to commit to a daily program, so I gave him a set of acupressure points to press on while he watched TV. He followed through diligently, and wonder of wonders, his nodules went away. I also asked him to cut back on his dairy, too—a tough proposition, since he was raised on an Iowa farm! He was in his seventies back then, and his hand problems went away until the age of 86, when he developed a heart valve infection. And he played tennis until he was 84!

Along with dairy, avoid these processed foods totally:

- Polyunsaturated vegetable oils, such as corn and soy
- Partially hydrogenated and hydrogenated oils (AKA trans fats) found in processed foods

- Processed foods containing artificial coloring and chemical preservatives

And if those dietary changes aren't giving you the results you want, try going on a Paleo-based diet like the one described in Part III of this book.

Spice Up Your Life

Your spice rack contains a few bottles that vie with pills for their ability to ease pain. Two important facts about using spices to augment osteoarthritis treatments: First, spices rarely have side effects. Second, spices don't work as quickly as drugs do, so you must use them regularly and frequently—or, better still, use them in cooking as well as in supplement form.

These three spices top my list for helping ease arthritis.

Turmeric (*Curcuma longa*). This spice is related to ginger; its most medically active compound is curcumin. This spice, that gives curry, ballpark mustard, and bread-and-butter pickles their brilliant golden hue, comes from the plant's rhizome (its underground stem connected to the roots). Curcumin is a compound that researchers have been studying for many years. It has several medicinal effects, not the least of which is its ability to reduce inflammation. You can use this exotically tangy spice to enhance your cooking. It adds a distinctive touch to scrambled eggs and curries, and it's a wonderful partner for butternut and other winter squash dishes. Just make sure the food you're adding it to contains a little fat to help your body absorb the curcumin. You can also take it as a supplement (see below.)

Ginger (*Zingiber officinale*). Ginger's spicy, warming flavor gives a nice sparkle to foods both sweet and savory—think smoothies, soups, stews, roasts, salad dressings, fish, vegetables, and even the occasional dessert. Ginger enhances most foods you add it to.

Beyond its flavor, ginger has been used in Chinese medicine since at least 2000 BC.

Among its many medicinally active compounds, are the diarylheptanoids (curcumin also contains these). [50, 51]

Black pepper *(Piper nigrum)*. You probably never thought of just plain black pepper as a healing spice, but in fact, it's also common remedy in Traditional Chinese Medicine. Pepper is packed with compounds that have many healthful actions—including anti-inflammatory properties. In a 2013 test tube study, researchers looked at the effects of piperine, an active pepper constituent. They pretreated human osteoarthritis chondrocytes (cartilage cells) with black pepper and then zapped the cells with an inflammatory protein. Through some very complex science, they learned that piperine inhibited the cells' inflammatory activity, leading the researchers to conclude that piperine could be an effective osteoarthritis treatment. To be sure, my suggestion that you spice things up with black pepper is certainly a long way from what these researchers found in the lab. However, as a physician who's studied Chinese herbal medicine, I'm very aware of black pepper's effects in dampening pain and reducing inflammation. It also increases the absorption of turmeric. So, I encourage you to increase your use of this tasty spice. One more word of advice: Do use a pepper mill to grind peppercorns freshly for each use. [52]

Acupuncture

I've been trained in acupuncture and have been using it since 1978. I've seen it benefit any number of conditions. It's been frequently studied and proved to be successful time and time again for arthritic pain and other conditions. One large Canadian study of 712 knee and hip osteoarthritis patients reported in the journal *Arthritis & Rheumatology* showed that clinical osteoarthritis severity and health-related quality of life improved markedly in patients receiving acupuncture, as opposed to controls. After months of treatment, a measurement of the severity of osteoarthritis (WOMAC score) had improved 17.6 points, and the controls had only improved 0.9 points. The changes maintained through 6 months. [53]

At present, quite a few insurance policies cover acupuncture treatments. To find a licensed, qualified practitioner, visit www.nccaom.org.

Supplements

I frequently recommend dietary supplements to my patients who have osteoarthritis. Some of these I consider to be an essential part of everyone's plan. Certain supplements work better for some people than others, depending on their individual conditions. Here are the supplements I use and why.

Fish oil/omega-3 fatty acids. If you think of your arthritic joints as squeaky hinges that quiet when you oil them, you can see how "lubricating" your joints by taking fish oil might be a helpful solution. Beyond the too-easy metaphor, however, is scientific evidence that the right kind of fish oil supplement, at the correct dose, can help ease osteoarthritic pain because of its ability to decrease inflammation.

Dose	*NOW Foods Ultra Omega 3, one capsule a day.* [54, (Altshul, 2014 #389)]

Glucosamine/chondroitin. Studies have delivered somewhat differing results on this combination of naturally occurring substances. But many people find the combination useful for helping ease their arthritis pain, and the good news is that some studies show that it can help rebuild cartilage. You need to take this supplement for at least 2 to 4 months before experiencing improvement, though some people do feel better sooner.

Dose	*1.5 grams a day, taken once or in three 500-milligram doses.* [54, (Altshul, 2014 #389)]

Curcumin. We mentioned turmeric as a spice you can to add to your food regularly for its anti-inflammatory benefits. In addition, I recommend that my patients consider taking it in supplement form. In a recent study, taking curcumin was as effective a pain reliever as ibuprofen, but caused less abdominal distress.

Dose	*Two 500-milligram capsules a day. It may be better absorbed when taken with a meal containing some fat and a dash or two of black pepper.* [54, (Altshul, 2014 #389)]

SAMe (S-adenosylmethionine). This is a compound found naturally in every cell of the body. It's key to your body's production of the neurotransmitters dopamine and serotonin as well as cartilage components. In studies, SAMe has proven effective for the joint pain and stiffness of osteoarthritis, and several studies show that its benefits lasted longer and had fewer side effects than NSAIDs. [55]

In one 8-week-long 2009 study, 134 patients were randomly assigned to one of two groups: One group got 400 milligrams of SAMe three times a day; the other group got 1,000 milligrams of nabumetone, an NSAID, once a day. At the end of the study, patients rated the SAMe as equally effective for pain treatment to the NSAID. [56]

Exercise, Slowly but Surely

"Use it or lose it" is a great reminder about getting up and walking, especially when you have osteoarthritis. Yes, the pain can be enough to turn you into a couch potato, but I can tell you that's absolutely the worst thing you can do for yourself. We know that physical activity is proven to ease OA symptoms. I don't recommend to my patients that to feel that they need to go to the gym, but I do want them to be up and moving rather than spending hours at a time sitting. See Part III for some easy walking, strengthening, and stretching programs. Stretching is excellent for helping ease arthritis pain—especially if you've been inactive for a while. Your gym or Y might have a special class specifically for people with osteoarthritis. Many even have pool programs, which combine the warmth of the pool water with gentle exercises that put no pressure on your joints. Exercise in warm water is very good for osteoarthritis.

EFT

For an explanation of the power of EFT, turn to Part III! You might not think about pain as a stressor, but in fact, it's one of the most significant stressors the body can face. You also may not think of stress or past trauma as a contributor to joint pain, but it can be. Many people have found EFT to be an effective way to deal with the chronic pain of arthritis. See the EFT description in the Stress Reduction section of Part III.

Clinical Pearls for Osteoarthritis

1. Try a Paleo-type anti-inflammatory diet: No grains, sugars, dairy, or alcohol, and plenty of high quality protein, fresh fruits, and vegetables. If this eliminates most of your pain, consider getting tested for delayed-type food allergies. (One of the reasons for testing is that you may be able to eliminate specific food to get the same effect with fewer restrictions.) That said, you may want to follow the Paleo way of eating for the rest of your life, since you feel so good.
2. Get some good physical therapy, find an exercise program tailored for you, and try exercise in warm water.
3. Do a trial of at least two supplements—glucosamine/chondroitin sulfate and turmeric. If you are already on medications, find a health care practitioner who will supervise you.
4. Try acupuncture.
5. Try one or more of the stress-reduction methods in Part III.

CARDIOVASCULAR DISEASE

Cardiovascular disease is a term that refers to disease that affects the heart and blood vessels. Since the heart is the main "pump" that circulates blood throughout your body, and the blood vessels are the "pipes" that carry oxygen and other nutrients to every cell, tissue, and organ in your body, when your heart or blood vessels are in trouble, so are you.

Though your genes and your family history can influence whether you become a candidate for disease, your lifestyle is a far more significant factor. One thing I know for certain: The first line of defense against heart disease is preventive changes in your lifestyle. The end results of the plan described here could be that you (a) might prevent cardiovascular disease, (b) might be able to reduce your pills if you already have it. The answer depends on your personal health factors and how closely you follow the plan.

Cardiovascular disease also refers to the several intertwined problems that lead to one in four deaths in America every year. The condition called atherosclerosis is common. A sticky substance called plaque builds up on artery walls. Plaque buildup narrows and stiffens the arteries, restricting blood flow. Plaques that rupture and break away from artery walls become blood clots that can stop blood flow and cause heart attacks when they form in the heart's blood vessels, or strokes when they form in the brain's blood vessels. [57, 58]

The Truth About High Cholesterol

What is cholesterol? It's the most common steroid found in the human body. It has two key roles: to help the body produce such life-sustaining compounds as vitamin D, progesterone, estrogen, and other hormones; and to help cells absorb nutrients and release waste products. When levels of certain kinds of cholesterol—low-density cholesterol (LDL) and triglycerides—are too high, cholesterol can build up on artery walls, reducing blood flow and setting the stage for heart attacks and strokes.

Until recently, we've believed that lowering our blood levels of cholesterol via low-fat diets would keep our hearts healthy. As I said in Part I, this mistaken notion triggered food companies to pump out tons of low-fat and fat-free processed foods that were laced with salt, sugar, and, often, heavily processed grains to compensate for the lack of flavor and "mouth feel" that fat delivers. As a result, Americans became more obese—and less healthy. Now we have discovered that diets rich in omega-3 fats, and low in sugars and starches, such as the Mediterranean diet and the Paleo diet are far better ways to keep cholesterol levels within a healthy range. [59, 60]

In 2013, the American Heart Association and the American College of Cardiology did something that many medical experts found shocking: They issued new cholesterol guidelines that suggested that millions of otherwise healthy Americans should start taking statin drugs to lower their cholesterol. Two eminent physicians, John D. Abramson, M.D., on the faculty of Harvard Medical School, and Rita F. Redberg, M.D., a cardiologist at the University of California, San Francisco Medical Center and the editor of *JAMA Internal Medicine,* took issue with those guidelines in a *New York Times* editorial in November 2013.

Here's what they said: "This announcement is not the result of a sudden epidemic of heart disease, nor is it based on new data showing the benefits of lower cholesterol. Instead, it is a consequence of simply expanding the definition of who should take the drugs—a decision that will benefit the pharmaceutical industry more than anyone else." [61]

My opinion? I think statins are a good example of the pharmaceutical industry strong-arming the medical community (and patients) into believing something that isn't true. To understand what I mean, you need to understand the medical research term *number needed to treat.* This refers to the number of people who must take a drug for a single person to benefit from it.

For statins, the "number needed to treat" is huge. In a 2011 review of statin research, the study author reported that when it comes to statins, *1,000 people would need to be treated for 1 year to prevent one heart disease–related death.* That means many people would have to cope with statins' side effects (not to mention, they would also have to shell out for the cost of the drugs) to prevent the death of one person from heart disease. [62]

Interestingly, researchers who conducted a gigantic 2013 *BMJ* analysis of studies comparing drug treatment for heart disease to exercise pointed out that our national cholesterol education program used to advise taking statins only after lifestyle changes had failed. Then, noted the researchers, we changed our national cholesterol program—we lowered the threshold for drug treatment, which meant that doctors were encouraged to prescribe statins to more and more people than ever. [63]

My bottom line: I believe that this is dysfunctional math, and that using statins as a primary method, without lifestyle changes, to lower heart disease risk is simply not good medicine.

Cholesterol by the Numbers

Here's what your cholesterol numbers should be, as far as I'm concerned. I use the older guidelines because the new ones have yet to be proven. Like many other doctors, I believe that the new guidelines, which lowered the cholesterol treatment threshold, may have been put in place to increase the number of cholesterol-lowering drug prescriptions.

Total cholesterol	Less than 200 mg/dL
LDL (bad) cholesterol	Less than 130 mg/dL

HDL [64] cholesterol	Above 40 mg/dL for men, 50 mg/dL for women
Triglycerides:	Less than 150 mg/dL [65, 66]

Conquer Heart Disease with Diet

Studies confirm the benefits of diet, and especially the Mediterranean diet and the low carb Paleo-based for besting all the components of heart disease—so many studies, in fact, that listing them would take more space than we have! In fact, researchers began linking diet to its effects on heart disease as far back as 1935. And now we even have proof that the right diet can equal the benefits of certain pills for lowering heart disease risks—without pills' side effects.

For example, in one landmark study published in *JAMA* back in 2003, researchers proved that a diet rich in fruits, vegetables, and nuts delivered about the same results as did a common statin drug. Both drug and diet effectively lowered C-reactive protein (an inflammation marker implicated in raising heart disease risk) and heart-unhealthy LDL cholesterol by about 30 percent. [42]

What's more, it doesn't take long for a heart-healthy diet to improve heart health. In just three months, eating a Mediterranean-style diet reduced the risk of heart disease by 15 percent, when compared to a low-fat diet, according to a 2005 study published in the *American Journal of Clinical Nutrition*.

"It's never too late," says Bonnie Spring, Ph.D., professor in preventive medicine at Northwestern University Feinberg School of Medicine in Chicago. Dr. Spring and her team recently studied data from 5,000 participants in a lifestyle study and learned that by adopting healthy lifestyle strategies—such as maintaining a healthy weight, eating a healthy diet, being physically active, and not smoking—people could improve the health of their coronary arteries. [8]

According to Dr. Spring, her team's discoveries helped debunk two myths held by some health care professionals: One, that it's nearly impossible to change a patient's behavior. (About 25 percent of the people in her study made changes on their own.) And two, that once damage has been done to coronary arteries, it's irreversible. It turns out that you can reverse the damage. Though the people in her study were young adults, Dr. Spring says that reversing heart disease is possible at any age—it just takes a commitment to making a lifestyle change. [8]

What is a heart-healthy diet? It's simple—high in fiber, low in sodium (none of those sodium-bomb processed foods, for example), low in sugars and refined starches, and loaded with fruits, vegetables, and good fats. A diet like this is one of the healthy habits that can control and potentially even reverse the natural progression of coronary artery disease, according to a 2014 study published in the journal *Circulation*.

Do Eat These Foods!

One trick to creating a diet your heart will love is to keep it varied, says Arthur Agatston, M.D., the renowned cardiologist who created the South Beach Diet. Eating many different types of organic, rainbow-colored fruits and vegetables, eggs, wild fish, and grass-fed meats means you'll get the widest possible assortment of heart-healthy phytochemicals, antioxidants, and good fats. But even among those great choices, some foods give your heart an even healthier edge, like these:

Wild salmon. This succulent powerhouse fish is rich in omega-3s and the potent antioxidant selenium, which studies show protects the heart.

Extra virgin olive oil. Swap this beautiful oil in for less healthful vegetable oils—it contains higher levels of good fats and antioxidants to help unclog your arteries. Another good fat choice, though pricey, is avocado oil, which in a 2005 study proved to help decrease hardening of the arteries. [67]

Walnuts and almonds. Again, it's the omega-3s that make these nuts such wonderfully powerful heart foods; both are great sources of fiber.

Brussels sprouts (along with its cruciferous cousins, broccoli and cauliflower) reduce inflammation in the cardiovascular system and improve the health of your blood vessels.

Spinach and asparagus are rich in the B vitamin folate, which lowers homocysteine levels. Homocysteine is an amino acid that plays a role in heart disease, stroke, and peripheral artery disease. Up to half of all people with heart disease have high homocysteine levels, compared to just 5 percent of healthy people. High homocysteine levels are implicated in severe atherosclerosis. What's more, we suspect that homocysteine promotes vascular problems by damaging blood vessel linings and enabling blood clot formation. [68]

Garlic. Cooking with garlic reduces heart attack risk in three ways: It makes red blood cells less sticky, thus reducing blood clot risk; it prevents damage to arteries; and it discourages cholesterol from lining those arteries and making them so narrow that blockages are likely. But here's a trick: First, make sure to chop, slice, or mash it, because doing so combines two garlic compounds into the potent allicin, which is responsible for garlic's health benefits. Then, let it sit for 10 minutes. Add it close to the end of the cooking time to preserve garlic's power. [69]

Chia seeds. Emerging research points to chia seeds' ability to lower cholesterol, triglycerides, and blood pressure, according to the Academy of Nutrition and Dietetics. [70]

Blueberries and strawberries. Eating three or more half-cup servings of blueberries or strawberries a week can lower your heart attack risk by 34 percent, according to a 2013 Harvard School of Public Health study that reviewed data from more than 90,000 women over 18 years. [71]

Apples. Rich in polyphenols, which protect cholesterol from free-radical damage, these crunchy fruits also contain pectin and fiber, which block cholesterol absorption and help clear it from the bloodstream. And they just may, as the old saying goes, keep the doctor away! Tips: Vary the kinds of apples you enjoy and leave the peels on—they contain most of the fruits' antioxidants.

Avocados. They are laced with monounsaturated fats, the good fats that help lower cholesterol and reduce the risk of blood clots. And try avocado oil, which can help modify fatty acids in the tissues that surround the heart. [67]

Don't Eat These: Scratch Trans Fats Off Your Menu

Trans fats are among the unhealthiest fake food ingredients ever created. The food industry concocted trans fats years ago via a process that adds hydrogen to liquid vegetable oils to create a solid fat. They're cheap and easy for processors to use, and they give processed foods a taste and mouth feel designed to make them addictive. On food labels, these killers are listed as "hydrogenated fats" or "partially hydrogenated fats."

Trans fats raise levels of unhealthy LDL cholesterol and lower levels of healthy HDL cholesterol. The American Heart Association says that trans fats boost your risk for heart attacks and strokes. [67]

The good news is, if you stick to a heart-healthy diet, you won't be eating trans fats, except for the tiny amount that naturally occurs in grass-fed, organic meats. What's more, the addition of trans fats to foods has become less frequent since the FDA took away their "generally recognized as safe" designation in 2013. Still, they haven't disappeared entirely, so read labels carefully. And keep this in mind: The ability of your cells to absorb nutrients and eliminate wastes depends on the quality of the fats in their membranes. Those disgusting trans fats stick around (pun intended) for *120 days.* That's four months! What do you want your cells to have: nice clear fats like organic olive oil, or fake trans fats, which are like the congealed fat on your stove? [72]

Healthy Heart Supplements

I often recommend these six key supplements to patients. In studies—and in my experience—they have been found to help guard against heart disease.

Fish oil. The two omega-3 fatty acids found in fish oil, eicosapentaenoic and docosahexaenoic acids (EPA and DHA for short), have an impressive body of research proving their therapeutic role in protecting the health of your heart. I like NOW Foods Ultra Omega-3. I recommend that my patients take one a day.

Folate. Folate (vitamin B9) is a key heart-health nutrient. As we noted above, folate (along with B6 and B12) helps lower high levels of homocysteine, an amino acid that promotes blood vessel problems. (Folic acid is its synthetic form.) Women who get at least 400 micrograms of folate a day have a 20 to 30 percent lower risk for heart disease, according to studies. [68]

Vitamin D. A study presented at a 2014 meeting of the European Society of Cardiology showed that vitamin D deficiencies worsen brain function following a heart attack—and lead to a sharply higher risk of death following a sudden heart attack. In the study of 53 patients, three times as many patients with vitamin D deficiencies had poor brain function 6 months after their attack as did people with normal D levels. What's more, nearly one-third of the people with low D levels died within 6 months after their heart attacks, compared to none of the patients with normal D levels. I recommend at least 1,000 IU of vitamin D42 for most adults, but

keep in mind that a recent study showed that at least 50 percent of adults over the age of 60 need 2,000 IU a day. That's five times the "minimum daily requirement" of vitamin D, which is still 400 IU, though many of us hope for this number to be raised.

CoQ10. This antioxidant coenzyme is a must, especially if you're taking statin drugs. One potential cause of the muscle pain that is a known side effect of statins is the fact that these drugs deplete blood levels of CoQ10. I recommend 100 to 300 milligrams a day for my patients. [73]

Aged Garlic Extract. If you're not eating garlic regularly (you should be!), consider taking an aged garlic extract supplement to reduce your risk of developing blood clots and to keep arteries healthy. Take 600 milligrams twice a day. [73]

Magnesium. Magnesium plays a role in keeping blood pressure stable. If you have low blood levels of magnesium (ask your practitioner to check), 100 to 400 milligrams of magnesium every evening can help. Take magnesium glycinate, not magnesium citrate to avoid digestive upset. Note: It's best to take minerals, especially calcium and magnesium, at night. [73]

Foods, Supplements and Activities That Lower Cholesterol

Walnuts. Adding about 1½ ounces of walnuts a day to your diet can lower "bad" cholesterol by about 10 mg/dL, which is a significant reduction, according to a 2014 study published in the journal *Metabolism*. [74]

Wine. Drinking a glass of red wine is a relaxing strategy I particularly love—and it helps lower cholesterol. "Antioxidants contained in red wines such as Cabernet Sauvignon, Merlot, and Pinot Noir help slow down the oxidation of HDL and LDL cholesterol," says Vincent Rifici, Ph.D., of the Robert Wood Johnson Medical School in New Brunswick, New Jersey. [75]

Walking. A 30-minute walk at any time of the day, done regularly on at least 5 days a week, will help lower your cholesterol. But strolling after dinner offers even better benefits, according to a 2014 Chinese study of 330 people. The study revealed that taking an evening walk drops cholesterol numbers a bit lower than a morning walk does. [76]

Red Yeast Rice. This natural supplement, long used in Traditional Chinese Medicine, is made by culturing rice with a strain of yeast. It's chemically similar to statin drugs, though at weaker concentrations. "I recommend RYR to people who haven't had a bypass, stent, or previous heart attack and for people who'd rather not take statins for high cholesterol," says David Becker, M.D., a cardiologist in Philadelphia who has published several RYR studies. Most people with moderately high cholesterol do benefit from RYR, but it may not be strong enough for people with cholesterol higher than 190 mg/dL, says Dr. Becker. I like NOW Foods brand and recommend that my patients start with 600 milligrams a day. [73]

Policosanol to Raise Levels of Good Cholesterol

One type of cholesterol, HDL (for high-density lipoprotein), is healthy for your heart—you want to raise your HDL number if it's too low. Ideally, your HDL levels should be above 60; if they're below 40, you need to act. Policosanol is a sugar cane compound proven to safely lower "bad" cholesterol and can raise HDL cholesterol by a healthy 17 percent, according to one study. In a study of 437 patients, those who took policosanol experienced a 28 percent increase in HDL cholesterol. You can find this supplement at most drugstores. [77]

Niacin. Niacin, (Vitamin B3) is a top choice for normalizing blood lipid levels. It can raise HDL levels by up to 40 percent, while reducing total cholesterol 10 to 25 percent and triglycerides by 50 percent. Thomas Lee, M.D., Editor in chief of the *Harvard Heart Letter,* warns not to take no-flush niacin, which doesn't contain nicotinic acid or nicotinamide. He recommends taking an intermediate release niacin called Niaspan and taking it at bedtime to minimize the flushing. It is also flushed from the body after 12 hours, protecting the liver. NOTE: Do not take niacin if you are taking Lipitor or another lipid-lowering drug. [78]

Preventing Stroke by Lowering Stress, Hostility and Depression

A 2014 study confirms that stress, hostility, and depression play as big a role in your cardiovascular health as do your cholesterol levels, blood pressure, and whether you smoke tobacco, says Susan Everson-Rose, Ph.D., lead study author and associate professor of medicine at the University of Minnesota in Minneapolis. In her study of more than 6,700 adults, ages 45 to 84, she learned that those with the highest levels of stress, depression, and hostility were sharply more likely to have a stroke or transient ischemic attack (TIA) than happier, less stressed people.

Compared to people with low stress, low depression, and low anger scores, those with the highest scores for these states of mind were:

- 86 percent more likely to have a stroke or TIA for high depressive scores
- 59 percent more likely to have a stroke or TIA for the highest chronic stress scores
- More than twice as likely to have a stroke or TIA for the highest hostility scores [79]
- Many strategies in this book can help you combat depression, stress, and hostility. Cognitive behavior therapy is a good place to start. I often refer people who deal with crazy-making amounts of stress to the works of my friend, Loretta LaRoche. She wrote the book *Life Is Not a Stress Rehearsal.* It's funny and irreverent, and a great way to gently jolt you into a healthier frame of mind. To learn more, visit www.lorettalaroche.com.

Exercise Beats Pills for Heart Disease

You know that your heart is a muscle. Like other muscles in the body, when you don't exercise it, it gets flabby. And a flabby heart does your vigor and longevity absolutely no favors at all.

If you're not a fan of taking pills, you'll be especially interested in the results of a recent review of more than 57 clinical trials that focused on exercise; it included nearly 15,000 people. The study was published in the renowned UK journal *BMJ* in 2013.

What did this study reveal? Exercise is about as effective as some heart drugs (statins, beta blockers, antiplatelet drugs, and ACE inhibitors) for preventing heart disease deaths. Here's what the researchers said: "Exercise and many drug interventions are often potentially similar in terms of their mortality benefits." They concluded that exercise should be considered as an alternative to— or at least recommended alongside—drug therapy. But the sad truth is that only about 33 percent of primary care docs prescribe the "exercise pill." [63]

If you really want to do your heart some good and lessen your chances for having to take drugs (or potentially be able to reduce the amount you take, or even stop taking them, under your doctor's supervision) you could choose to follow the walking interval exercise program like the one in Part III. Aerobic interval exercise has been proven to improve heart health in people with coronary artery disease. Just make sure you are "cleared" for exercise by your doctor before you start your program, and if you have heart disease, you might want to start with exercise tailored for you, in a cardiac rehab center. [80]

High Blood Pressure

We call high blood pressure a silent killer because this central component of heart disease causes no outward symptoms—your first indication of a problem is likely to be when your doctor straps the cuff around your arm and delivers the unwelcome news.

Staggering Stats

We're terrified of cancer and cower before scary, news-making epidemics like Ebola. Though heart disease doesn't often hit the headlines, it certainly should: It beats cancer as the leading cause of death in the United States, according to these 2011 statistics from the Centers for Disease Control and Prevention.

Disease Deaths in 2011	
Heart disease	596,577
Cancer	576,691
Chronic respiratory diseases	142,943
Stroke (cerebrovascular disease)	128,932
Accidents	126,438
Alzheimer's disease	84,974
Diabetes	73,831 [81]

Blood pressure numbers are a measurement of the force of the blood that pushes against artery walls as your heart pumps. If your blood pressure remains high over time (a condition called hypertension), it damages your heart, your arteries, and other organs. One in three Americans has high blood pressure. Blood pressure is measured in two numbers: systolic (the first number) and diastolic (the second). In a normal blood pressure reading, numbers should be less than 120/80. People are considered to have "pre-hypertension" when pressure reads 120 to 139/80 to 89. Physicians diagnose Stage 1 hypertension at 140 to 159/90 to 99; Stage 2 is 160 or higher over 100 or higher.

But blood pressure isn't static. It's lower when you're asleep or in a deeply relaxed state—when you're meditating, for example. It rises when you're awake, active, excited, or nervous. [82]

That's why it's so important to spend periods of time in a relaxed state as often as possible. It gives your cardiovascular system a much-needed rest and allows your circulation to flow freely. The following steps (along with the other suggestions in this section) can help prevent you from having to rely on medications as your only solution for lower blood pressure.

Master a form of meditation. Researchers who searched medical studies for evidence about meditation's effects on heart disease and blood pressure discovered that several forms of meditation had positive effects. They learned that mindfulness-based stress reduction, transcendental meditation, progressive muscle relaxation, and stress management courses effectively help lower blood pressure. [83]

Chair massage. Massage is much more than a luxurious indulgence reserved for special occasions. Even a 10- to 15-minute chair massage helps lower high blood pressure or pre-hypertension. Here's the science: Iranian researchers studied the effect of massage on 50 women with pre-hypertension. Twenty-five of the women got 10 to 15 minutes of Swedish massage three times a week for 10 sessions; the other 25 spent the same amount of time relaxing. After the 10 sessions, the systolic blood pressure of the women in the massage group dropped from a mean of 128 to 116. The blood pressure of the control group went up about a point. The results persisted at least 3 days following the last massage. What's nice about this study is that it shows even a few chair massage sessions can work wonders to lower blood pressure. Results of this study were published in 2013 in the *International Journal of Preventive Medicine.* Other studies have confirmed massage's positive impact on lowering blood pressure. [84, 85]

Blueberries. Eating just one serving of blueberries a week can drop your risks of having high blood pressure by 10 percent, according to research published in the *American Journal of Clinical Nutrition* in 2011. Blueberries are loaded with powerful antioxidants known as anthocyanins. This compound also occurs in strawberries and raspberries, so be sure to enjoy these sweet treats as well. [86]

Probiotics. In their 2014 study released by the American Heart Association, Australian researchers examined nine high-quality studies involving more than 500 people that measured the effects of taking probiotics on high blood pressure. They concluded that taking probiotics can lower blood pressure. My favorite is Renew Life Ultimate Flora capsules that contain either 30 or 50 billion of these "good bacteria." Generally, the older you get, the more probiotics you need. [87]

Put two dates on your calendar

People with high blood pressure who check in with their doctors twice a year are three times more likely to keep their blood pressure under control.

Check Your Drugs

Prescription, over-the-counter, and recreational drugs can cause high blood pressure. Among them:

- Amphetamines, ecstasy, and cocaine
- Corticosteroids
- Cyclosporine Erythropoietin
- Estrogens (including birth control pills) and other hormones
- Migraine medications
- Nasal decongestants
- OTC drugs—especially cough/cold and anti-asthma medications
- Alcoholic beverages can also increase blood pressure [88]

Clinical Pearls for Cardiovascular Disease

1. Make sure you have your diet, exercise, and stress reduction plan in place (see Part III).

2. Review your prescriptions with your doctor and consider getting a second opinion for an additional review. Find a practitioner who will supervise the use of supplements.
3. Drink one cup of beet juice or use one scoop of powdered organic beets in water or juice every day. This is the probably the best food for the linings of your whole vascular system—all your blood vessels! Beets increase the production of NO (nitric oxide). Dark chocolate is another way to increase nitric oxide and lower your blood pressure. Karin Ried and other researchers from the University of Adelaide in Australia found that chocolate lowered blood pressure by increasing nitric oxide because of its high polyphenol and bioflavonoid content. [89]

CFS/ME (CHRONIC FATIGUE SYNDROME/MYALGIC ENCEPHALOMYELITIS) AND FIBROMYALGIA

Chronic fatigue syndrome can leave you feeling too tired to get through the tasks of your day. It can make you so intolerant to exercise that you are exhausted after crossing a room or taking a shower. It has been called "yuppie flu" and many people who have had it have been told by their doctors that it's all in their heads. It's not. Chronic fatigue is a very real, burdensome illness. Fibromyalgia is another illness that has a history of being misdiagnosed, with patients getting told there is nothing wrong with them, that they should take an antidepressant or get counseling therapy and nothing more. I have seen many patients with CFS/ME, fibromyalgia and other illnesses who have visited a primary care practitioner or two, a rheumatologist, an endocrinologist, and a neurologist and still did not get a correct diagnosis. *Wrong Diagnosis—They Get It Wrong, You Get Blamed* could be a title for a whole additional book on this subject!

CFS/ME

Fatigue, even exhaustion, often comes with the territory of 21st-century life. You may be a breadwinner or a co-breadwinner with a demanding job, and on top of that, a mother or father, supportive spouse, daughter or son of aging parents, or the go-to support person for close friends. You may feel as if you're the tent pole that holds your extended family together. It's no wonder you're exhausted from time to time.

But when your exhaustion lasts longer than 6 consecutive months and interferes with your daily activities, and you've enlisted your doctor's diagnostic skills and still can't connect your fatigue to a medical condition, you could have the debilitating condition known by several names: CFS-Chronic Fatigue Syndrome or CFIDS-Chronic Fatigue Immune Deficiency Syndrome in the U.S., and CFS/ME Chronic Fatigue Syndrome/Myalgic Encephalomyelitis in the UK. The UK term is a little more accurate because it at least implies that there is truly something wrong with your brain and muscle function—and there is! For the rest of this section, I am adopting the UK terminology-CFS/ME because I believe it is a better one. Its symptoms include:

- Severe, chronic fatigue that lasts longer than 6 months
- Fatigue that significantly compromises your daily life, plus four or more of these symptoms:
- Post exertional fatigue lasting more than 24 hours
- Unrefreshing sleep
- Difficulty concentrating or remembering
- Headaches unusual in frequency or duration
- Muscle pain
- Joint pain
- Sore throat
- Tender lymph nodes [90]

Here is a brilliant description of the effects of the illness from Darcell Rockett's *Chicago Tribune* article about the CFS/ME documentary, *Unrest*.

"If you had to live your life knowing that you have only 20 percent of your energy to expend on any given day, how would you ration out your days? How would you make your decisions if hours and days of pain followed, while trying to recharge?"

That's what people who suffer from myalgic encephalomyelitis, or chronic fatigue syndrome, must contend with. ME/CFS is a systemic neuroimmune condition characterized by a severe worsening of symptoms, like profound cognitive and neurological impairment, tachycardia that prevents many from maintaining an upright or sitting position, immunological dysfunction, and an abnormal response to ordinary exertion. The effects leave 25 percent of patients housebound and/or bedridden. Up to 91 percent of those with ME have not been diagnosed, according to the Open Medicine Foundation, which supports ME research.

Jennifer Brea, a former doctoral candidate at Harvard University, was stricken with the disease in 2011. As a way to make sense of her diagnosis, Brea made the documentary "Unrest" from the confines of her bed. It took four years and creatives around the globe to make it happen, but the Sundance-award-winning film captures the experiences of those living with the disease around the world. Brea hopes change comes from her endeavor—more awareness, research, and more empathetic care from medical practitioners.

In "Unrest," Jen and her husband, Omar Wasow, confront an uncertain future in the face of chronic illness... "I want people to know that there are millions suffering invisibly because science and medicine do not see us, because our disabilities are invisible, or because we are trapped in homes and bedrooms and therefore invisible to our communities,' she said. 'How could medicine ignore a disease this common and this devastating? I believed that if the world could see what the experience of this disease was really like... then things might begin to change." [91]

Not so long ago, if your doctor couldn't diagnose your symptoms, she might have suggested they were psychosomatic—that is, all in your head. But 16 years ago, in 2001, acclaimed author Laura Hillenbrand, wrote a best-selling book, even though, like Jennifer Brea, she was suffering with extreme CFS/ME symptoms. Hillenbrand, now 34, can barely enjoy the fruits of her runaway success. She deals with night sweats, fevers, and extreme exhaustion, and for days at a time, she can't leave her home in Washington, DC. Though as of this writing, no treatment has proved effective for Hillenbrand, she says that, "Writing this book was a matter of dignifying my place in this world. I wasn't going to let CFS defeat me." I am shocked that so little has been done to help with CFS/ME in the 16 years between the book and the film, and that health care practitioners are still saying "it's all in your head." [92]

Fortunately, about 75% of people with CFS/ME have milder symptoms. Still, you may have good days and bad days; symptoms can swing from mild to severe from morning to evening for no apparent reason.

Commonly, CFS/ME can overcome a previously fit and active person following an infection of some kind (Hillenbrand's started with a bad case of food poisoning). One theory is that a severe infection can cause a type of immune dysfunction that drastically lowers the ability of the cells to produce energy. Less common triggers include exposure to VOCs, pesticides, or other chemicals; a major trauma or stress (a bad accident, for example); surgical procedures; and even pregnancy. Sometimes, you can't pinpoint a cause: Your energy just starts flagging—you begin feeling tired and ill and no one knows why.

Some experts link CFS/ME to the Epstein-Barr virus or cytomegaloviruses, but viral links certainly aren't apparent in all people with CFS/ME. However, the symptoms of long-term, relapsing Epstein-Barr virus look very much like many of the symptoms of CFS/ME, which include:

- Impaired concentration or short-term memory
- Muscle pain
- Joint pain without swelling or redness
- Headaches of new type, pattern, or severity
- Tender lymph nodes in the armpit
- Frequent or recurring sore throat

There is still no test to prove definitively that you have CFS/ME. However, there are a few preliminary studies that confirm that there may be measurable markers for the disease. In one study, published in the January 2016 Scandinavian Journal of Immunology revealed that CFS/ME sufferers had a lower than normal count of NK (natural killer) cells. [93]

A 2015 study at Griffith University in Australia, has found possible genetic markers for CFS/ME, called SNPs—single nucleotide polymorphisms. They are seeking to partner with a company to produce a laboratory test for the disease. [94]

When I see a person with CFS/ME, I review their diet and environment and see if they are reactive to any of the common allergenic foods and airborne allergens. I advise them to get help to do a clean-up of their living space. I check to see if they have had viruses like EBV or CMV, which may still be sapping their immune systems. I make sure they have no underlying conditions like hypothyroidism. I also check for deficiencies in key vitamins and minerals. A carefully constructed exercise program can be helpful. And as a beginning stress reducer, guided imagery can be a good start. And, I usually recommend at least a trial of the supplements I have described below—NADH and Co-Q10. I would probably not prescribe pills, such as antidepressants or sleeping pills, as a first-line treatment. [95]

Supplements for CFS/MENADH and Co-Q10 for Chronic Fatigue

NADH increases energy at a cellular level. It is a "co-factor" that helps cells produce more ATP (adenosine triphosphate), which is a basic energy source for all cellular activity. Co-Q10 is also a cellular energy co-factor that increases the efficiency of NADH.

A groundbreaking 2015 study from Barcelona, Spain has shown that giving the supplements NADH and Co-Q10 in combination to CFS/ME patients improved their energy and their blood levels of important markers. Here is part of the abstract of the study:

> "We conducted an 8-week, randomized, double-blind placebo-controlled trial to evaluate the benefits of oral CoQ_{10} (200mg/day) plus NADH (20mg/day) supplementation on fatigue and biochemical parameters in 73 Spanish CFS patients. ...A significant improvement of fatigue showing a reduction in fatigue impact scale total score (p<0.05) was reported in treated group *versus* placebo. In addition, a recovery of the biochemical parameters was also reported. NAD+/NADH (p<0.001), CoQ_{10} (p<0.05), ATP (p<0.05), and citrate synthase (p<0.05) were significantly higher, and lipoperoxides (p<0.05) were significantly lower in blood mononuclear cells of the treated group. These observations lead to the hypothesis that the oral CoQ_{10} plus NADH supplementation could confer potential therapeutic benefits on fatigue and biochemical parameters in CFS."

The bottom line is that 20 mg of NADH and 200 mg of Co-Q10 significantly reduced the CFS/ME sufferers' fatigue, increased their blood levels of NADH and ATP (markers of cellular energy production), and lowered levels of lipoperoxides (markers of oxidation). [96]

I believe it would be worthwhile for all people who have a diagnosis of CFS/ME to do at least an 8-week trial of 20 mg of NADH and 200 mg of Co-Q10. Of course, you must make your own decision about that, and consult with your health care practitioner. Source Naturals makes a good sublingual 10 mg NADH and Precision Naturals makes a highly absorbable 100 mg Co-Q10 tablet. The correct dose, according to the study, is two of each, once a day in the morning.

Antiretrovirals can be helpful in CFS/ME if it is determined that a viral illness was part of the cause. Antiviral herbal medicine can also be beneficial. The "name of the game" is to clear your diet and environment of anything that you react to, add energy with diet and supplements, and do your best to avoid expending so much energy that you cause an energy "crash." I attended a showing of the film *Unrest*. The husband of the chronic fatigue sufferer in the film spoke and answered questions at the end of the performance. He said his wife had been helped by having an electric scooter to use, instead of trying to walk all the time.

FIBROMYALGIA

If having chronic fatigue syndrome makes you exhausted, fibromyalgia makes you hurt. It's a chronic pain syndrome whose additional symptoms include fatigue and specific body points that are tender to the touch.

The latest common thinking on fibromyalgia is that it may have a genetic component, and that stress plays a role: It often surfaces after you've experienced significantly stressful events— physical or emotional.

In my clinical experience, fibromyalgia is often associated with inflammation from undiagnosed food allergies, and clinical or subclinical hypothyroidism. If you have been diagnosed with fibromyalgia, be sure to have these checked!

Too often, instead of considering all the other potential factors for your problem, including hormone imbalances, vitamin and mineral deficiencies, and undiagnosed food allergies, physicians diagnose fibromyalgia and prescribe a drug. It appears that the number of fibromyalgia diagnoses is on the rise thanks to the major marketing campaign by the makers of the widely promoted fibromyalgia drug pregabalin (Lyrica). Unfortunately, this drug doesn't come without the potential for some negative side effects.

Pregabalin Side Effects

This anti-seizure medication might be the first thing that comes to your doctor's mind when she's weighing treatments for your fibromyalgia. But Pregabalin has been associated with some disturbing and dangerous side effects.

Ten percent of people experience:
- Dizziness or drowsiness

Between 1 and 10 percent of people experience:
- Visual problems
- Lack of coordination of muscle movements
- Memory problems
- Speech problems
- Constipation
- Dry mouth
- Loss of sex drive/erectile dysfunction
- Weight gain
- Rare side effects:
- Serious, even life-threatening, allergic reactions
- Suicidal thoughts or actions
- Swelling of hands, legs, and feet [97]

If the side effects of a drug like pregabalin don't convince you to try safer, nondrug therapies, maybe the math will. The odds that a drug such as pregabalin or an antidepressant will ease your symptoms are pretty low, says Winfried Häuser, M.D., associate professor of psychosomatic medicine at the Klinikum Saarbrücken in Saarbrücken, Germany. Dr. Häuser is a world-renowned fibromyalgia researcher and expert. [98]

According to Dr. Häuser, out of every four to six people who take an antidepressant or pregabalin for fibromyalgia, one person will experience about one-third less pain. "No drug is very good when it comes to easing any kind of chronic pain condition," says Dr. Häuser. However, there is good news: Two therapies offer sustained relief for fibromyalgia—and are better than drugs, he notes. Aerobic exercise and cognitive behavioral therapies are scientifically proven as effective fibromyalgia treatments and are safe, according to Dr. Häuser. [99]

Supplements for Fibromyalgia

In the case of fibromyalgia, reducing your pain means making sure that your muscles receive the nutrients they need to perform optimally. I advise most people to take a good high-potency multivitamin with minerals, fish oil, and a probiotic. In addition, some studies over the past few years have yielded positive news about the benefits of certain supplements for easing symptoms of fibromyalgia. Here's what we know.

Vitamin D. We know that low blood levels of vitamin D are common in people with severe pain and fibromyalgia, but until 2014, researchers hadn't studied whether taking vitamin D supplements might help. In a study published in the journal *Pain,* 30 women with fibromyalgia were given either a placebo or enough vitamin D to raise their blood levels of the vitamin to sufficient levels. After 24 weeks, the women given vitamin D reported that their pain decreased significantly. Since most people have vitamin D deficiencies, especially those living in the northern half of the United States, I recommend that my patients take a daily supplement of 1,000–2000 IU per day. [100]

Co-Q10. A deficiency of this pro-energy coenzyme has been linked to fibromyalgia. Researchers gave 20 people with fibromyalgia either 300 milligrams of Co-Q10 a day or a placebo for 40 days. At the end of the trial, the participants in the Co-Q10 group reported less pain, fatigue, and morning tiredness than did the people in the placebo group. What's more, the people who'd taken Co-Q10 had fewer "tender points" and less inflammation than those who took a placebo. I recommend that my patients with chronic fatigue syndrome and fibromyalgia take a daily Co-Q10 supplement of 200 to 400 milligrams. [101]

I also recommend **NADH** in combination with Co-Q10 for fibromyalgia as I do for Co-Q10. (See above.)

Acetyl-l-carnitine. This so-called non-essential amino acid is found in red meat and dairy products. It plays a role in the production of acetylcholine, which is a key neurotransmitter; some experts recommend it for memory problems. In a 2007 study, 102 people with fibromyalgia were given either two capsules a day of 500 milligrams LAC or a placebo. Researchers tested them at 6 weeks; tender points were reduced in the LAC group, along with other problems including stiffness, fatigue, and depression.

SAM-e (S-adenosylmethionine) is a supplement with antidepressant properties, that also supports liver function. It can be helpful for both CFS/ME and fibromyalgia. The usual beginning dose is 200 to 400 mg, but sometimes a larger dose is needed—as much as 800 milligrams daily.

Food and Exercise and Stress Reduction Plan for CFS/ME and Fibromyalgia

A diet full of fresh fruits and vegetables, high quality proteins, and good fats—the diet in Part III of this book—is especially beneficial for people with chronic fatigue syndrome and fibromyalgia because it's rich in antioxidants. These are particularly important for fighting both conditions, because antioxidants neutralize free radicals. This helps prevent cell damage and inflammation that can contribute to the exhaustion and pain caused by CFS and fibromyalgia.

Make sure to add these super antioxidants to your daily diet. All must be organic.

- Green, black, hibiscus, and rooibos teas
- Berries of all colors—blueberries, raspberries, strawberries, blackberries
- Red, purple, and blue grapes
- Dark green veggies [102]

In addition, what you leave out of your diet counts! A Paleo-style, low-carbohydrate higher-fat diet like our Alive and Well Food Plan omits these inflammatory foods: grains, sugars, dairy, and alcohol. Freeing your body from having to process these inflammatory foods is very helpful for more energy and less pain.

Note: For most people, an occasional treat such as a fast-food meal or a pizza, for example, won't be a problem. But even one such diet departure could worsen symptoms of fibromyalgia and CFS/ME. People who have one of these conditions may be more reactive than others to food additives, pesticides, gluten, corn, and soy. If you have CFS/ME or fibromyalgia, and you have tested reactive to any of these foods or food additives, it pays to be extra vigilant about your diet to avoid any potential triggers.

Finally, be aware that unrefreshing sleep is a hallmark problem for CFS and fibromyalgia. Please see the Insomnia paragraphs of this section (below) where I outline strategies to help you learn better sleep habits. After some weeks of practice, you will probably begin to get the deep, restful slumber that can ease symptoms of both conditions.

Exercise

When you have fibromyalgia or CFS/ME, probably exercise is the last thing on your mind. You're exhausted, and you may be in pain. And you also may fear that exercise will worsen your symptoms. Many people with CFS/ME experience something called post exertional fatigue, which means that your symptoms might worsen within 12 to 48 hours after you exercise. If you have either of these illnesses, you probably already know that there seems to be an invisible "line" when it comes to exercise—stay under that line and you can keep going. Go over it, and something in your body "snaps" and you need to lie down.

Start slowly. At first, start with just a few minutes of gentle movement and build from there. If possible, find an exercise coach who specializes in working with people who have chronic fatigue or fibromyalgia.

Move, then rest. Try following every 1 minute of exercise with 3 minutes of rest. Then increase your exercise sessions slowly by 1 to 5 minutes each session.

Spread it out. Don't feel you have to do all your exercise at once. It's generally better for you to spread two or three sessions out during the day.

Try warm water exercise. Warm water exercise is proven to help ease pain in people with fibromyalgia. Your local YMCA may have pool classes for people with arthritis, which are perfect. If not, try other pool-based exercise programs or check out aquatic physical therapy.

Avoid getting out of breath. While you're exercising (our walking program in Part 3 is a perfect way to start), you should be able to speak normally without losing your breath.[103]

Cognitive Behavioral Therapy, EFT, and Guided Imagery

One of the problems with recommending any kind of counseling therapy or antidepressant medication for people who suffer from CFS/ME or fibromyalgia is that they are so (rightfully) disgusted with being told their very real illness is all in their head. Any suggestion of psychologically-based treatment seems to them to be another way of dismissing their illness. Here is the problem with that: These very real, physical illnesses take their emotional toll. There are diagnostic categories called "Depression, reactive to illness" and "Anxiety, reactive to illness." Counseling therapy and medications may be needed just to manage the stress of the major and often catastrophic life changes brought on by these two chronic diseases.

Cognitive behavioral therapy is a talk therapy that helps you change thinking and behavior. It's been proven as one of the most effective ways for helping people with fibromyalgia feel better—and many experts also believe that this therapy can be a powerful tool for people with chronic fatigue syndrome, too. A 2013 review of 23 studies involving 2,031 people revealed that after 12 weeks, CBT slightly reduced pain, negative mood, and disability, and improvements continued for at least 6 months after therapy ended. Remember, this is far from another way of saying it's all in your head. It is a way to ease the very real stresses that are bound to be a part of your life if you have CFS/ME or fibromyalgia. To find a therapist near you, visit academyofct.org. [104]

EFT is a therapy based on the acupuncture system. To learn more, see the section about stress relief in Part III. EFT can help heal past trauma and present stresses, which may be a contributing factor in these illnesses.

Guided Imagery can also be helpful for many aspects of CFS/ME and fibromyalgia. For more about these methods, see Part III.

DEPRESSION AND ANXIETY

Anxiety and depression are serious and potentially dangerous health disorders that affect both the mind and body. And though many effective natural therapies exist to treat these disorders, unfortunately, the current treatment of choice—despite the many side effects—is usually a pill.

Anxiety occurs more often than depression—18 percent of Americans have a diagnosed anxiety disorder, compared to 6 percent who've been diagnosed with depression. Depression is the most disabling of all the mental and behavioral disorders. [105, 106]

What is the difference between being chronically anxious and chronically depressed? It's not as black and white as you'd suspect. You might think that anxious people are high-strung and fidgety, and that depressed people have low energy and seem sad. But these are stereotypes that cloud the reality and perpetuate the misunderstandings that surround these illnesses.

Although anxiety and depression are different medical disorders, they share several similarities. People with depression often feel hopeless and angry. Ordinary daily tasks overwhelm them, and they tend to have low energy levels. People dealing with anxiety can also be overwhelmed by life's responsibilities and may face normal life situations with fear or panic. They, too, can feel chronically exhausted. In fact, many people have aspects of depression *and* anxiety. Both depression and anxiety can interfere with your ability to work or maintain relationships. In severe cases, you may even be unable to leave your house. In conventional medicine, anxiety and depression are usually treated similarly with pills—various antidepressant and anti-anxiety medications. [107]

Depression

Unfortunately, despite all the dramatic drug ads showing depressed people becoming "happy" again once they take the advertised pills, the fact is that 55 to 65 percent of people either don't respond fully to antidepressants or they experience side effects, including insomnia, sexual problems, weight gain, restlessness, and memory lapses. Rarer but even scarier side effects include suicide, violence, psychosis, and abnormal bleeding.[108]

There's no one-size-fits-all when it comes to depression. You're certainly familiar with the feeling of being sad, unhappy, or even downright miserable. Usually, in someone who doesn't have a diagnosable mental illness, sad feelings are caused by an upsetting event—a death or divorce, a serious illness (yours or a loved one's), a change in financial circumstances, or an "empty nest." The feelings can last a few days, weeks, or a couple of months. But when sadness doesn't go away, and when it interferes with your daily activities, then your depression needs to be addressed. Symptoms of clinical depression include:

- Low mood, most of the time
- Loss of pleasure in daily activities
- Early morning waking
- Trouble sleeping, or sleeping too much
- Changes in appetite—either weight gain or loss
- Exhaustion
- Feelings of worthlessness, self-hate, and guilt
- Difficulty concentrating
- Feeling hopeless
- Suicidal thoughts [108]

Anxiety: When Worry Is Winning

Anxiety comes in many variations. At one end of the spectrum is the garden-variety anxiety that we all know so well and experience nearly every day—usually, several times a day. Realities such as the traffic jam, the deadline, the angry boss, the bounced check—any of these can generate anxious feelings. But for most of us, most of the time, these feelings are fleeting— and are part of our daily stresses. I describe the effects of stress and discuss several effective stress-relieving methods in Part 3.

True anxiety, on the other hand, isn't just stress caused by a rotten day. True anxiety happens when your stressful feelings become overwhelming, or nearly so, and chronic. You begin to feel as if your life is just one fierce worry after another. That light at the end of the tunnel? You're afraid you'll never see it.

When worry like this consumes you, especially when your worries are unrealistic (your house will burn down during your vacation; the bridge you're driving across will collapse; your airplane could crash; terrorists will bomb your city; you might contract Ebola), then you're edging into the territory of an anxiety disorder. Officially known as Generalized Anxiety Disorder (GAD), this is a very real condition characterized by an inappropriate level of worry. When such worry interferes with your daily life, and you've experienced it on a chronic basis for at least 6 months, that is classified as GAD.

Some 6.8 million adults will experience GAD in any given year, according to the Anxiety and Depression Association of America; women are twice as likely as men to be affected. We don't know exactly what causes GAD, but we suspect that genetics, family background, and life experiences, particularly stressful ones, play a role. [109]

Throughout your life, your anxiety levels will shift up or down. If your anxiety levels fall mostly on the mild side of the spectrum, you can enjoy a normal work, family, and social life, though you might find yourself avoiding situations that make you especially anxious (think parties or travel, for example). People with more severe GAD will have trouble dealing with even simple everyday activities. [109]

You may also develop certain physical symptoms, including:

- Muscle tension
- Fatigue

- Restlessness
- Difficulty sleeping
- Irritability
- Edginess [110]

Panic Disorder

Having a panic attack is a truly terrifying experience. Your heart races; you might have trouble breathing; you break into a sweat—you may even feel chest pain and worry that you're having a heart attack.

Not everyone who experiences a panic attack has a panic disorder—you can have just one attack and never have another. Panic disorder affects some 6 million people—twice as many women as men; it may be an inherited condition.

Left unaddressed, panic disorder can make you afraid to leave the house (a condition called agoraphobia). Unfortunately, it can be a difficult condition to correctly diagnose. On the good news front, however, once it's diagnosed, panic disorder often responds to treatment, especially to cognitive behavioral therapy and EFT. [105]

When Trauma Lingers: Post-Traumatic Stress Disorder (PTSD)

People who have experienced horrific ordeals—combat veterans, victims of violent crimes, survivors of child abuse, or people who've lived through natural disasters, for example—may develop PTSD, which affects nearly 8 million Americans. Marked by flashbacks of the event, nightmares, and frightening thoughts, PTSD often causes its sufferers to lose interest in activities they once enjoyed, to become depressed and even feel guilty, and to avoid situations or places that trigger memories of the event. People with PTSD tend to startle easily, have angry outbursts and trouble sleeping, and feel anxious. As with panic disorders, cognitive behavioral therapy (CBT), EFT, or EMDR (Eye

Movement Desensitization and Reprocessing) can be extremely helpful. Standard talk therapy may not work well for PTSD because it may retraumatize rather than help the person. For more about this, read Belleruth Naparstek's superb book, *Invisible Heroes* (Bantam, 2007). [111]

The Medication Situation: One of America's Top-Selling Drugs Is an Antipsychotic

I admit it: I was stunned to learn that the drug Abilify (aripiprazole) had become America's top-selling drug in 2013, with sales of $6,293,801,000. The drug is meant to be prescribed for schizophrenia and bipolar disorder. However, it is also often prescribed with antidepressants for people diagnosed with depression. Although millions of Americans are currently taking Abilify, we don't actually know how it works. In 2012, Richard A. Friedman, M.D., professor of psychiatry at Weill Cornell Medical College in New York City, expressed his concern in a *New York Times* article. He wrote that Abilify and similar drugs are increasingly prescribed for people with less serious conditions, such as depression and anxiety—conditions for which they may not be appropriate. I agree. These drugs may have their place in treating serious psychiatric disorders, but I can't imagine the circumstances that would have me prescribe them for less debilitating emotional problems. [112-114]

Even without the "off label" prescribing, antidepressant drugs carry serious risks. A September 2017 study published online in the journal *Psychotherapy and Psychosomatics* found a 33% increase in risk of death from all causes, and a 14% increase for new cardiovascular events from antidepressant use. Both the newer serotonin reuptake inhibitors (SSRIs) and the older tricyclics were tested. The above numbers are for the SSRIs, but the study revealed almost equal risk for the tricyclics.

"In general-population samples, antidepressant use increased the risk for death from any cause by 33% (hazard ratio

[HR], 1.33; 95% confidence interval [CI], 1.14 - 1.55) and the risk for new cardiovascular events by 14% (HR, 1.14; 95% CI, 1.08 - 1.21)." The study did point out that this increased risk did not apply to people with established cardiovascular disease. They speculated that this effect might be caused by the blood-thinning effects of the antidepressants. [115]

Lead researcher Paul W. Andrews, Ph.D., J.D., of the Department of Psychology, Neuroscience and Behavior, McMaster University, Hamilton, Ontario, Canada, told *Medscape Medical News:* "The common wisdom is that antidepressants are safe and effective, and by treating people with depression with antidepressants, we can save lives. However, research over the last decade has shown that antidepressants are much less effective than we had thought. Our research is part of a body of research that suggests that antidepressants are much less safe than we had thought." [116]

All too often, physicians and others in our medical system assume that "chemical imbalance" or "faulty brain wiring" or "deficient neurotransmitters" are the sole causes of mental disorders. However, that kind of thinking fails to consider other, easily addressed causes, such as underlying vitamin and mineral deficiencies, allergic reactivity, hormone imbalances, or family dynamics. In my opinion, these all need to be addressed and corrected. Drugs may be needed too, but not as an isolated solution.

I do understand that for some people, medication can play a valuable, even life-saving, role when properly prescribed. A prescription may be needed to address the symptoms while all other factors are being examined, and for some people, regular, long-term use of medication is necessary even when all the other factors that can affect anxiety or depression have been addressed. Here is more information on the medications frequently prescribed for depression and anxiety.

Selective serotonin reuptake inhibitors (SSRIs). These are the drugs with the 33% greater risk of death from all causes. These drugs are designed to relieve symptoms by blocking the reabsorption (reuptake) of serotonin by certain nerve cells in the brain. That allows more serotonin to circulate, which may improve your mood; doctors prescribe these drugs for both anxiety and depression. SSRIs include citalopram (Celexa), escitalopram (Lexapro), fluoxetine (Prozac), paroxetine (Paxil), and sertraline (Zoloft). Among the more common side effects linked to SSRIs are insomnia or its opposite, sleepiness. They're also known to cause weight gain and sexual dysfunction. [115, 117]

Serotonin-norepinephrine reuptake inhibitors (SNRIs). These pills, including venlafaxine (Effexor) and duloxetine (Cymbalta), increase levels of serotonin and another neurotransmitter, norepinephrine. They are considered an appropriate first-line treatment for anxiety disorders, though they're also prescribed for depression, according to experts at the Anxiety and Depression Association of America.

Both drugs come with a dramatic warning for children, teens, and young adults up to 24 years of age. During clinical studies on antidepressants such as venlafaxine and duloxetine, a small number of people in those age groups became suicidal. We don't know whether that's a side effect of the drug, or if depressed young people are simply at higher than normal risk for suicidal thoughts. Still, both drugs are associated with a very long list of side effects, all of which could make a person feel worse rather than better. [118, 119]

Benzodiazepines. They're prescribed for short-term anxiety treatment because, unlike SNRIs and SSRIs, they act quickly to make you feel relaxed. But these drugs, which include alprazolam (Xanax), clonazepam (Klonopin), diazepam (Valium), and lorazepam (Ativan), also trigger dependence and addiction, and you can develop tolerance to them, meaning that you'll need increasingly higher doses to achieve the same effect.

These drugs have a huge potential for side effects such as confusion, sleepiness, and even depression. What's more, they're responsible for deadly effects when people drink alcohol while they're taking benzodiazepines (and opioid pain killers), which happens all too frequently.

According to the Centers for Disease Control and Prevention, alcohol was involved in about one in five deaths related to abuse of opioid pain relievers or benzodiazepines in 2010. Here's what CDC and FDA researchers found in an analysis of data on drug-related ER visits and deaths.

- Alcohol was involved in 19% of the 440,000 ER visits related to opioid abuse and in 27% of the 410,000 visits related to benzodiazepine abuse.
- Alcohol was involved in 22% of the nearly 4,000 opioid-related deaths and in 21% of the 1,500 benzodiazepine-related deaths.

My take on this class of drugs is pretty much to avoid them if possible. Of course, as with everything in medicine, there is the exceptional patient in extraordinary circumstances for whom a short-term treatment with these drugs might be appropriate—a physician might prescribe them correctly for someone who has experienced a terribly traumatic event, for example, and then only with appropriate support. The bottom line in my opinion: The use of these drugs should be very carefully considered—and infrequent.

A Non-Pharmaceutical Approach to Relieving Depression and Anxiety

Though you wouldn't know it from the drug company advertising you see on television and in magazines, the truth is that diet along with exercise and several other natural therapies can help ease your symptoms of depression or anxiety. Studies show that some of these therapies are every bit as effective as pharmaceutical antidepressants.

The Man Who Felt He Was Going to Die—All Because of Dye!

It is important for anyone with depression to check the basics: diet is first—including looking for vitamin and mineral deficiencies as well as reactions to foods, additives, and dyes. In my experience, just as food sensitivities can trigger physical problems, they can also play a role in emotional problems—especially if you're regularly eating foods, dyes, and additives to which you react. A patient came to me with severe anxiety, depression, and mental confusion, as well as weight loss and digestive problems. Several doctors told him they could find nothing wrong with him. His medications weren't working. He and his family were convinced he might die. It turned out that he was allergic to food dyes and had a habit of constantly eating orange Tic-Tacs. Unfortunately, none of his other health care practitioners had taken a complete enough history (or suspected the damaging power of food dyes) to discover this. Luckily, after quitting his Tic-Tac habit, he recovered completely.

Paleo-style diet for depression and anxiety—Low sugar, high Omega 3s

One key benefit of a Paleo-style diet when it comes to depression and anxiety is this: It's extremely low in sugar. Why is this so important if you're dealing with mood issues?

Because eating sugar can make you feel like you've hopped on a mood roller coaster. Eat that sugary doughnut for breakfast or a mid-morning snack and the next thing you know, your mood is going up and down right along with your blood sugar. Soon after downing the doughnut, you're feeling happy as can be. But just a few hours later, you crash into the doldrums. One key to maintaining a balanced mood is to keep your blood sugar balanced, and that's exactly what a Paleo-type diet will do for you. After all, if this type of diet plus exercise, supplements, and stress reduction can reverse

Alzheimer's disease, as I described earlier, imagine what it might do to relieve your anxiety and depression!

Another key benefit is that a Paleo-type diet contains fish. As we've noted before, fish is rich in omega-3 fatty acids, which studies have shown can ease depression. Aim for at least four servings a week. One 3.5-ounce serving of wild salmon provides about 1,000 to 2,000 milligrams of EPA and DHA, which are the key omega-3s shown to benefit depression. Since most studies show you need to take about 2 grams of fish oil a day, I also recommend that my patients take a good fish oil supplement. [120]I've seen several studies that point to the mood-lifting benefits of the B-vitamin group. So, concentrate on eating plenty of foods that contain B6, B12, and folate. You'll find these in leafy green veggies, organic eggs, and organic fish, chicken, and meat. [121]

Talk Therapy for Depression and Anxiety

For many of my patients who have anxiety or depression (or both), once I work on identifying any food allergies and help them structure a more appropriate diet, I usually suggest they also engage in some form of talk therapy. One of the best studied and most effective of these is cognitive behavioral therapy.

Cognitive behavioral therapy (CBT)

CBT has been proven effective in hundreds of clinical trials for many different mental disorders. It's different from the psychotherapy you probably think of first—lying on the couch, Freudian style, pouring out your past experiences to a therapist over months or years, seeking the moments that help you understand why you behave the way you do. Instead, a CBT therapist will teach you how to create new and more useful thought and behavior patterns. The therapist will also help you to identify your distressing thoughts and to figure out whether those thoughts are distorted— and will show you how distorted thinking can affect your behavior.

Once the therapist helps a patient see that her thoughts are distorted, the therapist will help her learn to change the distorted thinking. When people think more realistically, say CBT experts, they feel better. The therapy then focuses on teaching you how to solve problems and create more helpful behaviors. [122]

The process is goal-oriented: Most CBT therapists will help you develop a goal list and decide which goals you'll work on yourself and which you'll work out in therapy. The therapist will also help you develop an "action plan" or homework to do during the week. To find a CBT therapist near you, visit academyofct.org. [122]

In a CBT study published in the September 2014 issue of *Lancet Psychiatry,* researchers analyzed 101 clinical trials, which included more than 13,000 participants. They compared the effectiveness of various pharmaceutical drugs and different psychotherapies for treating social anxiety disorder (the fear or anxiety of being in social situations). [123]

The research team concluded that one-on-one cognitive behavioral therapy might prove more effective than drugs for treating adults who have social anxiety disorder. What's more, they said, it has fewer side effects and "should be regarded as the best intervention for initial treatment" of the disorder.

Exercise for Depression

Exercise has been confirmed to be a major factor in relieving depression by studies known as the SMILE studies, done by a research group at Duke University. The study subjects had all been medically diagnosed with major depressive disorder (MDD). Here is a good definition of MDD, from an article "Is Exercise a Viable Treatment for Depression" by members of the Blumenthal group.

> "Depression is a term that refers both to a transient mood state and a clinical syndrome or disorder. Depression as a mood state is characterized by feeling sad, discouraged,

or unhappy, while depression as a clinical condition is a psychiatric disorder in which diagnostic criteria require five or more depressive symptoms, one of which must include either depressed mood or loss of interest or pleasure along with at least four other depressive symptoms including significant weight loss, sleep disturbance, psychomotor agitation or retardation, fatigue or loss of energy, feelings of worthlessness or excessive guilt, diminished ability to think or concentrate, and recurrent thoughts of death. Major depressive disorder (MDD) is distinguished from transient feelings of depression by both the severity and duration of symptoms: symptoms of depression must be present for all or most days of the week for at least 2 weeks, represent a *change* from a previous level of functioning, and be accompanied by somatic, cognitive, or affective symptoms." [124]

I have included this definition of MDD to emphasize that the people studied had serious, long term, medically diagnosed cases of depression. Yet what happened when they exercised? Their depression improved. Initially they studied 156 older adults and randomized them to three groups—medication only, exercise only, and medication plus exercise. At the end of the study it initially appeared that there was no significant difference between the treatments. But a 10-month follow-up revealed that not only were the exercisers less likely to relapse, people who had exercised during the 10-month period were 50% less likely to be depressed than non-exercisers. In a subsequent study and follow-up, the Duke research group confirmed this finding—that the people who continued to exercise in the follow-up period were the ones who were least likely to be depressed. Most studies also found that 30-45 minutes of exercise three times per week was enough to improve depression and prevent relapse, but there is still no clear, agreed upon finding about the exact "exercise dose" that is needed. But even without that, we know without a doubt that exercise is an effective treatment for depression. [124-128]

Traditional Chinese Medicine for Depression and Anxiety

Since I have been trained in Traditional Chinese Medicine (TCM), that is often one of my choices for treating anxiety and depression. Throughout this book, we'll discuss the effectiveness of acupuncture for several different conditions. You're probably aware that acupuncture is one of the therapies under the TCM umbrella. But TCM is much more—it encompasses medicinal herbs, massage, diet, movement, meditation, and breathing exercises.

In TCM, healers use herbs much differently than most Western herbalists do. Rarely are Chinese herbs used singly, nor are they typically used to treat single symptoms. That's because TCM practitioners believe that symptoms are caused by a variety of imbalances within your system that block the flow of vital energy, so herbs are blended into formulas intended to correct specific imbalances. Sometimes practitioners will make an individual formula for a patient; sometimes they will use classic Chinese herbal formulas.

For treating depression and anxiety, I often rely on a group of Chinese herbal formulas that belong to a category known as herbs that "nourish the heart and calm the spirit." I appreciate the names of these blends--Heavenly Emperor, Peaceful Spirit, or Restful Sleep-- they're an indication of how differently TCM views medicine. If you want to explore TCM and Chinese herbs, I recommend that you find a certified TCM practitioner—this is not a DIY therapy. Visit the National Certification Commission for Acupuncture and Oriental Medicine at nccaom.org. [129]

Supplements That May Ease Anxiety and Depression

Remember, I am talking about mild anxiety and depressed mood when I discuss supplements. If you have acute, moderate, or severe anxiety or depression--for example, a diagnosis of GAD (generalized anxiety disorder) or MDD (major depressive disorder), see your health care practitioner. None of these supplements work overnight, so when I give them to my patients, I tell them to take them for at least a few weeks to see if they help.

Theanine. L-theanine is an amino acid that's been studied for several different effects; most of the research centers on its effectiveness as an anxiety treatment. It's something I use first for many patients, especially because it doesn't interact with other medications they may be taking. Theanine is found mainly in green and black teas, and you can find it in supplement form at health food stores and some drugstores. In studies, it seems to relax the mind without causing drowsiness. In one study, taking 400 milligrams a day of theanine reduced anxiety among people with schizophrenia. A cup of black tea has about 20 milligrams of theanine. [130]

B vitamins. We know that vitamin deficiencies can cause mental problems. For example, thiamin, AKA vitamin B1, deficiency is directly connected with depression. Like other B-complex vitamins, thiamine is sometimes called an anti-stress vitamin because it may strengthen the immune system and improve the body's ability to withstand stressful conditions. Finnish researchers found that high to normal blood levels of vitamin B12 increased the effectiveness of drugs and therapy in 115 people with depression. Other studies suggest that getting enough vitamin B12 may prevent depression in the first place. NOTE: It is worth a trial to take a B-complex vitamin once a day. [131, 132]

Fish oil. The latest research shows that taking fish oil can increase certain white blood cells that get rid of inflammatory substances. And that might play a role in the fact that fish oil seems to be useful for easing depression, which some researchers suspect has an inflammatory component. I use NOW Foods Ultra Omega-3—it doesn't have a fishy aftertaste; it's mercury free; and it contains 2½ times the usual EPA/DHA dose in each capsule. Most fish oil capsules have 300 milligrams of combined EPA/DHA in a single 1,000-milligram (1-gram) capsule. Ultra EFA has 750 milligrams of EPA/DHA in one 1,000-milligram capsule. I believe it is well worth taking a fish oil capsule a day. [133]

SAMe: Depression relief equal to pharmaceuticals. Short for S-adenosylmethionine, SAMe is a naturally occurring compound made from an amino acid. Your body uses it to produce neurotransmitters, and it's possible that it may boost levels of serotonin and dopamine. In Europe, SAMe has been prescribed as a treatment for depression for more than 25 years. A recent report from the Agency for Healthcare Quality and Research analyzed the results of 28 studies and found that SAMe was about as effective as standard antidepressants, without the side effects. The one downside of SAMe, however, is its price. It could cost up to $200 per month, depending on the dose you need. On the bright side, it may also relieve arthritis and other forms of pain. Doses range from 400 to 1,600 milligrams per day, but most people do well on the 400-milligram daily dose. [133]

Curcumin: New research on its use for depression/anxiety. The potent antioxidant compound curcumin, which is found in the Indian spice turmeric, was recently proven in a clinical trial to be helpful for relieving depression. In this gold standard 2014 study, published in the *Journal of Affective Disorders,* 56 people diagnosed with major depressive disorder were treated with a curcumin extract (500 milligrams twice a day) or a placebo. Participants were asked to rate their depression levels on a standardized scale. By week 4, and continuing through week 8, curcumin was significantly more effective than the placebo in lowering their symptoms. What's more, noted the researchers, curcumin was even more effective in relieving symptoms of atypical depression, which they said is a more difficult disorder to treat. [134]

"Curcumin promotes the formation of new brain cells, a process called neurogenesis," says Ajay Goel, Ph.D., director of epigenetics and cancer prevention at Baylor Research Institute in Dallas. What's more, he says, curcumin inhibits monoamine oxidase, which helps boost the levels of various neurotransmitters to help fight depression. It might also play a role in easing anxiety, theorizes Dr. Goel. "I believe taking curcumin could help treat anxiety, because anxiety is also a consequence of altered levels of various neurotransmitters." The extract used in the study is known as BMC-95, which is available in several supplements, including Life Extension Super Bio-Curcumin and Curamin. [135]

German chamomile: Gentle relief from anxiety. Chamomile (*Matricaria recutita*) can be an appropriate herb for people whose anxiety upsets their digestion. It contains compounds that relieve spasms in the gut as well as volatile oils that have sedative qualities. In one 2012 University of Pennsylvania study, researchers gave 57 people diagnosed with anxiety, depression, or both, either a chamomile extract or a placebo for 8 weeks. The researchers concluded that chamomile effectively reduced their symptoms. The dose was four 220-milligram capsules a day. An extract similar to the one used in the study is Nature's Way Standardized Chamomile. It is important to avoid chamomile if you are allergic to ragweed. Chamomile and ragweed belong to the same plant family. [136, 137]

DIABETES

When you hear the words *terrifying epidemic,* the first thing you envision is a disease like Ebola, which was capturing daily headlines and nightly television news stories around the country three years ago. In December 2014, the *New York Times* reported that 10 people in the United States had been infected with Ebola; of them, two died. Also, in December, the Centers for Disease Control and Prevention, reported that worldwide, nearly 6,400 people, mostly from West African countries, had died.

Contrast that to diabetes. According to the ADA (American Diabetic Association) in 2010, diabetes was the seventh leading cause of death in the United States. Diabetes was listed as the cause of death on more than 69,000 death certificates, and as a contributing cause on 234,000 additional death certificates that same year. In 2012, almost 30 million Americans had diabetes. That's 9.3% of the population, nearly one in every 10 people. Of Americans 65 and older, almost 26 percent have diabetes. Diabetes contributes to blindness, amputations, heart disease, kidney disease, neuropathy, Alzheimer's disease, and dementia, among other painful and life-shortening conditions. That's what I call a truly terrifying epidemic. And the worst thing about those numbers? Type 2 diabetes, the far more prevalent form of the disease, is largely preventable.

Why this astounding epidemic of diabetes? We reviewed many of the reasons back in Part I. In a nutshell, it's our couch potato lifestyle married to our factory farm/big food/big pharma culture. We are taking the nutrition right out of our produce and our livestock. We are polluting our waters and our atmosphere. We are concocting processed foods out of unhealthy and downright harmful chemicals. Our jobs are largely sedentary, and we're addicted to sitting and staring into the screens of our TVs, computers, tablets, and cell phones.

And to the "rescue" comes the pharmaceutical industry with its expensive drugs, riddled with side effects, to treat illnesses like diabetes, that should be—and could be—prevented.

Don't mistake my message. I'm not saying that all drugs are harmful or that they aren't important tools for treatment of conditions. I am saying, however, that taking pills as the first and only line of defense for treating lifestyle diseases like diabetes makes no sense to me—especially when some of those pills may not help the disease significantly, may contribute to causing other diseases, and may never offer the hope of a cure. In fact, once diagnosed, and given medications without lifestyle changes, you're usually stuck with a lifetime of pill taking.

What Is Diabetes?

Type 2 diabetes occurs when your cells become resistant to the hormone insulin. Insulin, produced in a cone-shaped organ called the pancreas, is the key that "unlocks" your cells to let in glucose, or blood sugar, which cells depend on for energy. When cells start resisting insulin's action and don't "unlock," the pancreas pumps out increasingly higher levels of insulin. When you can't produce enough insulin to meet increased demands, blood sugar levels increase, and type 2 diabetes develops.

Here's how these higher blood sugar levels hurt you—they weaken the linings of your blood vessels and affect your heart. As an easy metaphor, think of sugar as a tiny sharp-edged diamond, scraping the insides of your blood vessels and damaging the interior walls.

The deadly combination of high blood sugar, high blood pressure and high blood fats leads to heart attacks, strokes, and peripheral artery disease. The constant presence of sugar against the interior walls of the vulnerable vessels of the kidneys and the eyes gradually shuts them down, causing kidney failure and loss of vision. Left untreated, diabetes compromises your entire circulatory system, which in turn slows wound healing, makes infections more difficult to overcome, and eventually creates the kind of circulation problems that can lead to nerve damage, diabetic ulcers, and even amputations.

Type 1 diabetes, which accounts for about 5 percent of all diabetes cases, is an autoimmune disease. With this type of diabetes, your immune system attacks and destroys the beta cells in the pancreas, which produce insulin. People with type 1 diabetes must monitor blood sugar carefully and give themselves insulin injections or use an insulin pump.

Pre-Diabetes

You're in your doctor's office, and she's going over the results of your recent checkup, which included routine blood tests. She has some news that you're not too happy to hear. Namely, that you've gained some weight since your last checkup, and your levels of blood sugar, cholesterol, and your blood pressure have edged above normal limits. According to your doctor, you have prediabetes.

A prediabetes diagnosis occurs when your fasting blood sugar levels measure 100 to 125 mg/dl, or your A1C (a measurement of blood sugar levels over time) is 5.7 to 6.4. If your blood sugar levels are 126 mg/dl or above, or your A1C is 6.5 or above, your diagnosis is type 2 diabetes.

If you're wondering why your doctor is diagnosing you with a condition before you even *have* that condition, you're not alone. You might think it means that you're at extremely high risk for developing diabetes—to the extent that maybe it makes good sense to take a pill now in hopes of staving off the disease.

The truth is, less than 50 percent of all people who are diagnosed with prediabetes develop diabetes within 10 years. And yet, a pill, usually metformin, is often the first line of defense in this diagnostic category. If you have gotten a prediabetes diagnosis, what do you do?

Here's the wrong reaction to getting a prediabetes diagnosis, says Matt Longjohn, M.D., M.P.H., who is the national health officer for the YMCA of the USA: "Whew, at least I don't have diabetes." And he adds, "Your reaction really should be, 'Wow—I need to do something about this *right now*.'" And what you need to do immediately is to change your lifestyle, not just take a pill!

One smart and scientifically proven way to stop prediabetes in its tracks, and prevent it from becoming the "real thing," is to join a coach-led weight loss program called the Diabetes Prevention Program. Conducted at YMCAs around the country, the program can prevent nearly 60 percent of people with prediabetes from developing diabetes. If you're over age 60, that number rises to 71 percent, says Dr. Longjohn.

People in the YMCA program typically meet for 16 weekly hour-long classes, led by a specially trained lifestyle coach. The coach helps instill healthy, diabetes-protective behaviors, including how to eat more healthfully and teaching that exercise is vital to preventing diabetes. **In the studies, people either took the YMCA program or took metformin. Twice as many people who took the course prevented diabetes, compared to the metformin group.** To find a program near you, check the YMCA website, or, <u>NOTE</u>: visit the CDC.gov website and type "diabetes prevention program" into the search box. [138-140]

Who Is at Risk for Type 2 Diabetes and Prediabetes?

Researchers don't fully understand why some people develop prediabetes and type 2 diabetes and others don't. It's clear that certain factors increase the risk, however. Here is a list of risk factors for prediabetes and Type 2 diabetes from the Mayo Clinic.

Weight. More fatty tissue gives you greater insulin resistance.

Inactivity. The less active you are, the greater your risk. Physical activity helps you control your weight, uses up glucose as energy, and makes your cells more sensitive to insulin.

Family history. Your risk increases if a parent or sibling has type 2 diabetes.

Race. Although it's unclear why, people of certain races—including blacks, Hispanics, American Indians, and Asian-Americans—are at higher risk.

Age. Your risk increases as you get older. This may be because you tend to exercise less, lose muscle mass, and gain weight as you age. But type 2 diabetes is also increasing dramatically among children, adolescents, and younger adults.

Gestational diabetes. If you developed gestational diabetes when you were pregnant, your risk of developing prediabetes and type 2 diabetes later increases. If you gave birth to a baby weighing more than 9 pounds (4 kilograms), you're also at risk of type 2 diabetes.

Polycystic ovary syndrome. For women, having polycystic ovary syndrome—a common condition characterized by irregular menstrual periods, excess hair growth, and obesity—increases the risk of diabetes.

High blood pressure. Having blood pressure over 140/90 millimeters of mercury (mm Hg) is linked to an increased risk of type 2 diabetes.

Abnormal cholesterol and triglyceride levels. If you have low levels of high-density lipoprotein (HDL), or "good" cholesterol, your risk of type 2 diabetes is higher. Triglycerides are another type of fat carried in the blood. People with high levels of triglycerides have an increased risk of type 2 diabetes. Your doctor can let you know what your cholesterol and triglyceride levels are.[141]

Look at this list carefully. It mentions weight but says nothing about the risk factors of a diet that causes you to gain weight. Unfortunately, it's not a surprise to me that the most obvious diabetes risk factor is missing from that list.

The missing risk is what many practitioners like to call the SAD diet—an acronym for the Standard American Diet. It is the way most Americans are eating now, and as we saw in Part I of this book, it has even gotten worse over the last 20 years!

More than a decade ago, leading researchers from Harvard University published a study proving that our "Western-style diet" has increased the incidence of diabetes, and, NOTE: a 2013 study published in the *American Journal of Medicine* confirms the connection: Following a "Western-style diet" leads to greater risk of diabetes, heart disease, and premature death, said study author Tasnime Akbaraly, Ph.D., a research fellow at University College London [142, 143]

The Downside of Diabetes Drugs

I'm not alone in worrying about the problems that come from medicating people with diabetes, especially when they're in the early stages of the disease. A 2014 study published in the journal

JAMA Internal Medicine, found that for many people, the benefits of taking diabetes medications are so small that they're outweighed by the minor harms and risks associated with treatment. The authors of that study strongly urge us to change the root causes of diabetes rather than to medicate otherwise healthy patients who meet the criteria of so-called prediabetes. [144]

"Ultimately, the aim of a treatment is not to lower blood sugar for its own sake, but to prevent debilitating or deadly complications" of the disease, says John S. Yudkin, M.D., the study coauthor and emeritus professor of medicine at University College London.

How old people are when they begin taking diabetes pills, plus the difficulties and side effects of the treatment, are important factors that contribute to benefit from taking a drug. That's the conclusion Dr. Yudkin and his team came to after their 20-year study, involving more than 5000 people, of type 2 diabetes treatments in the United Kingdom.[145]

Unfortunately, the medical industry has not paid any attention to this medical advice from "across the pond." The top-selling diabetes drug, metformin, is considered the frontline treatment for type 2 diabetes, and in a 2012 study published in *Diabetes Care,* researchers suggested that doctors should also expand the pool of people who should take metformin to those diagnosed with prediabetes.

Here's one of the problems with that: In a 2013 study also published in *Diabetes Care,* researchers linked metformin use to impaired cognitive function. [146, 147]

How to Prevent Diabetes

You have probably already guessed that diet and exercise are a "dynamic duo" for diabetes prevention. The ideal diet for preventing diabetes or reducing its severity is a low carb, Paleo-style diet. New science proves that low-carb diets like this plan should be the first line of attack for treatment of type 2 diabetes and should also be used (in conjunction with insulin) for people who have type 1 diabetes, according to the findings of a July 2014 study published in the journal Nutrition. [148]

A team of 26 physicians and nutrition researchers reviewed mountains of previously published research and came up with key points that highlight why low-carb diets can reliably reduce high blood sugar, slash diabetes risk, and reduce the risk for heart disease. Here are just some of those points released by the research team based on their study.

- People with type 2 diabetes on low-carb diets can reduce and frequently even eliminate their medication. People with type 1 diabetes on low-carb diets usually require less insulin.
- Compared to the side effects of pharmaceuticals for diabetes, lowering blood sugar levels via a low-carb diet has no side effects.
- High blood sugar is the most important feature of diabetes. Restricting carbohydrates has the greatest effect on reducing blood glucose levels.
- Our obesity and type 2 diabetes epidemics have occurred because calorie increases in our diets are almost entirely due to increased carbohydrates.
- You don't even have to lose weight—restricting your carbohydrate intake is enough to achieve health benefits.
- Although weight loss is not required for the diabetes benefits, carbohydrate restriction is the best diet for weight loss.
- A low-carb diet for people with type 2 diabetes is at least as good as other diet interventions, and frequently is much better.
- Replacing carbs with proteins is generally beneficial to people with diabetes.

- Dietary total and saturated fats do not raise the risk of heart disease.
- Carbohydrates have more to do with raising triglyceride levels than do dietary fats.
- A low-carbohydrate diet is the most effective method of reducing triglyceride levels and raising levels of healthy HDL cholesterol.

The following is a good example of what diet changes can do, even in advanced, insulin-dependent diabetes.

No More Needles for Mary Zuk

In February 2015, Mary Zuk, 73, came to see me in Chicago. I am using her real name—Mary encouraged me to tell her story in case it could help someone else. She was a long way from her hometown in Ocean Isle Beach, North Carolina. She had a long list of worrisome issues: Her diabetes was out of control, she had abdominal pain, and she had bouts of diarrhea after eating. A previous doctor told her she was "lactose intolerant," but the recommended Lactaid milk didn't help.

She was an insulin-dependent diabetic. Despite the insulin and an oral anti-diabetic pill, her blood sugar was "all over the place"—it could swing from 94 one morning to 290 the next. We tested her for allergies and learned she was reactive to aspartame, MSG, sulfites, grain alcohols, cane sugar, corn, gluten, and dairy.

I advised her to avoid all her allergenic foods and additives and recommended a Paleo-style low-carb diet and exercise. I gave her the corn-free multivitamin Perque 2, NOW Foods Ultra Omega-3 fish oil, and a Renew Life probiotic with 50 billion organisms in each capsule. We set up a phone consult for March 26, after she was back home.

When we spoke in March, just one month after our first visit, Mary was happy. By removing additives, dyes, artificial sugars, cane sugar, corn, dairy, and gluten from her diet, she found that her fasting glucose had gone from 299 to 69 in a month. Her doctor in North Carolina was amazed. She was still taking one oral anti-diabetic pill, but no longer needed her insulin. Plus, she'd lost 8 pounds.

Mary called again on April 17. She said, "It's been fabulous. You have changed my life." Her A1C (a measure of long-term glucose levels) was down from 8.5 to 7.0. She was still taking just one anti-diabetic pill, and no insulin.

I called Mary again on October 10 to follow up. She said, "I feel really good if I follow my diet." Her A1C had stayed down at 7.2 despite a bout of pneumonia. She said she had lost a total of 60 pounds, was still off insulin, and was taking her one anti-diabetes pill. She said, "It's like a miracle. People keep telling me how wonderful I look."

My Own Pre-Diabetes Story

I was searching through my records to find a patient who would be an excellent example of my overall preventive approach for people who have chronic illness, and it turned out to be my own encounter with "pre-diabetes!" One reason I am such an enthusiastic advocate of the Paleo-style diet is that it worked for me.

What kind of health problems could a doctor like me have, what with all my knowledge about disease prevention and healthy eating? Good question.

Some "roots" of illness are genetic, and in my case, I inherited something called polycystic ovary syndrome (PCOS) from my mother (her sister also had the condition). PCOS produces higher estrogen levels and insulin resistance, and it predisposes women who have it to infertility, diabetes, and hypothyroidism, among other things. Happily, I took hormone treatment and gave birth to two wonderful children. I think the treatment, and the births, probably put me into remission. The only problem I dealt with was a tendency to have low blood sugar if I didn't eat often enough. I was fine through menopause (a time when problems often crop up), but then I broke my foot. I blamed my unwilling but necessary inactivity for the fact that in 2 years, little by little, I gained more than 20 pounds. Then my fasting blood sugar started to creep up too.

That was enough for me. As a doctor, I knew just how much damage high blood sugar can do. My diet was already pretty good, but I eliminated all starches and cane sugar. I even put myself on Metformin for a few weeks, but then I thought, "What am I doing?" I'd never let one of my patients go down this route! I let go of my fears and followed my own best advice.

I'd heard about the popular Paleo diet, which eliminates grains, sugar, dairy, legumes, and alcohol. What attracted me wasn't the notion of eating like a person from paleolithic times. The science behind it is what made me want to try it.

I added some interval exercise work because science showed interval training can reduce fasting blood sugar and A1C, a measure of blood sugar taken over time. Instead of sugary snacks, I added nuts—especially pistachios, which studies show can lower blood sugar. And I took the blood sugar–lowering natural supplements I recommend to patients: berberine and bitter melon. And I changed the timing of my meals. (See "When You Eat" in Part III.) In just 4 months, I'd lost 24 pounds, and my blood sugar was—and still is— normal, with a completely non-pharmaceutical approach.

More Food Tips for Diabetes

Vinegar with starchy meals. Though you won't be eating many high-glycemic foods while you're on a Paleo-style plan, there's always the chance that you'll want to splurge when you are invited over for lasagna Bolognese on your birthday. When you indulge, you may be able to keep your blood sugar from spiking so badly by having a tablespoon of vinegar in a green salad that you eat along with a starchy entrée, or even in a quick vinegar shot (mixed with seltzer, it makes a refreshing spritzer). A Greek study published in *Journal of Diabetes Research* in 2015 showed that vinegar can lower post-meal blood sugar by as much as 42%. [149]

Coffee! It turns out that people who drink the most coffee have the lowest diabetes risk—if you drink three or more cups a day, you have a 37 percent lower risk than people who drink just one. [150]

Nuts and strawberries. A 2014 study published in the journal *Nutrition* compared people who ate a couple of servings of pistachio nuts a day to non-nut eaters. People in the pistachio group lowered their markers for metabolic syndrome and reduced inflammation levels. I love to use pistachios as "croutons" in my salad! In other tasty news, almonds and walnuts have also been studied and proven to help lower blood sugar. [151]

Strawberries are sweet, low in sugar—and they pack a little blood sugar lowering power, too, according to two 2012 studies. Because strawberries are a powerhouse antioxidant fruit, they also lower markers of inflammation. Choose deeply colored, organic-only strawberries and enjoy. Ounce for ounce, they contain more vitamin C than oranges. [152]

Supplements That Lower Blood Sugar

Many supplements promise that they can help lower your blood sugar. These are the supplements that have scientific evidence to show that they work.

Alpha lipoic acid

Here's the story on alpha lipoic acid from University of Maryland Medical Center.

Overview

Alpha-lipoic acid is an antioxidant made by the body. It is found in every cell, where it helps turn glucose into energy. Antioxidants attack "free radicals," waste products created when the body turns food into energy. Free radicals cause harmful chemical reactions that can damage cells, making it harder for the body to fight off infections. They also damage organs and tissues.

Other antioxidants work only in water (such as vitamin C) or fatty tissues (such as vitamin E). But alpha-lipoic acid is both fat and water soluble. That means it can work throughout the body. Antioxidants in the body are used up as they attack free radicals. But evidence suggests alpha-lipoic acid may help regenerate these other antioxidants and make them active again.

In the cells of the body, alpha-lipoic acid is changed into dihydrolipoic acid. Alpha-lipoic acid is not the same as alpha linolenic acid, which is an omega-3 fatty acid that may help heart health. There is confusion between alpha-lipoic acid and alpha linolenic acid because both are sometimes abbreviated ALA. Alpha-lipoic acid is also sometimes called lipoic acid.

Diabetes

Several studies suggest alpha-lipoic acid helps lower blood sugar levels. Its ability to kill free radicals may help people with diabetic peripheral neuropathy, who have pain, burning, itching, tingling, and numbness in arms and legs from nerve damage. Researchers believe alpha-lipoic acid helps improve insulin sensitivity.

Alpha-lipoic acid has been used for years to treat peripheral neuropathy in Germany. However, most of the studies that have found it helps have used intravenous (IV) alpha-lipoic acid. It's not clear whether taking alpha-lipoic acid by mouth will help. Most studies of oral alpha-lipoic acid have been small and poorly designed. One study did find that taking alpha-lipoic acid for diabetic neuropathy reduced symptoms compared to placebo.

Taking alpha-lipoic acid may help another diabetes-related condition called autonomic neuropathy, which affects the nerves to internal organs. One study of 73 people with cardiac autonomic neuropathy, which affects the heart, found that subjects reported fewer signs of the condition when taking 800 mg of alpha-lipoic acid orally compared to placebo.
For more, check out www.umm.edu.

Berberine

A study was published in the journal Metabolism in 2008, comparing the efficacy of the supplement Berberine with the drug Metformin. I am quoting the entire abstract of the study here for two reasons: 1) the results are impressive 2) I am often confronted with the assertion "there are no double-blind studies" when I am discussing use of supplements or other methods in integrative medicine. That is just not true. There are many of studies, and good ones. They are generally free of bias or suppression of data, which is more than I can say for some of the studies funded by the pharmaceutical industry. Also, you have probably noticed that anything I have included in this book is backed up by at least one study. Here is the report of the study:

> "Berberine has been shown to regulate glucose and lipid metabolism in vitro and in vivo. This pilot study was to determine the efficacy and safety of Berberine in the treatment of type 2 diabetic patients. In study A, 36 adults with newly diagnosed type 2 diabetes were randomly assigned to treatment with Berberine or Metformin (0.5 g

t.i.d.) in a 3-month trial. The hypoglycemic effect of berberine was similar to that of metformin. Significant decreases in hemoglobin A1c (HbA$_{1c}$; from 9.5% ± 0.5% to 7.5% ± 0.4%, $P<0.01$), fasting blood glucose (FBG; from 10.6 ± 0.9 mmol/L to 6.9 ± 0.5 mmol/L, $P<0.01$), postprandial blood glucose (PBG; from 19.8 ± 1.7 to 11.1 ± 0.9 mmol/L, $P<0.01$) and plasma triglycerides (from 1.13 ± 0.13 mmol/L to 0.89 ± 0.03 mmol/L, $P<0.05$) were observed in the berberine group. In study B, 48 adults with poorly controlled type 2 diabetes were treated supplemented with berberine in a 3-month trial. Berberine acted by lowering FBG and PBG from one week to the end of the trial. HbA$_{1c}$ decreased from 8.1% ± 0.2% to 7.3% ± 0.3% ($P<0.001$). Fasting plasma insulin and HOMA-IR were reduced by 28.1% and 44.7% ($P<0.001$), respectively. Total cholesterol and low-density lipoprotein cholesterol (LDL-C) were decreased significantly as well. During the trial, 20 (34.5%) patients suffered from transient gastrointestinal adverse effects. Functional liver or kidney damages were not observed for all patients. In conclusion, this pilot study indicates that berberine is a potent oral hypoglycemic agent with beneficial effects on lipid metabolism."

This abstract emphasizes that berberine lowers fasting blood sugar, lowers HbA1c (a blood test that reflects longer-term blood sugar levels), and lowers cholesterol as well! The dosage used in the study was 500 mg. three times a day. [153]

Bitter Melon

Bitter melon is another effective supplement for lowering blood sugar. According to a review of human studies of the effects of bitter melon (also known as momordica) published as a chapter in the book, *Bioactive Food as Dietary Interventions for Diabetes,* 10 of 13 studies showed effectiveness of bitter melon in lowering blood sugar. Bitter melon is available both as a food or a supplement. Most

Americans would probably not want to make bitter melon part of their diet, so the best alternative is the supplement, and the usual dose is 500-1000 mg. per day. It is less effective than Berberine or Metformin. It is contraindicated for use during pregnancy or if you are trying to get pregnant because though there is conflict about this point, some studies show that at high doses, bitter melon has abortifacient properties. It is also contraindicated in G6PD deficiency. [154]

Magnesium. This mineral is a key player in metabolic functions ranging from protein synthesis to blood pressure regulation. What's more, it can improve sensitivity to insulin and can lower blood sugar in people with type 2 diabetes.

Usual Dose	200 to 250 milligrams twice a day; avoid in advanced kidney disease. [73]

Alpha-lipoic acid. Alpha-lipoic acid is an antioxidant that performs triple duty for people with diabetes: It can improve numbness and nerve pain, which eases diabetic neuropathy, and it can lower blood sugar and help with insulin control.

Usual Dose	300 milligrams twice a day.

Fish oil. The latest research shows that taking fish oil can increase certain white blood cells that consume inflammatory substances. NOW foods Ultra EFA, which has 750 milligrams of EPA/DHA in one 1,000-milligram capsule, is a reliable brand which is mercury free, and will not make you burp up a fish taste. It is also very convenient because it is concentrated. One gel contains 2 ½ times the amount of EPA/DHA contained in most fish oil gels.

Resveratrol. Resveratrol, a compound found in red wine, improves blood sugar levels in people with type 2 diabetes, as well as Hb A1C, blood pressure, and cholesterol, according to two recent studies. In one 2014 study, people who took 200 milligrams of resveratrol for

26 weeks lowered their A1C scores, compared to people who took a placebo. They also had better memory performance, which is certainly a nice bonus. In a 2012 study, after 3 months of taking a 250-milligram resveratrol supplement, people with type 2 diabetes had lower A1C scores, lower blood pressure (a drop of about 12 points, systolic), and lower cholesterol. [155][156]

Exercise

When it comes to beating diabetes, you'll need to combine the Alive and Well diet with exercise to maximize your chances for lowering the dosage of your medications or, better still, getting off the pills completely. In fact, exercise has been proven to be as effective as medication for beating type 2 diabetes. That's because when you exercise, glucose leaves the bloodstream and enters muscle cells as fuel. The more muscle you build, the more glucose your muscles can store—thus dropping the glucose levels in your blood. As an added benefit, once you add exercise to your daily schedule, you'll likely lose a few pounds, which will improve your insulin response, and that will also help lower blood sugar.

Here are two smart exercise strategies that are specifically designed to improve diabetes.

1. Focus on interval training. We mentioned this in Chapter 4, but it's especially helpful for people with diabetes. One study showed that when you alternate high-intensity bursts of aerobic activity for a couple of minutes with low-intensity rest periods for as little as 10 minutes of total activity (via an exercise bike, an elliptical machine, or good old-fashioned walking), you can lower glucose levels by 13 percent for up to 24 hours. Aim for 90 minutes a week.

2. Add some weight. People who do a combination of strength training and aerobics can lower their A1C by 1 percent— which translates to a 20 percent lower risk for developing

heart disease and a 40 percent lower chance of eye or kidney disease. No pill can do that!

No access to a gym or equipment? No problem! Just doing simple body weight exercises such as pushups, lunges, and squats can help. Aim to do one or two sets of each move at least twice a week for 20 minutes. [152]

If you are testing your blood sugars after exercise, and find that they are higher, your exercise may cause your body too much stress, and raise your cortisol levels. If that happens, try an easier exercise routine. Test and make sure it is lowering, rather than raising, your blood sugar.

ECZEMA AND PSORIASIS

Redness, itching, scaling, peeling, cracking—these are the painful signs of troubled skin. Two common skin problems responsible for symptoms like these are eczema and psoriasis. Both these illnesses cause irritation and discomfort for millions of people.

Eczema is an umbrella diagnosis for chronic red, itchy, scaling skin patches that have no obvious external cause. Psoriasis is a condition in which skin thickens and scales, and is inflamed—usually on the scalp, elbows, knees and additionally in the ears, and on the trunk, arms and legs. Up to 30 percent of people with psoriasis also experience joint pain. That condition is called psoriatic arthritis.

Standard initial medical treatment for both conditions can be similar and often starts with prescription steroid creams, though specific topical ointments, and pharmaceutical immune suppressants, and UV light treatments are used for psoriasis, but not for eczema.

When you start a topical steroid, your skin reaction can calm down for a while, but when you stop using the cream, the cause of the skin problem is still there and the rash returns. In addition, prolonged use of steroids has a harmful side effect: They can thin the skin. Another superficial treatment used is oat-based creams or bath products. These are generally not very effective and can even cause harm to people who have (mostly unknown) allergies to oats.

In my view, both eczema and psoriasis are most often skin manifestations of delayed type reactions to foods. Using steroids on the skin while you continue to eat foods you are reacting to is just like trying to put out a fire while you are pouring fuel on it at the same time. Using immune-suppressant drugs, such as cyclosporine or methotrexate, which are often prescribed for psoriasis, is even more inappropriate and dangerous, not to mention expensive— these can cost more than $10,000 a year!

Using ointments and creams on the skin or taking immunosuppressant drugs won't do the job, because they don't "treat the root." By now, you already know that the first thing I do when I see a person with eczema or psoriasis is to identify which food proteins—often casein (one of the proteins in dairy)—are responsible for the inflammation, and then help the person either start on an allergen-free diet or a Paleo-based diet. Since a Paleo-based diet is free from dairy, grains, sugar or alcohol, it eliminates both their allergens, and other common inflammatory foods. [157, 158]

A Plan for Healthy Skin

Over the years, I have successfully treated more than a hundred people with psoriasis, and more than a thousand people with eczema by identifying and eliminating allergens from their diets and surroundings. It makes sense that an anti-inflammatory diet and environment can be one of the best remedies for these skin conditions.

Rajani Katta, M.D., professor of dermatology at Baylor College of Medicine in Houston, has written a paper that explains the need for dietary modifications in skin diseases, and emphasizes the systemic nature and risks of many skin diseases, including acne, (she notes the connection with acne and dairy consumption) skin cancer, aging skin, and psoriasis.

She presents research documenting that people with psoriasis have increased cardiovascular risk and suggests a way to prevent it: Diet changes! And the diet she suggests is one with whole foods, fresh fruits and vegetables, and Omega 3 fatty acids. She says, "Dietary intervention should be recommended to patients as a foundational therapy for reducing cardiovascular risk." [159]

Foods That Help Relieve Skin Problems

Eat three to five daily servings of these carotenoid-rich fruits and vegetables: Carrots; deep green, leafy vegetables; mangoes; sweet potatoes; tomatoes, winter squash

Eat at least five weekly servings of omega-3-rich fish, including: Arctic char; black cod (sablefish); herring, mussels; oysters; wild salmon; sardines. If you do not like fish or are concerned about mercury content, you can take an Omega-3 supplement.

Supplement Strategies to Improve Your Skin

When I start working with someone who has eczema or psoriasis, I recommend that they take these four key supplements. The anti-inflammatory power these exert can help speed your way to clearer skin.

Probiotics. One of the first supplements I recommend for anyone with eczema or psoriasis is probiotics. That's because most people with these conditions have gut irritation from years of eating foods to which they have delayed-type food allergies. Taking probiotics can help restore function and health to the gut, and blunt inflammation. I like Renew Life Ultimate Flora, containing 30 billion culture-forming units. The usual dose is one capsule daily with a light meal.

Berberine. This plant alkaloid is found in Oregon grape, goldenseal, and barberry, among other plants. It has a long history of use in Ayurvedic and Traditional Chinese Medicine and is believed to have anti-inflammatory action. Studies show that ointments containing berberine help improve eczema and psoriasis. The usual dose is 500 milligrams of berberine capsules one to two times a day. [160, 161]

Fish oil. Several studies have shown that high doses of fish oil improve psoriasis, and at least one recent study shows that high-dose fish oil therapy significantly improves eczema symptoms as well. NOW Foods Ultra Omega-3 fish oil soft gel capsules contains 500 milligrams of EPA and 250 milligrams of DHA in each gel. For high-dose therapy, the usual dose is seven capsules a day—two with breakfast, two with lunch, and three with dinner.

Vitamin D. Since light (sunshine, too) helps improve skin conditions such as psoriasis and eczema, then it stands to reason that the "sunshine vitamin" might also help improve them. That's been confirmed, in a recent review of nutritional supplements for psoriasis. I recommend that my patients tested for their level of vitamin D and that they take 1,000 to 5,000 IU daily, depending on the results of their tests. The process of being tested for and taking Vitamin D needs to be monitored by a doctor. When you achieve normal levels of D, the doctor can change your dose to a maintenance level. [162]

Let There Be Light—Therapy

Several types of light therapy are prescribed for skin problems. One that I've seen work is UVB therapy (narrow band ultraviolet light B). I have a 65-year-old woman patient who had psoriasis lesions on her arms, legs, and trunk for many years. She'd used steroid creams, but they weren't very effective. Finally, I suggested she stop eating dairy, gluten, and corn, and begin UVB therapy. She also took some Ayurvedic medical detox treatments with herbs and sesame oil. Happily, this combination approach was highly effective for her—now, her skin is almost completely clear. She continues with occasional UV light treatments and follows a Paleo-based diet. You can get a prescription for UVB light devices for home use from a dermatologist. [163]

How to Find Safer Skin Care Products

Most drugstore or beauty shop body products are loaded with allergens and chemicals. Just read the labels on soaps, lotions, shampoos, and conditioners, and you'll see what I mean: most have a long list of potentially toxic chemicals like sodium laureth sulfate, methyl and propyl paraben, and PEG-polyethylene glycol.

Environmental Working Group, a nonprofit organization, has a website at ewg.org that helps you find out if your beauty products contain potentially allergenic or otherwise harmful chemicals. They even offer a handy smartphone app you can download and take shopping. [164]

Toxic chemicals aren't the only problem. For some people, even so-called natural ingredients can trigger skin reactions. Some beauty and skin care products contain common food allergens, such as hydrolyzed wheat protein, oat protein, milk protein, and corn syrup. If you have eczema or psoriasis, you need to avoid these.

I ask my patients to moisturize with simple oils such as organic coconut oil, or with allergen-free body products. My favorites are Andalou Naturals. Dr. Bronner's makes a great old-fashioned soap in either liquid or bar form. My favorite is their fragrance-free bar. I do not recommend to my patients that they use the scented bars.

Elaine's Clear Skin Plan

Dr. Elaine Rosenblatt (her real name) a Chicago area psychotherapist, was at her wit's end—nothing she tried would calm the red patches that inflamed her skin. The worst inflammation was right on her face, plus her eyes were crusted with yellow fluid. Medication, including antihistamines, had done no good. Along with her skin problems, she had sinus congestion, and nasal sprays weren't helping, either. She had tested positive for antinuclear antibodies (ANA), an immune marker, and her doctor suspected she could have an autoimmune disorder. He referred her to a rheumatologist. Instead, she came to see me.

I tested her and discovered that she had delayed-type allergies to many different foods—gluten, dairy, white potatoes, oats, corn and corn products (including white vinegar, which is made from corn) and cane sugar. We eliminated these from her diet. She ate strictly organic produce, grass-fed meats, and organic eggs. She added lots of sardines and veggies, plus she ate an avocado every day to make sure she would be getting plenty of healthy omega-3 fats, which I knew would improve her skin.

I also recommended that she take each of these supplements twice a day with food.

- Probiotics: Ultimate Flora, 30 billion CFU
- 400 IU vitamin E
- 1,000 milligrams vitamin C
- 600 milligrams calcium
- 250 milligrams magnesium plus
- 1,000 IU vitamin D (NOW Foods brands)
- 1,000 milligrams fish oil with 750 mg. EPA/DHA (NOW Foods Ultra Omega-3)

In addition, I recommended that Elaine begin her day with this nutrient-dense smoothie, which is packed with eczema-soothing ingredients.

Elaine's Breakfast Smoothie

The smoothie is a blend of aloe vera juice, water, flaxseeds, spirulina or chlorella powder, chia seeds, red pepper, cinnamon, blueberries, banana, kale or spinach, lemon juice, and tea. (If you decide to try this smoothie, you will need a powerful blender to mix it, and you will need to be sure that you do not react to any of the ingredients. For example, I react to flax and chia seeds, so this smoothie would not work for me.)

I also recommended to Elaine that she avoid makeup, and massage organic coconut oil on the affected skin several times a day.

Later, Elaine e-mailed me with some very happy news: Her skin had completely cleared up, and what's more, she had lost 19 pounds, virtually without trying. She was delighted with her new look!

Non-pharmaceutical Remedies for Irritated Skin

Beyond cleaning up your diet and using recommended supplements, these tips may help you feel more comfortable as your skin becomes healthier.

Moisturize. I advise people with eczema and psoriasis to be sure to liberally and regularly moisturize their skin—but not with any of the commercial and so-called natural skin creams that contain dairy or wheat proteins (hydrolyzed wheat protein), corn syrup, or other corn products (check www.ewg.org). These can worsen skin problems for many people. Instead, as I have already said, simple "one-ingredient" moisturizer I recommend is pure organic coconut oil. Apply it right after a shower while your skin is still slightly damp to lock in the moisture. Generally, you will need to apply it only twice a day, in the morning and before bedtime. Some people prefer apricot or avocado oil. Just make sure that you are not allergic to the oil that you use.

Choose organic fabrics and allergen-free laundry soaps. Wear non-itchy, strictly organic fabrics—cotton is best—and wash your clothes in mild, fragrance-free organic laundry soap.

Keep your cool. Hot, sweaty skin aggravates eczema and psoriasis, so stay as dry as you can and shower after you've exercised. [157, 158]

MIGRAINE HEADACHES

There are headaches, and then there are *headaches.*
Common garden-variety headaches trouble almost all of us every
now and then. Virtually anything can cause them, including stress,
caffeine withdrawal, dehydration, muscle tension, hangovers, and
being too tired or too hungry. Most of the time, a plain old headache
will quickly disappear all by itself—if we don't chase it away with a
couple of pills (such as ibuprofen, acetaminophen, or aspirin) first.

In this chapter, we're not discussing those common
headaches. We're talking about migraine headaches--painful enough
to prompt 45 million Americans to seek medical attention for them.

The Anatomy of a Migraine

If you've ever had a migraine headache, you'll know that it is
far more painful than a simple tension headache. Migraines can be
preceded by warning signals, which can include visual disturbances
called auras. You may experience tunnel vision, temporary blind
spots, seeing stars or zigzag lines, and blurring. You could also have
eye pain. These symptoms most often occur about 15 minutes
before the onset of the migraine, though they could strike anywhere
from a few minutes to 24 hours beforehand—or not at all. Not
everyone who gets migraines will experience an aura. Other
migraine warning signals can include yawning, difficulty
concentrating, trouble finding the right words, or nausea.

Once a migraine develops, you know it—the symptoms can
be extreme. What may start off as a dull ache can escalate within
minutes or hours to become severe pain, usually on one side of your
head. You may be dizzy or nauseated, and you might even vomit.
You could be exquisitely sensitive to light or sound and need to
retreat to a dark, quiet room. Some people sweat or feel chills,
fatigue, numbness, or weakness, or lose their appetites. The pain
can take you to the hospital.

Even after a migraine resolves, you could have lingering symptoms, including neck pain, sleepiness, or feeling dull or confused.

We know that some people are sensitive to certain migraine triggers. These include: Caffeine withdrawal, changes in sleep patterns or too little sleep, alcohol, stress or physical exercise, loud noises or bright lights, certain odors, missed meals, and high tyramine foods such as aged cheeses or figs. [165]

A Headache-Fighting Food Plan

One key to battling migraines is to identify any delayed-type food allergies you may have. Allergic reactions can be an even worse migraine trigger than the lists of foods commonly listed as migraine trigger foods. In my experience, getting people off allergenic foods or additives is often the main thing that is needed to alleviate their migraines, and even to make them go away and never come back. Dairy, gluten, corn, MSG, aspartame, sulfites, nitrites, nitrates and food dyes are prime food and food additive culprits.

Here's the connection between allergies and migraines: In the delayed-type reaction to foods or additives, antibodies attack the foods to which you are allergic. This creates highly irritating particles called antigen-antibody complexes that inflame the linings of your gut and your blood vessels. The blood vessels contract and expand erratically—and can trigger migraines.

Just as certain foods can trigger headaches, other foods can potentially help relieve them, or at least dull the pain when they strike.

Wild salmon, sardines, and herring. An international research team, including scientists from the National Institutes of Health, examined the effect of dietary fats on chronic headaches. They learned that eating more omega-3s, which are found in fish, reduced headache pain and improved quality of life for people who suffered from chronic headaches. The study was published in the journal *Pain*.[166]

Vegetables and fruits. The No More Pills Plan focuses on antioxidant-rich vegetables and fruit. For headaches, we won't single out specific varieties for you to enjoy—we want you to eat several servings of multicolored organic produce a day to make sure that you're getting the most complete range of inflammation-fighting antioxidants. Choose the most colorful, freshest (or frozen) organic produce you can find.

Ginger. This spicy rhizome helps blood vessels, which can help prevent migraines. Use fresh or powdered ginger liberally in cooking—its taste enhances most meals. Or use naturally-pickled Japanese sushi-style ginger (with no artificial color added). As an occasional treat, nibble crystallized ginger candy or make ginger tea: Pour boiling water over three thin slices of fresh gingerroot, cover, steep for 10 minutes, and add a few drops of honey. [167]

Migraine Trigger Foods

The basic Paleo-style diet is virtually allergen free, so that's the perfect place to start when you're dealing with headaches. The plan also bans food additives, which is great for headache sufferers, since many of those chemicals are linked to headaches. According to the National Headache Foundation, these additives can trigger headaches, particularly migraines, for some people: Aspartame, nitrates, nitrites, MSG, sulfites.[168]

Beyond chemicals, we previously mentioned that certain foods, known as high-tyramine foods (even some that may be included on this plan and are fine for people who are not vulnerable to migraines), may trigger headaches in some people. Foods commonly associated with headaches, particularly migraines, include:

- Aged cheeses
- Avocados
- Bananas
- Balsamic vinegar

- Caffeine
- Chocolate
- Citrus fruit and juices (1/2 cup a day usually is okay)
- Dried fruit, especially figs
- Peanuts
- Raw onions
- Red wine and wine vinegar
- Smoked or cured meat
- Sourdough and other heavily yeasted breads
- Soy nuts [168, 169]

Migraine Remedies

When you visit your doctor for migraine relief, she's likely to reach into her pharmaceutical toolbox to offer aid. That is probably not the first approach I'd take, depending on your medical history. Instead, you already know I'd examine your diet first and eliminate any food allergies. I'd also ask about your home and office environment to see whether you could be allergic to anything around you. I'd work with you on strategies for easing stress in your life. I might even ask you to keep a headache journal, so we could identify potential triggers.

Massage and Meditation

The therapies outlined in the Stress Reduction section of Part III can go a long way to helping ease the pain and stress of headaches, even if they are migraines. I also recommend that my patients try massage and meditation.

Massage. Two kinds of massage have been studied for its effects on migraines—with positive results. In a 2006 study, 47 migraine sufferers were treated with weekly 45-minute massage sessions for 5 weeks or were in a non-treatment control group. The massage was designed to relax muscle tension in the back, shoulders, neck, and head. Those who got the massage had fewer migraines and reported sleeping better, both during the massage trial and for 3 weeks afterward, compared to people in the control group. People who got the massage treatment had lower heart rates and levels of the stress hormone cortisol. They also reported reductions in their anxiety. [170]

A specific type of massage called craniosacral therapy is a gentle technique during which practitioners relax the soft tissues surrounding the central nervous system. In a small 2012 study, 20 people with migraines had six craniosacral massage treatments over 4 weeks. The researchers gave the participants a test that measures the effectiveness of headache treatments and learned that the therapy significantly lowered headache test scores. [171]

Meditation. In a small pilot study, researchers assigned 19 people with migraine headaches to one of two groups. The first group took an 8-week mindfulness-based stress reduction (MBSR) course that taught meditation and yoga. The other group received standard migraine care. At the end of the study, people in the MBSR group reported having one fewer migraine a month, and less severe headaches, than did people in the control group. The 2014 study was published in the journal *Headache.*[172]

Pain-Fighting Supplements

These supplements may help you with headache pain.

Triple therapy. Alexander Mauskop, M.D., a neurologist and acupuncturist who's been treating and studying headaches for some 25 years, is the director of the New York Headache Center in New York City. In his 2001 book, *What Your Doctor May Not Tell You about Migraines,* he describes this simple therapy for easing migraines:

> 300 to 400 milligrams magnesium
> 400 milligrams riboflavin
> 100 milligrams feverfew

Dr. Mauskop recommends breaking the dosage in half and taking it twice a day with meals. The formula is also available as Migrelief, available online and at health food stores. [173]

Butterbur. A review of studies that included 293 people with migraines showed that the herb butterbur reduced the frequency of migraine attacks after people took it for 3 to 4 months. Petasin is a compound contained in the plant; it's considered a major anti-inflammatory. "I've had patients get off their migraine prescriptions after taking butterbur," says Aaron Michelfelder, M.D., professor of family medicine and bioethics at Loyola Stritch School of Medicine. The supplement Petadolex contains the extract used in the studies. Follow label directions.

Feverfew. This is a centuries-old European herbal medicine for headaches and many other ills. The migraine-relieving activity of feverfew is likely due to its complex of compounds, including parthenolide; together, they relieve inflammation and help relieve smooth muscle spasms. Feverfew also helps prevent the constriction of blood vessels in the brain (one of the leading causes of migraine headaches) and inhibits the production of prostaglandin hormones, which can inflame blood vessels. Finally, feverfew makes platelets "less sticky" and normalizes blood flow, which may also help reduce migraine frequency and severity. Choose feverfew products standardized to 0.2 to 0.35 parthenolides; the dose is 50 to 100 milligrams daily. [174, 175]

Ginger. In a 2014 study, 100 people with migraines were treated either with 50 milligrams of sumatriptan, a migraine drug, or with 250 milligrams of powdered ginger. Before taking either medication, 22 percent of the people in the sumatriptan group and 20 percent of the people in the ginger group reported having severe headaches. Two hours after treatment, 64 percent of the people who'd taken the ginger and 70 percent of the people in the sumatriptan group experienced a 90 percent reduction in headache pain. In the sumatriptan group, 20 percent of people reported side effects that included dizziness, vertigo, and heartburn; 4 percent of people in the ginger group reported mild indigestion. [176]

Migraine Drugs

Sometimes, drugs are needed for migraines. My drug choices for migraines are informed, in part, by a 2013 study published in the *Journal of General Internal Medicine.* The researchers found that some FDA-approved medications, including beta blockers and angiotensin inhibitors, worked better than placebo and prevented 50 percent or more headaches in 200 to 400 people, per 1,000 treated. Those drugs had fewer side effects than did other drugs that are prescribed "off-label" for headaches, including antidepressants and anticonvulsants. [177]

Another class of drugs, called triptans, can head off a migraine if you catch it early on. However, they're not for people with known or suspected cardiovascular disease, as they may increase risk of heart attacks or strokes. In my experience, triptans can be especially helpful for menstrual migraines. [169]

IBS and GERD

People who have digestive problems may be among the most misdiagnosed and poorly treated people who I see in my office, after they have made multiple visits to other doctors. And from the increasing number of visits from people who have digestive complaints, it seems to me that the number of people with these illnesses is rising sharply. Recent statistics will back me up—as many as 20 percent of adults in this country have a digestive problem of some kind. [178]

Trouble in the Digestive System

Before we define the common problems that affect the digestive system, here's my opinion: I consider IBS and GERD to be among the most common, and most harmful label-only diagnoses. The problem with these diagnoses is that they belong in the "rule-out" diagnostic category. For example, an IBS diagnosis is usually made only after you've been in discomfort for at least three months, and after it has been determined that you have no other disease or injury that could be causing your symptoms. The diagnosis is only made after all tests—blood tests, celiac disease screening, bowel biopsies—have come back as "normal." [178, 179]

This means the doctor has ruled out cancer, celiac disease, full-blown inflammatory bowel disease, or any other known specific bowel disease. The doctor and you know what you *don't* have but have no idea what you *do* have. The problem with this is that label-only diagnoses lead to prescriptions of mostly ineffective drugs, and keep you in a gut-wrenching limbo, doing exactly whatever you were doing to bring about the problems in the first place. [179]

Those approaches fail all too often, because the symptoms, troubling as they may be, aren't the problem. The *causes* of the symptoms, most often delayed-type reactions to foods, are the problem, and that's what we need to address. Once you eliminate the cause, you'll eliminate the symptoms. Here's a good example.

Healing Carla's Constipation

I recently saw Carla Patton, a 66-year-old woman who came in with a lifelong history of constipation. She said it started when she was about 5 years old, and she recalled having "every kind of test," including a colonoscopy. She experienced bloating and gas after eating, along with the constipation. She practically lived on the laxative Miralax. She followed a gluten-free diet, had oatmeal every morning for breakfast, and ate a generally healthy diet. Still, she couldn't get rid of the constipation.

I tested her, and we discovered she was reactive to gluten, which she had been avoiding, but also reacted to buckwheat, oats, food additives and dyes, and red and white wine, and was borderline reactive to peanuts, almonds, cane sugar, corn sugars, and goat's milk. We removed all allergens except the "borderlines" from her diet, and I gave her a probiotic.

She came for a follow-up appointment two months later and was thrilled that her constipation had finally vanished. But two months after that, she called to report she was constipated again. Thinking she was safe, she had begun including some of the foods containing her "borderline" allergens, and I advised her to stop them. She did, and that resolved her problem. Labeling her illness "IBS with constipation" (see below) and giving her a prescription would have done nothing for her. A big bowl of oatmeal every morning would have been enough to keep her constipation going, perhaps for the rest of her life.

IBS: Many Problems, Many Symptoms

When your gut stops functioning in the way it's supposed to, all kinds of problems occur. In the past, doctors diagnosed these functional problems under such conditions as mucous colitis, spastic colon, nervous colon, functional dyspepsia, or spastic bowel. Various manifestations of IBS include changes in your bowel habits accompanied by abdominal pain, bloating, and cramps. Typically, people dealing with IBS experience constipation or diarrhea to one degree or another. In our current failed diagnostic system, we now divide the "label only" diagnosis of IBS into smaller labels. Four IBS "subtypes" are recognized: IBS with constipation, IBS with diarrhea, mixed IBS, and un-subtyped IBS. [179]

When your doctor diagnoses you with IBS, what she's really doing is telling you what you *don't* have; she is ruling out other types of bowel problems—cancer, infection, or inflammatory bowel disease such as Crohn's disease or ulcerative colitis. IBS is a "rule-out" diagnosis that means, "You're sick, and we know it's not cancer or any specific inflammatory bowel disease, but we don't really know why you're having digestive problems."

The Alive and Well Plan for Gastrointestinal Problems

When someone comes in to see me for help with their digestive complaints, you already know how I start—testing them for allergic reactivity to foods, and then putting them on a Paleo-type diet that eliminates both their allergens, and other inflammatory foods. Often, the problem is foods containing gluten; other people have problems with dairy, corn, or soy. Many people react to food additives, which is another reason why I urge my patients to choose organic, additive-free foods exclusively.

IBS and the Low-FODMAP Diet

A Paleo-style diet is already friendly to people with IBS, since it doesn't contain most of the key IBS dietary triggers, which include gluten, dairy products, legumes, additives, and artificial sweeteners. But even some of the healthy foods on the plan may trouble some people with IBS. This brings up the issue of the low-FODMAP diet. FODMAP stands for Fermentable Oligosaccharides, Disaccharides, Monosaccharides and Polyols. If you react to these saccharides and polyols that are elements of certain foods, then you will need to avoid these three types of foods: those which specifically cause you a delayed-type allergic reaction, FODMAP foods, and inflammatory foods in general.

You will need more than the list below if you are following a low FODMAP diet! It can be very complex, and it is not intuitive. For example, most IBS diets allow apples and pears, but prohibit citrus fruits. The low-FODMAP diet is just the opposite. If you think you need to follow it, you will need a skilled practitioner to diagnose and guide you. Be sure that all fruits and veggies are organic. Lean protein foods, including wild fish organic poultry, grass-fed beef, pork, and lamb, are generally digestible for most people on a low FODMAP diet. As for fruits and vegetables, make sure they are organic, and you will need to follow a FODMAP outline. Here is a brief one from the Cleveland Clinic.

Eat these veggies: Carrots, celery, green beans, spinach, squash, sweet potatoes, zucchini, eggplant.

Avoid these veggies: Broccoli, cabbage, cauliflower.

Limit these veggies: Artichoke, asparagus, brussels sprouts, leeks, onions, shallots.

Eat these fruits: Bananas, berries, cantaloupe, citrus fruits, grapes, kiwi.

Avoid these fruits: Apples, pears, watermelon, fruit juice, dried fruits. [180]

For more about avoiding the possible pitfalls of a low-FODMAP diet, check out this website:

https://aboutibs.org/low-fodmap-diet/five-low-fodmap-diet-pitfalls-and-what-you-can-do-to-avoid-them

Be Careful What You Drink

While my patients are dealing with IBS, I tell them that it's important to drink at least 48 ounces of pure, filtered water a day. Most can drink green or black tea as well as other unsweetened herbal teas. However, since caffeine can stimulate activity in the colon, which could worsen diarrhea, I often advise them to limit caffeinated beverages, or to switch to non-caffeinated teas, or water only.

Carbonated beverages can also worsen diarrhea—and so can alcohol. I recommend that my patients avoid alcoholic drinks altogether. If they feel they must drink at least some wine, I ask them to try drinking no more than one glass of red wine with food, on any one day, and no more than three times a week; cut back or stop completely if it makes symptoms worse; and of course, no wine if they have tested allergic to wine. [181]

The Stress/Gut Microbiome Connection

You know the reference to having a "gut feeling" about something? It's not just a cliché. There is, in fact, a brain situated in our digestive systems. As a matter of fact, there's an entire nervous system down there, called the enteric nervous system, situated within the lining of the digestive tract. It contains neurons that sense when food is moving through the gut, at which point the neurons signal muscle cells to start contracting and pumping the food along, breaking it down into nutrients and waste. During the process, neurotransmitters such as serotonin interact with the central nervous system. It's quite a miraculous process.

Even more miraculous is this: Your gut is a world of its own, populated by a microbiome of up to 1,000 distinct species of living bacteria and other organisms. A staggering 100 trillion bacteria and other microbes live in our gut—in fact, we contain 10 times more microbes than we do human cells! And research is revealing the intricate ways in which these microbes interact with our health— immune function, obesity, allergic diseases, and even neuropsychiatric disease could be linked to changes in the intestinal microbiota. Among the conditions linked to such changes are IBS and inflammatory bowel disease. [182-184]

Stress can upset your inner world of microbes. When you're under severe stress, your system releases a flood of stress hormones to slow or even stop digestion. That's nature's way of diverting energy to help you deal with the crisis at hand. The stress of an argument at dinner or a post-luncheon speaking engagement can also disrupt digestion, leading to cramping or other symptoms. It's entirely possible that stress hormones negatively affect your gut microbe balance and help produce the symptoms that cause so much discomfort. [185, 186]

So, it's easy to understand why stress-reduction techniques are high on my list of strategies for dealing with digestive problems. They play an important role in helping you learn to "disconnect" from stressful events and prevent the cascade of stress hormones from flooding your system and triggering the symptoms we call IBS. There's enough science behind each of these approaches to convince me that they're helpful for people with digestive problems.

Cognitive behavioral therapy (CBT). A 3-month study of people with IBS symptoms found that CBT was better than simple patient education and improved overall symptoms and well-being, though it didn't relieve pain.

Relaxation therapy. Several techniques, including progressive muscle relaxation (you consciously relax muscles in your toes and progress up your body, slowly and systematically relaxing all your muscles moving up your body, until you've relaxed the muscles in your face and head), can help blunt your reactivity to stress.

Hypnotherapy. A form of this practice is called gut-directed hypnotherapy, or GDH, and it's specifically designed for people with IBS and other digestive problems. What's more, GDH might be helpful for people whose symptoms aren't stress-related. In one study, people with severe IBS had 3 months of hypnotherapy treatments. In the treatments, they were directed to place their hands on their bellies while being asked to feel warmth and imagining they had control over their gastrointestinal functioning, reported the *Harvard Health Letter* in 2010. By study's end, the people in the hypnotherapy group reported significant symptom improvement, compared to people who were in a supportive psychotherapy group. And in another study, researchers reported that the benefits of gut-directed hypnotherapy could last for years. [185, 186]

IBS-Friendly Supplements

My first step when treating a patient with IBS is to target the cause of the symptoms. If it's a delayed-type allergy to certain food proteins, I recommend that the person avoid those foods completely. For most people, eliminating the allergens eliminates the symptoms. For those who want to lose weight, I recommend a Paleo-based diet. I'll also suggest these supplements for everyday use:

Probiotics. I list probiotics first because it is absolutely the most important supplement you can take for your gut—and that's confirmed by a 2014 review of more than 40 studies that concluded that taking probiotics eases pain, bloating, and flatulence. I recommend that my patients take one capsule a day of a probiotic product that contains a broad spectrum of 30 to 50 billion live cultures, such as my favorite, Renew Life Ultimate Flora. For any patients who have had a history of digestive problems, I recommend that they take probiotics every day from then on. Interestingly, the latest studies show that the brain has some of the same receptors as the gut, and that taking probiotics can even improve brain function, including memory.

Fish oil. Researchers recently discovered that people who have IBS also have deficiencies in their blood levels of long-chain fatty acids; fish oil helps fill that gap. In my view, fish oil is another "take it every day from now on" basic. I like NOW Foods Ultra Omega-3. Take one a day. [187]

Other Supplements that May Help IBS

Peppermint oil. According to a 2014 review of treatments in the *Journal of Gastroenterology,* enteric-coated peppermint oil is considered a first-line treatment for IBS cramps and pain. Take one or two capsules three times a day between meals. [188]

Curcumin. This phytochemical, responsible for the spice turmeric's brilliant yellow hue, reduced IBS symptoms by 50 percent in a study published in 2004. Curcumin supplements may help by reducing inflammation and abnormal muscle contractions in the bowel. Take 300 to 400 milligrams three times a day with a meal that contains some fat.

Slippery elm. This soothing herb, made from the bark of the slippery elm tree, can heal irritated digestive tract tissues. You can find slippery elm lozenges in health food stores and some drugstores. [189]

GERD: Another Digestive Problem with a Label-only

Diagnosis

GERD was formerly known as heartburn or acid indigestion, but these days, it's become an official disease, with a host of drugs designed specifically to treat it. GERD is another "label-only" diagnosis, that names the problem and finds the drug designed to treat it. I've learned over the years that GERD, like IBS, is often triggered by a delayed-type allergy to food proteins. I have had literally hundreds of GERD patients over the years who have been able to stop taking proton pump inhibitor drugs (PPIs) after they made appropriate dietary changes and avoid their well-known side effects.

In some cases, GERD can be a side effect of medications, including asthma drugs, calcium channel blockers, antihistamines, painkillers, sedatives, and antidepressants. Smoking, or being exposed to secondhand smoke, can also trigger GERD.

Though the main, and best-known, symptom of GERD is frequent heartburn, it also causes other less obvious symptoms, including: A dry, chronic cough, wheezing, asthma, recurrent pneumonia, nausea, vomiting, sore throat, hoarseness, difficulty swallowing, and chest pain. [190]

GERD and Delayed Type Gluten and Dairy Allergies

The sticky proteins in gluten (wheat, rye, barley, spelt), oats and corn (they have their own type of gluten), and casein (in dairy) are most often the cause of GERD. If you react to them, your immune system attacks the proteins in your allergenic food and turns the lining of your gut into an inflammatory war zone. It is just as if you were allergic to wool and you constantly wore a wool sweater. Pretty soon, the healthy skin of your arm would become a red, irritated, and possibly even infected mess.

If you stopped wearing the sweater and applied a healing balm to your arm, your skin would return to normal quite quickly. The same principle applies to the lining of your upper gut—the area that is affected by so-called GERD.

Easing Carl's GERD

I saw Carl P. (not his real name), a man in his fifties, for just two visits 2 years ago. Following his first asthma attack at the age of 15 months, he had had continual asthma attacks until his 10th birthday. Then his asthma abated when he started taking medication. But over the years, he developed GERD, headaches, and dizziness, and his sinusitis was so bad that two specialists had recommended surgery—he'd even lost his sense of smell some 25 years before. He didn't want surgery, which is why he came to see me.

With all his inflammatory illnesses, I of course suspected environmental and delayed-type food allergies. I found he was reactive to feathers, gluten, corn, and dairy, as well as bakers' and brewers' yeast. I told him how to clean up his environment, put him on an allergen-free diet, and he was diligent about sticking to it. He came back in a month and told me, "I feel like I'm at 9.5 on a scale of 10!" He was thrilled to report that his sense of smell had returned, a result that surprised even me, since it had been gone for 25 years. His sinuses were clear most of the time; his reflux was "almost nonexistent"; and he was down to taking his GERD pills only three times a week.

The solution to many digestive problems can be almost that simple. Find the foods and environmental allergens you are reacting to, remove them from your diet and environment, take some good probiotics and fish oil, and soon the inner linings (mucosa) of the esophagus and stomach return to normal. When you use probiotics for the upper gut, take them out of the capsule and swallow them with a spoonful of applesauce. In the capsule, they will bypass your upper gut. The probiotics will soothe your irritated esophagus and stomach. And don't take peppermint, as you might for IBS symptoms. For GERD, peppermint may act as an irritant and it will relax the lower esophageal sphincter, making it easier for reflux to occur.

Getting Rid of Susan's GERD and ADD

I saw Susan (not her real name), a young woman in her teens, in 2013. She experienced chronic abdominal pain above her navel and was diagnosed with GERD. Her doctor prescribed the GERD medication omeprazole. She'd also been diagnosed with attention deficit disorder [191]. I couldn't help but notice the dark bags under her eyes, which shouldn't have been there at that young age.

It turned out she was allergic to food dyes and gluten. I told her that after 21 days on her allergen-free diet, she could try tapering off the omeprazole. She came back for a follow-up visit 3 weeks later and told me she was feeling a lot better. She looked it! The bags under her eyes were gone; her stomach pains had vanished; she no longer felt bloated after eating; and she hadn't waited to start tapering off the omeprazole, she had already stopped it completely, with no problem.

What about her ADD? She said she was concentrating better and, as a matter of fact, had taken a retest and no longer needed an IEP (Individualized Education Program) at school. She's another perfect example of the many manifestations of the "great masquerader" food allergy, which shows up in so many different forms. She is living proof that inflammation from food allergies can affect every part of your body, even your brain.

Eating Out

If you are eating out and trying to avoid food allergens, do your best to steer the group to a restaurant that is already aware of allergies to gluten and dairy, or a restaurant that has Paleo entrees on the menu. Even some of the chains, like P.F. Chang and Outback Steakhouse, have gluten-free menus. And if you're in doubt, just order grilled fish, meat, or chicken; tell them to avoid any rubs, sauces, or marinades and cook it with only olive oil, salt and pepper. Make sure you don't use a commercial salad dressing and instead use squeeze of lemon and some olive oil. You can usually trust the olive oil in better restaurants, but in many of them, it can be adulterated with other oils or can be rancid. I have also been known to bring my own small bottle of good olive oil to restaurants. I also bring my own gluten-free soy or tamari sauce. You can also order grilled vegetables in many restaurants, and sweet potato is more common on menus now.

INSOMNIA

So many different elements can conspire to wreck your sleep that it can be tricky to figure out exactly what's keeping you awake. Risk factors include your sex (women are twice as likely to experience insomnia as men) and age (65 percent of people over age 65 have persistent sleep issues). Health problems are a factor—many can interrupt your sleep, especially if they are painful, cause breathing problems, or make you urinate frequently during the night. Finally, you might be taking a sleep-robbing pill. Antidepressants, B-antagonists, calcium-channel blockers, and some steroid medications all list insomnia as a side effect. [192]

Of course, that's just the beginning. There's also your sleeping environment: Is your mattress old and lumpy? Are you allergic to your pillows or bed linens, or to the detergent you use to wash them? Is the temperature in your bedroom too warm or chilly? Does your partner snore or thrash around? Do you have a pet that sleeps with you? Noisy neighborhood? Too much light in the bedroom? Undiagnosed sleep apnea? I could go on and on. Let's start with the basics.

Exactly What Is Insomnia?

Medically speaking, insomnia takes several forms: Sleep experts classify insomnia as *short-term insomnia,* when you've had trouble sleeping for less than 3 months; *chronic insomnia,* which means you lose sleep three or more times a week for 3 or more months; and *other insomnia,* which is any sleep problem that doesn't meet the short-term or chronic definition. Then there's *terminal* insomnia, which thankfully doesn't mean what it sounds like—it refers to waking too early and being unable to fall back to sleep. [192, 193]

What Happens When We Sleep?

What goes on during all those dark hours of downtime? Since we're not engaged in any of the activities that keep us busy while we're awake—thinking, talking, listening, moving, reading—you'd assume that our brains must be at rest, too, right? Well, not so much.

Your sleeping brain is a hotbed of action. During sleep, the brain's neural activity plays a role in maintaining memory, for one thing, which is why a lack of sleep can make you feel groggy and forgetful.

We pass through five sleep phases: stages 1, 2, 3, 4, and REM (rapid eye movement) sleep; each stage has its own function. Most people need a minimum of 7 to 8 hours of sleep a night to operate at their best.

Getting too little sleep is dangerous. Not only does it leave us drowsy and unable to focus properly the next day (which could cause accidents), it also affects our memory and even our physical performance. In one study of 15,000 people, researchers found out that getting an average of less than 5 hours of sleep a night over a few years resulted in a decline in memory performance that equaled two years of additional aging. During sleep, waste products from cellular activity are typically swept away; without enough sleep, harmful chemicals can build up and brain cells can begin to malfunction. Sleep may also be the period during which your brain exercises important connections that could otherwise waste away due to a lack of activity. [194]

Insomnia: It Can Start with Your Diet

I've had many patients who've had insomnia along with digestive symptoms and headaches. The first thing I do is put them on an individualized allergen-free diet, based on the results of ELISA or other types of testing. Once we've worked out what they're reactive to, and eliminate it, almost all my patients have been able to sleep well again.

I particularly remember one man who was reactive to gluten and whose only symptoms were anxiety and insomnia. Once he was gluten free, he began sleeping better and his anxiety resolved.

If you're wondering how it's possible that reactivity to gluten or to other foods could be related to sleep, let me explain. The first thing you need to know is that 80 to 90 percent of the neurotransmitter serotonin is manufactured in your gut. Serotonin affects mood, appetite, digestion, memory—and sleep—among many other things.

If your gut is inflamed due to food allergies, it can disrupt your body's production of serotonin, and that will absolutely impact your ability to sleep. For my patients who have insomnia, I recommend starting with a strict Paleo-type diet and giving it at least 3 solid, committed weeks. Meanwhile, I ask them to make sure their diet contains these sleep-supporting foods and drinks and eliminates the sleep-stealing ones. [195, 196]

Sleep-friendly Foods and Drinks

The top sleep-friendly foods are all lean protein. They are rich in tryptophan, which tends to support serotonin levels. They are: Blue crab; canned tuna (make sure it is in water or olive oil only. Tuna labelled as containing "vegetable broth" or "hydrolyzed vegetable protein" contains unlabeled MSG); chicken breast and skin; lobster; turkey breast and skin.

Antioxidant-rich foods, including green leafy veggies, citrus fruit, bananas, and tomatoes, are rich in magnesium and potassium, which help promote relaxation and circulation. In addition, a diet rich in calcium helps keep melatonin at sleep-promoting levels. Calcium-rich foods such as dark, leafy greens, nuts, and seeds maintain your blood level of calcium, which in turn maintain your melatonin level. [197]

Foods that help stabilize blood sugar overnight

If you find yourself waking in the wee hours and have trouble falling back asleep, it could be due to nocturnal hypoglycemia, or low blood sugar. When your blood sugar levels dip while you're asleep, it triggers the release of various hormones, including adrenaline, glucagon, and cortisol, which help bring blood sugar levels back to normal. But these hormones can also stimulate the brain and wake you up.

Complex carbs and good fats

To counter nocturnal hypoglycemia, I suggest that my patients make sure their dinner includes some complex carbohydrates, along with good fats. Some good foods with complex carbs are apples, pears, sweet potatoes, and winter squash. And the good fats in these nuts help keep serotonin levels stable overnight: almonds, cashews, pistachios and walnuts.

Kiwi helps you fall asleep and sleep soundly

In a 2011 study, when people ate 2 kiwifruit an hour before bedtime nightly for 4 weeks, it improved their sleep quality by 42 percent, improved their sleep soundness by 29 percent, and shortened the time it took them to fall asleep by 35 percent, compared to people who didn't get kiwi as a bedtime snack. What's more, people who ate kiwifruit enjoyed 13 percent more sleep than the control group. [198]

Sleep-friendly Drinks

Passion flower tea, and chamomile tea can both be helpful for sleep. Do not drink chamomile tea if you are allergic to ragweed-- it is a member of the ragweed plant family.

Sleep-destroying Foods and Drinks

Common sleep destroyers are foods in the nightshades family (tomatoes, potatoes, peppers and eggplant; aged cured smoked fermented and cultured foods (cheese, sauerkraut, salami, smoked meats); and refined carbohydrates like sugar and white flour.

Common sleep killers in the drink department are caffeine-containing drinks and alcohol. Another whole class of drinks is the "energy drinks" which are meant to keep you awake, so will harm your sleep.

Pharmaceuticals You May Want to Avoid

Many doctors rely on pharmaceuticals to treat insomnia—but this is a treatment that I believe should be avoided if possible. The side effects associated with many of these drugs can be severe.

Zolpidem. In 2013, the FDA released a warning about sleeping pills containing zolpidem. Brand names for pills that contain zolpidem are

Ambien, Ambien CR, Edluar, and Zolpimist. The FDA warning says that these drugs can impair driving and activities requiring alertness the morning after you take them. People who take insomnia drugs can experience mental impairment—even if they feel fully awake. The agency also slashed the recommended dose for these drugs. An even more dangerous zolpidem side effect is "sleepwalking." Under zolpidem's influence, people have been known to cook and eat food, wander around outside, and even take a spin in the car—while not fully conscious. They retain no memory of their frightening activities the next day. One of my patients took zolpidem by mistake in the afternoon. She started driving to a restaurant, remembers thinking the road looked a little tilted. The next thing she remembers is waking up in her car, in the parking lot of the restaurant. In the meantime, she had "sleep driven" to the restaurant, had gone in and gotten something to eat, and then had walked back out to the parking lot and gotten into her car. [199]

Benzodiazepines. These tranquilizing drugs, often prescribed for insomnia or anxiety, can increase your risk for developing Alzheimer's disease by 43 to 51 percent, according to a 2014 study of 9,000 people older than 66 who had ever used the drugs. The study was published in the *BMJ*.11 Benzodiazepines include lorazepam (Ativan), alprazolam (Xanax), temazepam (Restoril), chlordiazepoxide (Librium), and diazepam (Valium), among others. [200]

Aerobic Exercise for Insomnia

We've known for years that aerobic exercise plays a role in helping you beat insomnia. That was confirmed in a 2014 Brazilian study, which revealed that aerobic exercise not only improves sleep quality for people with chronic insomnia, but it also eases depression.

In the study, 21 sedentary middle-aged men and women with chronic insomnia were first tested on a treadmill to make sure they were medically able to participate in the study; then, they walked on treadmills at a pace deemed appropriately aerobic for them by the researchers. The participants walked on the treadmills 3 days a week for 50 minutes each session. Four months later, the researchers retested their sleep patterns. The researchers reported it took the participants 14 minutes less to fall asleep, their sleep time increased by 24 minutes, and their REM sleep time increased by a significant 2.5 percent. The participants reported being 30 percent less depressed, and their overall sleep quality improved by 40 percent. (*Tip:* Perform your exercise in the late afternoon or after work, not right before bedtime.) [201]

Meditation and Yoga

When you're stressed, as we've discussed many times in this book, your body releases a flood of stress hormones including cortisol and adrenaline. These activate and arouse your system, put your body on high alert, and make you more energetic—which, as bedtime approaches, is the very last thing you want to be. Practicing yoga can calm your arousal response, say Harvard Medical School researchers who studied yoga as an insomnia treatment in 2004.

Twenty participants, all diagnosed with chronic insomnia, learned how to perform a basic, easy hour-long seated yoga routine focusing on breathing and meditation techniques. They were instructed to practice it daily, preferably just before bedtime, for 8 weeks. At the end of the study, the participants reported that their total time awake during the night had dropped by about 50 percent and their sleep quality had improved, as did their total sleep time. [202]

Clean Up Your Sleep Act

These tips help many of my patients sleep better.
- Go to bed and wake up at the same time every day.
- Get the TV and all electronic devices out of the bedroom.
- Make sure your bedroom is dark, quiet, and cool.
- Use foam earplugs and a sleep mask, if necessary.
- Let pets sleep outside the bedroom if you can.

- Practice a wind-down ritual about 30 minutes before bedtime
- If you need to get up in the middle of the night, try not to turn on bright lights—rely on soft night-lights instead

Sleep-Supporting Supplements

If my patients have given the Alive and Well food plan a 30-day trial and are getting aerobic exercise but still have sleep problems, I suggest that they give these time-tested natural remedies a try:

- Melatonin, 1 to 3 milligrams 1 hour before bedtime
- L-theanine, 200 milligrams one to three times a day
- Fish oil: NOW Foods Ultra Omega-3 (Take one a day)
- Magnesium, 500 milligrams daily [203]
- Passionflower, tincture, 1/2 to 1 teaspoon in water 30 minutes before bedtime

Staying Away from Gluten Calms the Brain

In 1982, long before anyone recognized the links between gluten and emotional disturbances, I had already begun to observe the "food-mood connection." I saw an 8-month-old baby boy who had suddenly turned from a sweet little "easy baby" into a wild man who was irritable, hyperactive, and not sleeping through the night. I thought it might be his diet, since his parents had begun to give him a wider variety of baby foods. At that time, I did not have our current testing technology, so I tried an elimination diet. We went back to rice and bananas. It was like magic. The sweet baby was back! We added one new food every 4 days and made it safely through applesauce, chicken, and peas. Then we added sweet potatoes and boom! Wild man showed up again, and wild man also had a rash on his neck. So that was the end of the sweet potatoes, the wild man, and the sleepless nights, both for the little boy and his parents.

Cut to the mid-'90s. A couple came to visit our office so that the wife could be tested for her digestive problems. When her results came back, she did have some food allergies. The husband was not so sure he wanted to be tested because "all he had" was a little anxiety, plus some persistent insomnia. He didn't have a single digestive problem, no sinus congestion, no headaches—just the insomnia and anxiety. I was already aware that reactions to food proteins could trigger anxiety and told the husband I suspected his anxiety and insomnia might be from brain irritability caused by inflammation from a food. He agreed to be tested, and he was reactive to gluten. He became very exacting in removing gluten from his diet (much harder twenty years ago than it is now), and his anxiety and insomnia resolved completely. Since then I have seen many people whose insomnia, anxiety, and even ADD and ADHD improved or disappeared entirely when they removed allergenic foods from their diets.

Today, other physicians have become aware of the food-mood connection, most notably physician and author David Perlmutter, MD. Dr. Perlmutter is one of the few MDs who truly understand the medical importance of food. He is board certified both in neurology and nutrition, and as far as I know, he is the only physician in the United States to hold both these certifications. I share his belief that anxiety and insomnia can often be attributed to food protein reactions.

MENOPAUSE

A friend of mine who'd recently turned 50 loved enlivening her business meetings with a wisecrack or two. One day, she said that she had to stop joking around. When I asked why, she confessed that something bizarre was happening to her. "Every time I make a joke, my face turns beet red and I break out in an all-over sweat. It's like someone's turned the heat way, way up. It's humiliating, and people are noticing," she said.

I immediately recognized what was going on and knew it had nothing to do with her jokes—or the thermostat. She was having hot flashes.

Since my friend only felt the heat when she was laughing in the conference room, she didn't make the menopause connection. But her experience perfectly illustrates just how quirky menopause symptoms can be. By no means are they a one-size-fits-all set of problems, because menopausal symptoms can vary wildly from one woman to another.

Of course, women have been dealing with menopause forever. But only in relatively recent history have women been living decades beyond the "change of life." In the past, doctors often dismissed this natural transition. Their thinking was, "It's just a few hot flashes, and menopause doesn't last very long." Even now, at a time when women are at least somewhat more likely to discuss menopause, there's little mention of accompanying symptoms such as fatigue, arthritic pain, or anxiety—or the feeling of not being your old self. However, irritability may get a nod, as in, "I'm out of estrogen and I've got a gun."

The Age of Medicated Menopause

The prescription estrogen drug, Premarin, for menopause was introduced in 1942 and became wildly popular with doctors and patients around 1986. That's when the FDA announced that Premarin (named for the pregnant mare's urine from which it's made), NOTE, could effectively combat osteoporosis. Unfortunately, we soon discovered that many women who took it were getting endometrial cancer. Lesson learned: Giving estrogen without progesterone causes overgrowth in the lining of the uterus that can lead to endometrial cancer. So, progestin was added to Premarin; that drug was called Prempro. [204]

In 2002, researchers published the famous WHI (Women's Health Initiative) study; it included more than 27,000 postmenopausal women between the ages of 50 and 79. In my opinion, and that of other experts, it was a poorly designed study; the average age of the participants was 65. Unbelievably, the researchers took women, most who'd been in menopause for 10 to 15 years, and gave them large doses of hormones, referred to as hormone replacement therapy, or HRT. What a terrible idea! That's like taking a car that has been up on blocks for 15 years, putting bad gasoline in it, and trying to race it.

And in this case, the "bad gasoline" was the content of the hormones used in the study. But that was not all. The hormones were given orally and had to pass through the liver to enter the bloodstream. The hormones produced by our bodies are made of three types of estrogen: estriol, estradiol, and estrone. They are released directly into the bloodstream.

Now, consider Premarin and Prempro. Though these hormones are related to those in the human body, they are actually very different. They contain no estriol at all even though human estrogen is about 80% estriol; they contain 43% estrone, thought to be the most carcinogenic fraction of estrogen, while human estrogen is only about 10% estrone; and they contain a non-human form of estrogen—Equilin--from pregnant mare's urine, that should only be circulating in a horse, not a human. In addition, unlike your own hormones, which are secreted directly into the bloodstream, the "standard" hormone replacement is an oral medication that passes through the digestive system, making a "first pass" through the liver.

The table that follows compares how closely HRT options mimic human estrogen and how they enter your system. The closer, the better—that's my recommendation.

A comparison of human estrogens, bioidentical estrogens, and Premarin (CEE)				
Estrogen type	Human %	Tri-est %	Bi-est %	CEE %
Estriol	80	80	80	0
Estradiol	10	10	20	40
Estrone	10	10	0	43
equilin (horse)	0	0	0	17
route of entry	directly to bloodstream	directly to bloodstream (under tongue or on skin)	directly to bloodstream (under tongue or on skin)	Oral-first pass through liver

The results of the WHI study were startling to some people but not to me. Women who took Prempro increased their risk for stroke by 41 percent; their risk of having a heart attack rose by 29 percent; and their risk of developing breast cancer increased by 26 percent. A follow-up study of the women a decade later found that women who took Prempro also had an increase in breast cancer rates, and their cancers tended to be advanced and cause death. The people who did the study had not considered that the average age of the women in the study was 65. Even common logic says that women of that age, 10-15 years into menopause, should not be given hormone replacement at all.

The WHI statistics, compiled from a group of women mostly long past the appropriate age for receiving hormone therapy, do not warn us away from hormone replacement. They warn us away from giving hormones to women long past menopause, from giving hormones that contain xenoestrogens (foreign estrogens not normally found in the human body, like the Equilin in Premarin) and giving hormones by the oral route of administration, that must pass through the liver.

Today, we have more appropriate hormones. We call them bioidentical because they are structurally identical to the hormones that we produce in our bodies. It's worth noting that in the WHI study, even with the poor quality of the hormones, and the poor route of administration, many of the younger women benefited from the therapy.

Finally, in the fall of 2017, a review of the WHI study concluded that hormone replacement can be safe and beneficial, especially in early menopause. Here is their position statement:

"Hormone therapy (HT) remains the most effective treatment for vasomotor symptoms (VMS) and the genitourinary syndrome of menopause (GSM) and has been shown to prevent bone loss and fracture. The risks of HT differ depending on type, dose, duration of use, route of administration, timing of initiation, and whether a progestogen is used. Treatment should be individualized to identify the most appropriate HT type, dose, formulation, route of administration, and duration of use, using the best available evidence to maximize benefits and minimize risks, with periodic reevaluation of the benefits and risks of continuing or discontinuing HT.

> "For women aged younger than 60 years or who are within 10 years of menopause onset and have no contraindications, the benefit-risk ratio is most favorable for treatment of bothersome VMS and for those at elevated risk for bone loss or fracture. For women who initiate HT more than 10 or 20 years from menopause onset or are aged 60 years or older, the benefit-risk ratio appears less favorable because of the greater absolute risks of coronary heart disease, stroke, venous thromboembolism, and dementia. Longer durations of therapy should be for documented indications such as persistent VMS or bone loss, with shared decision making and periodic reevaluation. For bother-some GSM symptoms not relieved with over-the-counter therapies and without indications for use of systemic

HT, low-dose vaginal estrogen therapy or other therapies are recommended." [205]

In their statement, The North American Menopause Society still did not distinguish between types of hormones. They were still talking about "replacement" with CEE-Conjugated Equine Estrogen. As you saw in the table above, CEE contains a xenoestrogen, Equilin, with a molecule that is not identical to human estrogen; it contains a large proportion of estrone—thought to be the most carcinogenic estrogen fraction; and it contains no estriol, which is the most abundant fraction of human hormones, comprising about 80% of the normal circulating hormone supply. The only appropriate hormone in CEE is estradiol, and even that is compromised by its oral route of administration.

I understand that taking HRT is a choice. For those women whose menopause symptoms are excessive and severe, taking HRT for a few months to a few years right around perimenopause can provide nearly immediate relief. For my patients who do choose to take HRT, I recommend taking a bioidentical hormone replacement in the lowest dose possible, since we know that even low doses will protect your bones and ease your symptoms. I believe it is safest to avoid oral hormone therapy. There is currently a patch available, which is not entirely bioidentical because the progestin it contains is norethindrone acetate, rather than micronized progesterone. Although some of my patients have been able to take it safely, many of them have reacted to the adhesive of the patch. I believe it is best to find a doctor who has experience in prescribing sublingual or transdermal bioidentical hormone therapy. If you decide to do that, here are some helpful questions to ask:

- How long have you been prescribing bioidentical HRT?
- Were you specifically trained in using bioidentical HRT?
- Do you use creams or sublingual drops or pills?
- Is your compounding pharmacy certified?

Food for Menopause

In an Australian study of more than 6,000 women, followed by researchers for more than 9 years, the effects of six different diets on menopause symptoms were scrutinized. At the start of the study, which was published in the *American Journal of Clinical Nutrition,* the women were between 50 and 55 years of age. Forty percent of them experienced night sweats, 54 percent had hot flashes, and 42 percent were symptom free.

It turns out that the women who most closely followed a vegetable-rich Mediterranean-style diet were about 20 percent less likely to report hot flashes and night sweats than those who didn't stick to the diet. On the other hand, women whose diets were high in bad fats and sugar were 20 percent *more* likely to develop hot flashes and night sweats. Herber-Gast [206]

Menopause-Friendly Produce

Based on the above study, researchers said that fruits and vegetables were helpful for relieving menopause symptoms. Some on our list below are especially rich in antioxidants. Others contain phytoestrogens, a weak form of estrogen that occupies the estrogen receptors, potentially lessening symptoms. Make sure to enjoy several servings of these (organic only) veggies and at least two servings of fruit every day.

Vegetables: Asparagus, beets, bell peppers, carrots

Fruits: Apples, mangoes, melons, pears, pineapples, strawberries

Additionally, try tracking your food intake for a few days to see if you notice a link between certain items and hot flash frequency. Common triggers are caffeine, alcohol, and spicy foods; if these are problems for you, try avoiding spicy foods and limiting yourself to 200 milligrams of caffeine daily (about two 8-ounce cups of coffee) and three alcoholic drinks, with food per week (no more than one drink per day.)

Black Cohosh. A few well-designed studies show that this Native American herb eases hot flashes better than a placebo. I'm not entirely sure why, but there are theories that it could affect opioid receptors in the brain, act as an antioxidant, or have anti-inflammatory properties. The most tested product is Remifemin, available at most drugstores. Follow label directions. Another supplement that has worked well for some of my patients is a black cohosh-containing supplement called Herbal Equilibrium, from Women's Health Network.[207]

Exercise. Exercise is a critical component of the Alive and Well plan, and it's one that's especially crucial for relieving symptoms of menopause. Its benefits include helping prevent weight gain, strengthening bones, and increasing muscle mass. What's more, research tells us that exercise can also reduce menopause symptoms, say researchers from Victoria University in Melbourne, Australia, who published an in-depth investigation of research relating to exercise and menopause in 2014. [208]

Weight loss. Since you'll be changing your eating habits on this plan, losing a little weight will likely be a welcome benefit, especially if you're dealing with hot flashes. In one year-long study, women who lost at least 10 pounds (or 10 percent of their body weight) were 23 percent more likely to experience fewer or no hot flashes, according to researchers funded by Kaiser Permanente. Since fat locks in body heat, and since night sweats and hot flashes are your body's way of cooling you off, shedding a few pounds can help keep you cool and reduce your menopause-related symptoms.

Hypnosis. Hypnotic relaxation therapy reduced hot flashes and other symptoms by up to 80 percent after 12 weeks, according to a study from Baylor University in Waco, Texas. The researchers theorized that deep relaxation could calm brain regions responsible for heat regulation. What's more, hypnosis could improve memory decline, another frequent menopausal complaint. When the Baylor research team reexamined the data from their earlier study in 2014, they learned that hypnotic relaxation offered additional benefits, including improved sleep and mood. It's entirely possible that improving the sleep of menopausal women could also improve memory. [209]

Sage tea. Sage tea is a time-honored herbal remedy for reducing night sweats and excess perspiration. To brew a cup of this savory tea, pour 1 cup boiling water over 1 tablespoon fresh sage leaves (or 1 teaspoon dried). Steep, covered, for 5 minutes, and then strain. Add a little honey or lemon, if you'd like. Enjoy a cup of the tea two or three times a day. [210]

Take Care of Your Bones!

Osteoporosis (bone loss) and menopause can go hand in hand because losing estrogen plays a role in osteoporosis. After menopause, women tend to lose more bone than they build. That's why it's critical to make sure you're getting plenty of calcium (only 11 percent of American women get adequate calcium from their diets), along with other bone-building vitamins and minerals. Here are some important supplements: [211]

- Magnesium, 100-400 milligrams
- Calcium, 250-500 milligrams
- Vitamin D3, 800-5,000 IU
- Vitamin C, 1,000–5,000 milligrams
- Boron, 2–9 milligrams
- Zinc, 6-50 milligrams
- Manganese, 1-15 milligrams
- Copper, 1-2 milligrams
- Vitamin K, 70-140 micrograms
- Beta-carotene, 15 milligrams

Traditional Chinese Medicine for Menopause

As a practitioner of Traditional Chinese Medicine (TCM), I have case files that are full of menopause success stories. I believe that a combination of acupuncture treatments and Chinese herbal formulas, adjusted depending on each woman's needs, can offer excellent symptom relief. In fact, acupuncture was just proven effective for relief of hot flashes in a 2014 study published in the journal *Menopause.* Researchers analyzed the results of 12 studies that included 869 women, and they reported that acupuncture significantly reduced hot flash frequency and severity. Acupuncture also was proven to have long-term effects that lasted up to 3 months following treatment. [212]

I also use Chinese herbal formulas with wonderful, evocative names, including Free and Easy Wanderer, Two Immortals, Heavenly Emperor, Women's Precious, and Mobilize Essence, for example. These need to be prescribed by a qualified TCM practitioner; find one at the National Certification Commission for Acupuncture and Oriental Medicine—www.nccaom.org.

My Mother Regained Her Equilibrium—And Personality— with Hormone Replacement

I became interested in prescribing hormones because I saw firsthand over many years how much they helped my mother. She went into menopause when she was about 50, as I was graduating from high school. Her symptoms were a disaster. She had always been busy and generally positive. But she developed insomnia, had hot flashes so severe that she soaked through several changes of clothes a day, was irritable at best, and even had suicidal thoughts. It was as if she had developed a different personality. Our great old-fashioned family doctor, Dr. Kuhl, said that hormone therapy was probably her best shot at regaining her well-being.

Premarin had been on the market since 1942, so he tried that first. It made my mother so sick that she vomited constantly. Then he tried a new injectable estrogen-testosterone drug called Deladumone. It worked like magic—my mother was her old self again. She went for injections every 2 weeks, and that was it. It is interesting to note here that my mother's hormone replacement bypassed all the difficulties of the hormones given in the WHI study. Her replacement was timely, done early in menopause. The main hormone in her replacement was estradiol, with the same structure as the estradiol in the human body. There was no horse estrogen. And the hormones were injected, so they went directly into the bloodstream like our own circulating hormones.

Any time Dr. Kuhl tried to taper her off the hormone replacement, she'd react with extreme symptoms, so he kept her on it. And when the drug went off the market, he used injectable estradiol cypionate and testosterone cypionate, in the same dosage as the Deladumone. By the time he died, I had gotten my medical degree. I continued to prescribe the HRT for her. You should have seen my mother between the ages of 65 and 84! She sped around in her blue Buick, driving over the bridge from Iowa to Illinois to play tennis with women half her age. She had strong bones and played a mean game of tennis doubles.

Meanwhile, her book-club contemporaries were collapsing with arthritis, osteoporosis and other illnesses. And so was her oldest sister. Her story was completely different. My aunt elected not to take hormone therapy. She developed postmenopausal bleeding and had to have a hysterectomy. She gained weight. She was too tired to exercise and became diabetic. Then, she was diagnosed with breast cancer.

Obviously, the stories of these two sisters made a lasting impression on me. My mother, who took hormones, stayed healthy and did not get breast cancer. My aunt, who did not take hormones, suffered multiple disabling illnesses.

The hormones my mother took didn't contain Estrone or Equilin, and they were injected directly into the bloodstream without entering the digestive system, pretty much like the bioidentical hormones I take, and prescribe, today.

My mother enjoyed her life until she got a sinus infection and was given a pill by her new doctor. He failed to look at her chart and gave her penicillin, to which she was highly allergic. Of course, she got sick, so she stopped taking the pills. Several hours after she stopped taking the penicillin, she collapsed at home. My father called me, and I went racing out to Iowa to see her. She had gone into septic shock; a "super infection" had developed when she stopped taking the antibiotic. She died 20 years ago. My perfectly healthy, tennis-playing 84-year-old mother—whose own mother lived until the age of 93—died, I believe, years before her time. Because of a reaction to a medication she was allergic to, given to her in error.

But my mother had 35 years of a fabulous life thanks to a concerned doctor and a good medication—the injectable hormones. And that's what this book is about—a healthy lifestyle, coupled with wise, discerning use of medications, given only when necessary, after we've explored the *causes* for an illness. This book is a perfect memorial for her.

OBESITY

Obesity is the epidemic of this young millennium, and it's one that may end up hurting more people than any other plague on the planet. The sad truth is, we are getting fatter, and it's killing us.

In 2014, Stanford University researchers published statistics from 1988 to 2010, reflecting Americans' changes in obesity, belly fat, physical activity, and caloric intake. The news was grim. Our waists are expanding, and our bellies are getting bigger. Incredibly, the number of us who get no leisure time activity has more than doubled—in 1988, 19 percent of American women were inactive; as of 2012, that number skyrocketed to 52 percent. [213]

Fat is far more than a cosmetic problem. Being overweight is a life-threatening health risk. As the scale climbs, so do your odds for developing type 2 diabetes, heart disease, high blood pressure, nonalcoholic fatty liver disease, stroke, osteoarthritis, and cancers of the breast, colon, uterine lining, and kidney.

What's the Cause?

If you think people get fat because they eat too much and exercise too little, you're only partially right. The unfortunate truth? Part of the reason that we're growing fatter than ever, as we saw in Part I, is due to manufactured foods. We're eating out of boxes, bags, and cans, rather than from whole, natural foods we were evolved to eat over the millennia. In just the last 100 years or so, an evolutionary nanosecond, we've gone from farm to factory eating. There is simply no way our bodies can adapt fast enough to process the additives in these foods. Here is a review of just a few of them:

- Food dyes (made from coal tar)
- Artificial flavorings, MSG, sulfites, and aspartame
- Trans fats that block our absorption and elimination of nutrients at a cellular level by compromising the cell membranes
- Sugar content that is beyond anything in human history
- Brominated vegetable oil in sports drinks (also used as a flame retardant)
- Processed corn products, with their chemical residues and their genetically modified content, in most manufactured foods
- Pesticides, antibiotics, and bovine growth hormone in our milk

Not only is the nutrition processed right out of our mass-produced foods, and the additives put in, many of the additives make you fatter—artificial sweeteners and colors, emulsifiers, and other non-nutritive ingredients. Experts have named these chemicals obesogens.

Obesogens interfere with the way our hormone system works; they confuse insulin signaling; and they affect the way our fat cells function. Sad to say, these chemicals have been deliberately added to our foods to enhance food production, and to make them more addictive, not to improve our nutrition. Along with the additives, excess sugar, salt, and refined grains also play a role in the obesity epidemic. [214]

Ingredients That Fatten Us

Researchers from the department of medicine at Boston University Medical Center published a 2014 report on food additives linked to obesity. Here's a partial list.

- Salt
- Sodium benzoate
- Monosodium glutamate (MSG)
- Autolyzed yeast extract
- Sodium sulfite
- Hydrogenated and partially hydrogenated vegetable oils
- High-fructose corn syrup
- Sugar (all forms)

Beyond the chemicals that manufacturers deliberately add to processed foods, when environmental pollutants enter the food chain, they also can act as obesogens that contribute to our obesity crisis. These include:

- Bisphenol A (BPA), found in plastic bottles and canned foods
- Phthalates, found in plastic food packaging
- Organic pollutants and pesticides

- Organophosphates
- Carbamates
- Flame retardants
- Dioxins
- Arsenic
- Cadmium
- Lead
- Antibiotics (from animal feed) [214]

TV Makes You Fat

TV commercials that hawk food products are more than annoying—they can make you fat, especially if you are already overweight. It turns out that watching food-related commercials does just what the advertiser intended—they motivate you to eat, according to a 2014 study in the journal *Psychology and Health.* [215]

Losing the Weight, Keeping it Off

When it comes to weight loss, yo-yo diets are doomed to fail, and many times, to make you gain even more weight. To lose weight and keep it off, you need a satisfying eating plan that you can stick with for life, not some roller-coaster plan that you hop on and off.

A Paleo-type diet is free of all the kinds of foods that contribute to weight gain: no processed foods, no dairy, no sugar, no grain. And because I also recommend organic foods, my patients are already minimizing their exposure to environmental obesogens.

Here are a few simple tips I recommend to my patients:

- Enjoy 3 to 4 ounces of lean protein foods per meal.
- Limit nuts to two or three small servings a day (just enough to fill the hollow of the palm of your hand).

- Eat plenty of green, leafy vegetables. Enjoy these with lemon or organic vinegar and a teaspoon of one of the healthy oils in the Food section of Part III.
- Vinegar has been proven to lower blood sugar (see above in the Diabetes paragraphs).
- Have no more than two or three servings of low-sugar fruits per day
- Eat carbohydrate foods only at breakfast and lunch.
- Drink three to four cups of green tea a day.
- Spice up your food—a tiny bit of hot pepper can help reduce calorie intake by as much 16 percent and increase the feeling of fullness.
- Cucumber is the new cracker, celery is the new chip! They are great with salsa or small amounts of guacamole or hummus. [216]

Activity Is a Must

I will outline several possible exercise plans in the Exercise section of Part III.

Becoming active is an important success factor in weight loss, and interval exercise is a big key—we know, for example, that interval training can lower blood sugar. Be sure to follow the walking plan as outlined, and after a week or two, increase your pace during the interval portion and extend the "full-out" time by a few minutes each week.

Focus on De-Stressing

One terrible secret about stress is that it can sabotage even your most committed weight loss plans. Here's why: Whenever you're stressed out (a bad day at the office, an argument with your spouse, a financial worry), your body responds by releasing hormones. Suddenly, you get a shot of adrenaline so that you can spring into action, and a blast of cortisol prompting you to replenish the energy you haven't used. You probably already know that when people take steroids, they want to eat all the time, and they gain weight, especially around the waist. Well, when you're stressed, you're on your own steroids. Result? You feel the urge to eat.

Of course, you're probably not going to grab a celery stick. Instead, you'll want a sweet, salty, or fatty treat because you subconsciously know that eating something like that will release happy-making neurotransmitters that blunt your tension. Try these tactics the next time stress overwhelms you.

Try Mindful Eating. When you're stressed, you tend to eat faster, which usually means you'll eat more food than you need. So just slow down, savor each bite, and pay attention to your feelings of fullness. See more about mindful eating in Part III.

The Scary Side of Weight-Loss Supplements

First, let me say that when it comes to prescription drugs designed to help you lose weight, I believe that they cause more problems than they solve. Various side effects can range from fecal incontinence to heart problems. None of them help change eating habits or learn to eat more healthfully. I never recommend taking any of these.

But what about all those miracle-sounding weight loss supplements you see advertised? I'm a fan of those, either. When you see a headline about an herbal or other kind of supplement linked to illnesses or deaths, you're usually reading about a weight loss product. That's because makers of these products often skirt regulations and use sketchy and sometimes dangerous ingredients in their products.

As far as I'm concerned, the best way to burn off fat is to exercise and stay away from grains, sugars, dairy, most alcohol, and most manufactured foods. I think it's wise to avoid so-called natural weight loss products that promise a quick fix. Fall for the promise of "shed pounds like magic" and you might lose not only your cash, but also your health.

In a 2013 case involving OxyElite Pro, a "fat-burning" supplement containing the herb *Rauwolfia canescens,* the FDA notified USPLabs that its product was linked to dozens of cases of nonviral hepatitis and liver failure. The product also contained the stimulant DMAA, for which no required safety evidence was presented to the FDA. After receiving the FDA's notification, USPLabs voluntarily destroyed some $22 million worth of product.

"Women are often shocked when they end up in the ER and need urgent care for serious liver problems, especially when we trace the liver damage back to the 'herbal' weight loss pills they were taking," says Herbert L. Bonkovsky, M.D., professor of medicine at Carolinas HealthCare System in Charlotte, North Carolina, and the University of North Carolina at Chapel Hill. "They thought they were taking a safe, natural supplement that would magically help them shed pounds. Instead, it damaged their liver and made them deathly ill. Some have required liver transplants or have died."

Even when something innocuous, like green tea, is listed as the main ingredient, shape-shrinking products are bad news. "Read the claims," says Daniel Fabricant, PhD, who is the former director of the FDA's division of dietary supplement programs. "If they seem too good to be true, they probably are." [217]

Lynette's experience, described below, is a good example of weight loss without the dangerous weight loss supplements.

Lynette Loses Her Allergies—And 100 Pounds

I saw Lynette (her name has been changed) during the first 5 years that I began testing people for food allergies. Her case certainly made me understand that one of the major complications of delayed-type food allergies can be weight gain, and that the weight loss "cure" can simply be avoiding the offending foods. Lynette, then in her twenties, had come to me for help.

The first thing I noticed was that she was nearly 100 pounds overweight.

She was tall, 5 feet 10 inches, so her maximum weight should have been about 170 pounds. She weighed 265. We talked about what she was eating, and I decided to test her for allergies. When the results came back, we discovered that she was allergic to gluten, dairy, chicken, and eggs. She stopped eating those foods in the spring of 1994. By August, she was down to 188 pounds. By November, without doing anything but avoiding the allergenic foods, she had lost a total of 93 pounds and was down to 172.

I believe Lynette's dramatic weight loss was the result of removing the foods to which she was allergic, because doing so helped reduce her inflammation level. How does that help you lose weight? Let's look at a landmark study cited by Mark Hyman, M.D., the eminent functional medicine physician, and best-selling author.

The study was published in December 2007 and looked at two groups of children. The first group was overweight and the second was normal weight. The researchers measured three key factors connected to inflammation in both groups of children. First, they measured high-sensitivity C-reactive protein (CRP), a marker that shows the general level of inflammation in the body. Then they conducted ultrasound tests to measure plaque in the carotid arteries (the main arteries that supply the brain). Finally, they tested the children for delayed-type food allergies.

Here's what they found: The overweight kids had three times the level of CRP and had much thicker carotid arteries, which signal early atherosclerosis and heart disease. They also had higher rates of food allergies, which the researchers linked to the inflammation and obesity. As they explained in the study, inflammation from any cause can lead to insulin resistance and higher insulin levels. Because insulin is a fat storage hormone, when levels are consistently high, you end up storing more fat—particularly around the belly.

Lynette's experience dramatically illustrates what I have observed clinically in thousands of people over the last 35 years: Eliminating the foods that cause delayed-type food allergies is an effective strategy for treating obesity, along with a low-carb Paleo-type diet. It's not so much about limiting calories, although portion control is important. As I have already said, it's about avoiding the foods you react to, inflammatory foods, manufactured foods, refined starches and sugars, and chemical additives.

Coping with Emotional Eating

When you eat because you're sad, tired, angry, stressed, or bored, or when you think you deserve a special treat, you're eating emotionally. It's a problem for some 2.5 million people who eat to control their emotions. If you're among them, you're going to have trouble controlling your weight. I've treated many "emotional eaters" in my practice, and I've found there are strategies that can be powerfully effective for helping people blunt the emotional messages that prompt them to eat.

Emotional eating is a challenge, especially here in the United States. Our "food culture" is so ruled by food marketers that they can be impossible to escape. And eating is at the center of our culture—we have entire cable television channels and network TV shows devoted to the celebration of food—in fact, being a "foodie" is the latest craze. We've got *Cake Boss, Cupcake Wars, Chopped, Master Chef, Top Chef,* and *Iron Chef America,* to name just a few.

So, you're surrounded. Now, how to stop?

First, if emotional eating is really an out-of-control issue for you, you won't respond to the traditional advice, such as: eat according to your nutritional needs, make your own decisions about food, disconnect food from emotional triggers, eat mindfully, and keep triggering foods out of the house. None of that is going to do you a bit of good.

You will need to treat your emotional eating like an addiction—because it is! If it were a matter of being able to talk or discipline yourself out of it, you would have done that already. For more about emotional eating, see Part III, Why You Eat.

I follow the principles of Traditional Chinese Medicine when it comes to emotional eating; I focus on the root of the problem, not its symptoms. And the roots here are your own emotions, emotional triggers, and past unresolved emotional trauma. I have seen people who ate to fill up the hole of rejection from their parents. I have had clients who ate to calm the trauma from abuse, and who kept eating in a subconscious belief that fat could be their shield against being abused again. I have seen people who were given food instead of attention as children who now use food as a way of giving themselves love and attention. And of course, I have seen anorexia and bulimia.

I've found the following strategies help even deeply-rooted cases of emotional eating.

Emotional Freedom Technique (EFT). I describe this easy and surprisingly effective therapy in depth on page 311. It's especially good for emotional eating because it helps you deal with past trauma, which in my experience can often trigger emotional eating. EFT relies on bringing your unhealthy old beliefs or habits about food that you took on as a child to the front of your mind, as you tap acupressure patterns on key acupuncture points. Doing so actually changes your habitual neurological pattern. Many people find that working with a trained EFT coach in the beginning is extremely helpful; many do online sessions via Skype. Find a coach and learn more at eftuniverse.com or naturallythinyou.com.

Overeaters Anonymous (OA). If your eating truly feels like an addiction, you could try Overeaters Anonymous, a 12-step program modeled on Alcoholics Anonymous. In OA, you follow a food plan and use the group support and the 12-step methods to keep you on track. I have seen it work well for quite a few people, and it is widely available and free.

Cognitive Behavioral Therapy (CBT). Cognitive behavioral therapy is an individual short-term talk therapy (see more on pages 116 and 129) that aims to change your unhelpful behaviors. The therapy focuses on changing patterns of thought and action in a way that allows you to reach your goals.

Are You an Emotional Eater?

Signs of emotional eating are:

1. You eat when you are already full or think about food when you are full.

2. You eat when you are bored or tired.

3. You eat when you have either negative or positive emotions— when you are angry, sad, disappointed, anxious, or happy, and you describe food with emotional words like decadent or sinful.

4. You eat when you are stressed about getting something done for work or school—you gather your food and then sit there and munch it absent-mindedly while you work, almost without even realizing it. And surprise, all of a sudden, the big bowl of chips or candy is gone.

5. You have food cravings.

6. You can't stop yourself from eating even if you want to. You binge eat. You are out of control.

7. You eat food to feel good, and use it as a substitute for love, comfort, and security.

If two or more of these describe you, you have an issue with emotional eating. If three describe you, consider addressing your problem, and if four or more describe you, you may want to get some assistance.

When Might Bariatric Surgery Be the Answer?

Here are the guidelines regarding bariatric surgery from the Cleveland Clinic.

"Research supports the benefits of weight loss surgery for those with a Body Mass Index (BMI) between 35 and 39.9 with obesity-related health conditions such as type 2 diabetes, obstructive sleep apnea, high blood pressure, osteoarthritis, and other obesity-related conditions. You could be a candidate for surgical weight loss if you meet any of the following criteria:

- You are more than 100 pounds over your ideal body weight.
- You have a Body Mass Index (BMI) of more than 40.
- You have a BMI of more than 35 and are experiencing severe negative health effects, such as high blood pressure or diabetes, related to being severely overweight.
- You are unable to achieve a healthy body weight for a sustained period of time, even with medically supervised dieting.

"Research is proving that bariatric surgery can be the most effective way to treat obesity and may even cure type 2 diabetes. In fact, if you're obese, it could reduce your risk of developing diabetes by up to 80 percent, according to a 2014 study funded by the UK National Institute for Health Research. On the plus side, having surgery gives you an excellent chance of being able to reduce and even stop taking many of the medications you're now on for diabetes, high blood pressure, and high cholesterol. On the downside, you face the side-effects that come with any surgical procedure, and you'll have to learn to eat in a completely different way. Following surgery, you'll only be able to eat tiny portions of food. All in all, I still think surgery is something to consider for the person who is obese and has tried and failed at diet after diet."

SINUSITIS

When you're struck with sinusitis, your face can feel like a punching bag. Your cheekbones hurt, your eyes hurt—even your eyebrows ache. Blame it on your poor sinuses. You'd probably been coping with allergies or a cold, which eventually inflamed these air-filled spaces around your nose, eyes, and cheeks. Now your sinuses are infected and congested. And you're too weak to fight back because you may also have a fever, all-over body aches, and bone-melting fatigue. Sinusitis, which medically speaking means sinus inflammation, is bad enough—but if your sinuses become infected, you're in for a nasty, lingering problem. [218]

Three kinds of sinusitis exist:

- Acute: lasts up to a month or so
- Subacute: lasts from 4 to 12 weeks
- Chronic: lasts for more than 12 weeks and may continue even for years
- Recurrent: when you have several attacks in one year

An Environmental Clean-Up Plan for Sinusitis

Of course, first thing I do when someone comes to see me with sinusitis is help them figure out what environmental items or foods could be causing their problems. I recommend testing for food triggers and to see whether the patient is allergic to anything in the immediate environment—including pets, feather pillows, furniture, carpeting, even laundry detergent. Once we've identified the triggers, we eliminate them, and very often, that's the end of a person's sinus problems. You have already read a lot about that process in the Allergy section.

Removing just one or two offending environmental items can be almost unbelievably effective. For example, consider the amount of time you spend in your bed—for most people, it's somewhere between a quarter and a third of their lives. But if you're allergic to feathers and house dust, and you're spending that much time head down or even face down on a feather pillow that has collected months to years of dust mites, then it's no wonder you're congested. For clean-up guidelines, see the Allergy section here in Part II.

Anti-inflammatory Foods

By now you know that this plan is essentially an allergen-free way of eating. Still, some foods possess extra anti-inflammatory power, which is why I recommend that you focus on eating plenty of the following foods:

- Wild salmon, black cod (sablefish), sardines, and herring
- Tart cherries
- Avocados
- Organic eggs
- Dark, leafy greens
- Green tea
- Pineapple
- Berries
- Spices: ginger, basic, turmeric, red pepper, and horseradish

And even though they're included in most healthy food plans, there is some evidence that avoiding mushrooms, pickled foods and wine can help relieve sinusitis. [219, 220]

Other Treatments for Sinusitis

Most primary care doctors have a stock response for treating sinusitis that includes antibiotics to treat the infection, steroid inhalers to reduce inflammation, and antihistamines or decongestants to help dry up the congestion. I will occasionally prescribe antibiotics for people when I believe that a bacterial infection is raging, although even then, I may choose Traditional Chinese Medicine herbal formulas instead. One thing I won't do is prescribe antibiotics for a bad cold. Not only are they useless against colds, they're also harmful. They're useless because colds are caused by viruses, and antibiotics don't kill viruses; they're harmful because of their side effects, and because they add to our universal antibiotic resistance crisis.

But I'm unlikely to recommend the other drugs often prescribed for sinus problems. I don't believe that they're called for, in most cases, and I'm not happy with their side effects. As I've said, once we've removed allergenic foods and environmental triggers, sinusitis symptoms are likely to go away on their own.

Mary: Too Busy for Allergies

Mary first came to see me in June 2001. The then 44-year-old designer had a punishing schedule and cared for two young children; one was autistic. That child often woke around 2:00 a.m. and stayed up until 7:00 a.m. Mary started her day between 6:30 and 7:30 a.m. so she could get her kids to school, then she'd come home, where she did her design work.

Her work was a challenge: She needed 30 hours a week to finish her work, and she had a 4-hour window to get it done while the kids were at school. She worked nights and weekends to complete her assignments. The time after school was packed with therapy appointments 5 days a week for her autistic child, and lessons and sports for her other child.

Time for her own care or to de-stress was limited, to say the least. But Mary was resourceful. She hired a babysitter one night a week, and she and her husband traded off being with the kids so that they could each go to yoga or the gym once a week.

Mary's physical problems included congestion and chronic allergic sinusitis. She had known allergies to mold and cats, and she was already using air conditioning and an air filter in her bedroom. She wanted to get off antihistamines—they made her feel tired, and she just couldn't afford that with her schedule.

I put her on a mold-free diet, gave her homeopathic drops for the congestion, did some acupuncture to clear her sinuses and lower the stress, gave her a Chinese herbal formula, and sent her to be tested for food allergies.

She was allergic to dairy, eggs, and wheat. She came back for a follow-up visit in November, and we discussed ways to manage her allergen-free diet. I gave her enzymes and probiotics to take with each meal. She said she felt a lot better on the diet, and she stopped taking the antihistamines.

I didn't see her again until April 2007. She hadn't stuck with the allergen-free diet—she had edged back to a "normal" diet because her life was so stressed and busy. Also, she had recently broken out in hives from head to toe. She was still eating wheat—a piece of toast every morning—and I also suspected she had become allergic to more foods. I was right—testing revealed she now had allergies to food dyes, dust, mold, and the following foods: gluten, dairy, eggs (her previous allergies), plus corn, oats, cane sugar, and coffee. I gave her some acupuncture and Chinese herbs to calm the hives and cautioned her to strictly avoid all of her allergens.

She came for a follow-up visit 1 month later. She was working hard on her diet and told me that she'd figured out an additional cause for her hives—she'd been spending time in a friend's house who had cats, in a space with a hyperbaric oxygen chamber that they both thought was free of cat hair. But apparently, Kitty had been using the chamber as a playroom! At that visit, we also did more testing and found allergies to citrus, guar gum, sunflower seeds, and chickpeas.

She visited again in October that year, saying that now her worst problem was fatigue. She'd stuck to her diet and stayed away from the cat, and as a result, her hives had disappeared entirely in September. She'd lost 25 pounds and felt great about that. Her diet was:

Breakfast: Rice cereal or fruit and rice toast

Lunch: Large salad with chicken

Dinner: Meat or chicken, vegetables, potato

Snacks: Raw cashews or fruit

We discussed ways to increase her calorie intake a little bit so that she would not lose any more weight, and I gave her an adrenal supplement for her fatigue.

She came for one more follow-up visit a few weeks later. Her sinus congestion had improved dramatically, and she was feeling much less tired.

I didn't see her again until almost 7 years later, in March of 2014. Her now 19-year-old autistic child still needed plenty of her time, but her other child had graduated from college and was home helping. Now Mary was taking the tranquilizer Klonopin for her stress, which she wanted to stop, and she was also in menopause. Her muscles were tight and sore, despite weekly chiropractic treatments and massage. I suggested we try an Emotional Freedom Technique (EFT) session for her stress. We did one session and I referred her to an EFT practitioner for more. I also gave her an herbal formula for menopause. Additionally, I recommended a Paleo-style diet.

She came back to me in April and said that she was doing regular EFT sessions and that it eased her stress from caring for her son. But Klonopin caused unwanted side effects, and her menopausal symptoms had worsened—hot flashes, night sweats, and insomnia. I gave her a prescription for bioidentical hormone replacement therapy, and we talked about how to taper off the Klonopin.

We talked on the phone in September 2014, and it was all good news. She was off the Klonopin, her menopause symptoms had resolved, and she was feeling generally well, able to manage, and at last, felt she was really enjoying life.

Sinus Support

You may not be able to eliminate all your symptoms, even after removing allergens from your diet and environment—after all, it's a big world out there, and you don't want to live in a bubble. But these natural treatments can help provide relief for even stubborn sinus problems.

Probiotics. Probiotics are "good" bacteria that help strengthen your immunity and shield you against allergies. My favorite brand is Renew Life Ultimate Flora. It's available in several strengths, from 15 to 100 billion organisms in each capsule. For most people, I recommend either 30 or 50 billion live organisms, one capsule daily, with food.

Sinupret. This is a combination European herbal medication that's been clinically tested and proven effective for treating sinus conditions; it is also a natural antibiotic. It contains the herbs cowslip, yellow gentian, black elderberry, common sorrel, and vervain. Combined, these herbs clear congestion, ease inflammation, and are natural antibiotics. Find it in health food stores and online. Follow label directions. [221-224]

Environmental Hazards

In addition to dust and mold, many other household items can irritate your sinuses and clog up your head. For a list, check the Allergies section here in Part II.

Robert's Recovery from Sinus Problems

Robert (not his real name) first came to see me in 2005. He had recurrent sinus infections and congestion. After testing, we learned that he was allergic to tree pollens, gluten, peanuts, and coffee. He was careful about following his new allergen-free diet and did his best to avoid tree pollens. It worked! His sinus congestion vanished.

But 10 years later, I heard from him again. He called to say he had another sinus infection. Because it had become a full-blown infection, I prescribed an antibiotic, and it solved his sinus problems for a while. I gave him a refill, so he could take the antibiotics right away if he developed another infection. But when he needed a third round of antibiotics a few months later, I called a time-out.

Pills were obviously not the answer for Robert. We had to figure out what else was going on with him. I asked him to come in to get tested again. It turned out that he was now allergic to feathers, dust, and mold, along with the tree pollens. And he admitted that he'd been eating a little gluten, to which he was still allergic; on top of that, he'd also become reactive to buckwheat, oats, and dairy. (He had been eating an oat-based breakfast bar.)

Further, he was renovating his Michigan cottage, which was full of dust and mold. As if that was not enough, he was also riding his bike in a wooded area that had a lot of soil molds. It was a perfect storm of sinus killers—pollens, dust, molds, gluten, oats, and dairy. No wonder the pills didn't work—poor Robert was lucky to be breathing!

Here was the plan for Robert:

- Wear a filter mask while biking.
- Wear a filter mask during cottage rehab.
- Continue to avoid peanuts and coffee.
- Strictly avoid gluten grains, buckwheat, oats, and grain-based alcohols.
- Strictly avoid dairy.

The plan worked! Several weeks after he started our five-point plan, his sinus congestion and infections cleared up. And when he follows his plan and stays away from his allergens, Robert is free from sinus problems.

PART III: Preventive Health Care Strategies

SECTION 1: The Alive and Well Paleo-Based Food Plan

Before We Begin

There are countless books on the market with Paleo foods and recipes. Think of this section of the book as a guide, with some inside information, from a person with a medical background who has followed a Paleo-type diet for many years now, and who helps hundreds of other people do it. In this section, you will learn:

- What to eat and drink
- What not to eat and drink
- What you may safely add to the classic Paleo diet, including supplements
- Reasons to avoid "staff of life" foods like wheat and dairy
- How, why and when to eat

I have chosen a Paleo-based food plan for myself and my patients because it is easy to find good foods and create fresh, varied, tasty meals; it is also easy to find good free recipes on the web—they are so abundant, it's a case of "so many recipes, so little time"; it is possible to find good restaurants that have Paleo-friendly menus; it is not necessary to measure foods or count calories to maintain the Paleo way of eating; this way of eating is sustainable, long-term; and the good fats keep you from getting hungry between meals.

Many of my patients enjoy a modified Paleo, or what I call a Paleo-plus diet. That's a classic Paleo diet with the addition of some servings of rice and potatoes. It is perfectly possible to live in a healthy way with a Paleo-plus diet, if you are not trying to lose weight. If my patients want to adopt that diet, I show them how to modify their rice so that it has a lower glycemic index and doesn't cause blood sugar spikes. I teach them to get organic white basmati rice (no arsenic, and a moderate glycemic index of 58) and then lower the glycemic index as much as 50% by cooking it with added coconut oil, refrigerating it for 24 hours, and then reheating it to eat it. And I teach them to eat a small serving of organic potatoes (steak fries, roast potatoes, baked potatoes) earlier in the day, rather than a huge serving of mashed potatoes at dinner.

I have used the word "food plan" as much as possible instead of "diet." Why? To me, and to many of the people I see, the associations with that word are about the same as their associations with the word "jail." Too many Americans have been on the end of the yo-yo string, bouncing up and down in weight—never really losing it and keeping it off. And a "diet" really is a lot like jail. You get shut in and restricted, you count the days, and then you celebrate by having two doughnuts instead of one (after all, you've lost all that weight, right?) And then you pretty much go back to the way you were eating before, which is the very thing that made you gain weight in the first place! Getting the concept of changing the way you eat, making it a lifelong change, and finally tossing out the "low fat" diet—all this can be easy with the Paleo-style food plan, and it keeps the weight off. Here's a simple outline of the dos and don'ts of a classic Paleo-based diet.

What and What Not to Eat on a Paleo-Based Diet

DO EAT	DON'T EAT
Vegetables, fruits, lean meats, seafood, nuts and seeds, healthy fats (avocado, organic unprocessed coconut, olive, sesame, sunflower)	Dairy, grains, starches, sugars, legumes, alcohol, processed foods, food additives, food dyes

That was easy, wasn't it! Easy to say but challenging to accomplish in our manufactured food minefield. Then why do it? The theory is, humans were basically evolved over tens of thousands of years to eat hunted or gathered foods. Agriculturally-grown foods are a recent addition in the long run of evolutionary life, representing about 5% of our time on earth, and we really haven't adapted to them yet.

What about current research on the nutritional value, weight loss potential, and metabolic outcomes of a Paleo-based diet?

There are many studies confirming the benefits of a Paleo-based diet. For a "tour" of 23 of them, check out Kris Gunners' article, "23 Studies on Low-Carb and Low-Fat Diets—Time to Retire the Fad." The fad he is referring to is the low-fat diet. [225]

I have chosen two studies as good examples of three specific outcomes of the Paleo-based diet: the diet works, even for people who are severely obese; the diet lowers the blood test values that are markers for metabolic syndrome; and even without calorie restriction, it works better than a calorie-restricted low-fat diet.

One of my favorite studies was published in the New England Journal of Medicine. 132 severely obese subjects (BMI of 43) were randomized to a low-carb or low-fat diet for 6 months. The low carb group lost an average of 12.8 pounds, while the low-fat dieters only lost an average of 4.2 pounds, 1/3 as much as the low-carb group.

Here are the results of their blood tests:

The low-fat dieters lost more of their ability to produce insulin—their insulin levels went down 27%, while the low-carb dieters remained stable.

Fasting blood sugars went down only 5 mg/dL in the low-fat group, while the reduction in the low-carb group was an impressive 26 mg/dL.

Insulin sensitivity is the ability of cells to be sensitive to the insulin levels in the bloodstream, and transfer blood sugars into the cells instead of letting them circulate in the bloodstream. It got slightly worse in the low-fat dieters but improved in the low-carb dieters.

Triglycerides (a type of fat) went down only 7 mg/dL in the low-fat group. The average reduction in the low-carb group was more than five times that number—the triglyceride level went down by 38 mg/dL.

It is important to note here that only the low-fat group was calorie-restricted. The low-carb group was not, but still got the better results. [226]

In the next study, both the low-carb and low-fat groups were calorie-restricted. 40 people who had risk factors for cardiovascular disease were randomized to the two groups for 12 weeks. The low-fat group lost 11.5 pounds, while the low-carb group lost almost double that amount—22.3 pounds. The low-carb group also did much better lowering the lipid markers of metabolic syndrome.

Triglycerides	Low carb Down 107 mg/dL
	Low fat Down 36 mg/dL
HDL [64] cholesterol	Low carb Up 4 points [64]
	Low fat Down 1 point
Apolipoprotein B	Low carb Down 11 points
	Low fat Down 2 points
LDL size	Low carb Increased [64]
	Low fat Stayed the same [227]

Not every study showed results quite this spectacular, but in even the less favorable studies, weight loss results of low-carb diets were at least equal to low-fat diet results.

So that's part of the "why" of adopting a Paleo-based diet. In general, you are more likely to lose weight and prevent chronic illnesses like diabetes and metabolic syndrome on a Paleo diet. What are the good qualities of the diet that produce those results?

Anti-inflammatory, hypoallergenic. A Paleo-type diet eliminates all the common allergens, like gluten grains, corn, soy and dairy. These foods have always been common allergens and have become more allergenic over time (see below.) If you have allergies to these foods, they are a guarantee of chronic inflammation. And even if you don't, they can still cause inflammation and congestion. In a person with delayed-type allergies, inflammation can be life-threatening. I have had two-food allergic patients in their forties who have had strokes at that young age. One was reactive to gluten and dairy, and one was reactive to gluten, dairy and corn. In addition to inflammation in the gut lining, their allergic reactions to foods inflamed the lining (endothelium) of their blood vessels and set the stage for stroke. Now that both are on allergen-free diets, they've recovered from their strokes and are living healthy lives.

High protein. The Paleo-type diet is rich in protein—organic chicken and eggs, wild and organically-farmed seafood, and grass-fed, and naturally-lean meats make up about 30 to 40 percent of the diet. Diets high in protein are proven to make you feel fuller and more satisfied, and to help you burn calories more efficiently. What's more, a 2008 study suggested that high-protein diets can also improve heart disease risk factors. [228]

Low carb, low glycemic. A Paleo-type diet is free of grains and gluten, and it's extremely low in sugars. Carbs and sugars are responsible for rapid rises in blood sugar. The glycemic index (GI), developed by researchers at the University of Sydney in Australia, is a ranking of carbohydrates on a scale of 0 to 100, based on how high a food raises your blood sugar levels after you eat it. Foods with a high GI value are absorbed rapidly and quickly affect your blood sugar. The "blood sugar roller coaster" brought about by high-glycemic-index foods gradually causes insulin resistance and moves you in the direction of diabetes.

Foods with a low GI value are more slowly digested and absorbed, so blood sugar and insulin levels rise slowly. Research from the Harvard School of Public Health clearly links higher risks for type 2 diabetes and heart disease to diets with higher GI levels. To find out what a food's GI value is, visit glycemicindex.com, the web site that the University of Sydney maintains and updates listing the GI values of foods. [229]

How else do low glycemic index foods help you? A major 2014 study, published in the *Annals of Internal Medicine,* concluded that low-carb diets effectively lower your risk for heart disease. What's more, said the researchers, low-carb diets were better than low-fat diets for helping you lose weight. [230]

High fiber. You might worry about whether you're getting enough fiber once you purge your diet of cereals, breads, and other grain and gluten-containing foods. Rest easy—you'll be getting plenty of fiber on a Paleo-based diet. The vegetables you'll be eating, including various members of the squash family, leafy greens, and green veggies, and fruits, such as apples and pears, will provide more than enough fiber to keep you healthy. Recent research has linked high-fiber diets to a lower risk of heart disease. In fact, researchers who reviewed 22 studies published between 1990 and 2013 reported that the more fiber in your diet, the lower your chances for having a heart attack. [231]

More and better fats. Remember the days when we were told that cutting fat from our diets was a smart health move? Well, as we know now, that was terrible advice. In fact, when the food industry jumped on that bandwagon, the packaged foods they pushed as "low fat" usually replaced the fat with lots of sugar, salt, and other unhealthy ingredients. In the end, going "low fat" made us gain more weight and upped our risks for diabetes, heart disease, and other illnesses. Now we know better—that healthy diets can contain up to 30 or even 40 percent healthy fats. I'm talking about omega-3 fats. Some omega-3s, called EPA and DHA, are found in flaxseed, walnuts, sardines, and wild salmon. Another type, ALA, comes from Brussels sprouts, kale, spinach, and salad greens. Research has shown us that omega-3 fatty acids protect against heart disease; newer studies suggest they may also help protect against cancers, inflammatory bowel disease, and autoimmune conditions like rheumatoid arthritis. What's more, the grass-fed, organic meats you'll enjoy on this plan contain a fat called conjugated linoleic acid, or CLA, which helps reduce body fat and increases lean body mass. And if you elect not to eat red meat, you can always take a CLA supplement. [232, 233]

Nutrient-dense, not calorie-dense. How does this aspect of the food plan help you? Some of the conditions you may take pills for are caused by vitamin or mineral deficiencies, and your prescription drugs do nothing to change that. In fact, in a landmark study published in the *Journal of the American Medical Association,* deficiencies of several key nutrients, including D, E, and B vitamins, were linked to several diseases including colorectal, prostate, and breast cancer; heart disease; osteoporosis; and bone loss.

A Metabolic Game-changer. When you stop eating all grains and sugars, it changes your metabolic process. Instead of using starches and sugars as fuel and storing the excess around your waist as fat, your body burns fat as fuel. That is part of the reason why you lose weight so easily on this specific type of diet. I believe it is also part of the reason why generic "low carb" diets in some of the studies had different results. If study participants still consumed grains and sugars, no matter how low and amount, results could easily have varied. Even a low proportion of grains and sugars in a diet prevents the "metabolic magic" from happening. This is also one of the principles, and reasons for success, of the ketogenic diet. If that diet appeals to you, you can try it, but I have chosen the Paleo because I believe it is easier to follow, and therefore more likely to be followed by more people.

Now that you know more about the qualities of a Paleo diet and the studies that support it, here is an expanded list of Paleo foods, and a few modifications for eating a Paleo-type diet over a long period of time.

What to Eat: The Longer List

Proteins: Organic, grass-fed beef, bacon (uncured, no nitrites or nitrates); organic chicken, duck and eggs; elk; wild-caught or responsibly-farmed fish; lamb and goat; organic, additive and antibiotic-free deli meats; organic pork; pheasant and quail; shellfish; turkey; veal; venison.

Fresh or frozen organic vegetables—all veggies except peas are on the list. Enjoy these starchy vegetables: sweet potatoes, yams, and the many different squash varieties. (Spaghetti squash or zucchini "noodles" make a satisfying pasta substitute!) Here is a list: Artichoke, arugula, asparagus, beets, bell peppers, box choy broccoli, brussels sprouts, cabbage, carrots, cauliflower, celery, chili peppers, cucumber, eggplant, endive, escarole, garlic greens—collard, mustard, turnip, green beans, kale, kohlrabi, leeks, lettuce, mushrooms, nori seaweed, okra, onion, parsnips, pumpkin, radish, snow peas, spaghetti squash, snap peas, summer squash—zucchini, yellow, all varieties, sweet potatoes and yams, tomatoes, tomatillos, turnips, winter squash.

Fresh organic fruits. Choose fruits with lower fruit sugar content and higher fiber content, such as berries, apples, pears, or peaches. High-fiber fruits have the least impact on raising your blood sugar. Eat tropical fruits and watermelon very sparingly or avoid them, because their sugar content is much higher. Here's the list. Apples, apricots, bananas, blackberries, blueberries, cantaloupe, cherries, cranberries, dates, figs, grapefruit, grapes, honeydew melon, kiwifruit, lemon, lime, mandarin oranges, mangoes, nectarines, oranges, papaya, peaches, pears, pineapple, plums, pomegranates, raspberries, strawberries, tangerines (including clementines), watermelon.

Nuts and seeds: (not peanuts, which are legumes). Almonds, Brazil nuts, cashews, chestnuts, hazelnuts, macadamia nuts, pecans, pistachios, walnuts; chia, flax, pumpkin, quinoa, sesame, sunflower seeds and pine nuts.

<u>Healthy oils</u>: cold-pressed organic olive, coconut, avocado, sesame, walnut, macadamia. If not reactive to dairy, organic, grass-fed ghee (clarified butter.)

<u>Sweeteners</u>: Small amounts of local honey or 100 percent pure, preferably organic, maple syrup, or pure stevia (not blends with processed corn sugar—erythritol) as sweeteners

Eat Occasionally

If you are not trying to lose weight, you may have these:

- Once or twice a week, enjoy one small potato or half a larger one—preferably with blue, purple, or golden flesh and eaten with its skin.

- Two or three servings a week of organic quinoa, wild rice, or cooked, cooled and reheated basmati rice, preferably for lunch and not for dinner.

- One glass organic, non-sulfited wine, 2 to 3 times per week, with food.

- One or two squares of dark chocolate a day. Go Raw makes a good, agave-sweetened version.

Remember, these additions stop the "metabolic game changer" aspect of the Paleo-type diet. If you notice that you start to gain weight, either slowly or rapidly, by making these additions, cut them out again, and go back to the classical Paleo diet. If you have had a history of metabolic syndrome or prediabetes, don't add them. [234]

Herbs and Spices

Aromatic and flavor-rich herbs and spices are key additions to the foods you'll enjoy with your Paleo diet. Not only do they add a "flavor shot" to everything you eat, but many also offer significant phytochemicals that, together with foods, can deal a blow to chronic diseases. Make sure to add fresh or dried organic herbs and spices to your cooking. Try these for starters: Parsley, oregano, rosemary, turmeric, ginger, cinnamon and garlic.

In a study of people with type 2 diabetes, German researchers found that cinnamon can reduce blood sugar levels by 10 percent, possibly because compounds in cinnamon activate enzymes that stimulate insulin receptors. The sweet spice has also been shown to help lower levels of cholesterol and triglycerides, blood fats that may contribute to diabetes risk. [235]

People who consumed lots of garlic had lower rates of ovarian, colorectal, and other cancers, says a research review in the *American Journal of Clinical Nutrition.* Garlic contains more than 70 active phytochemicals, including allicin, which many studies have shown decreases high blood pressure by as much as 30 points. Garlic may help prevent strokes as well by slowing arterial blockages, according to a yearlong clinical study at UCLA. It's best to chop or crush fresh garlic and let it stand for 10 minutes—that way, its cardiovascular and cancer-fighting benefits will withstand cooking. [236]

Paleo-friendly Prepared Foods

I know that the classic Paleo diet has no processed foods. However, doing everything "from scratch" can be challenging in a busy life. Here is a list of Paleo-friendly prepared foods that we have developed as a "handout" in our office.

Breakfast foods

- Birch Benders Paleo Just-Add-Water Pancake and Waffle Mix (these are grain-, gluten-, soy-free and paleo! They are a favorite around my house. My grandchildren love them.)
- Siete grain free tortillas

- Kitchfix or Paleonola granola
- BHU Fit Bars

I have looked at many kinds of breakfast bars. Most of them either have grains (usually oats), cane sugar, or are made from dried fruits that have too many fruit sugars and calories and not enough protein. There is one exception: BHU Fit bars. They are non-GMO, gluten-free, USDA-Certified Organic. Their protein is vegan organic pea protein, and they are sweetened with monk fruit. A sample nutrition breakdown for the chocolate chip cookie dough flavor bar is: 13 grams protein, 2 grams sugars, 11 grams fiber. Very impressive!

Sweeteners and Gum

- Sweet Tree or Wholesome brand organic palm (coconut) sugar
- Date sugar. Note: All beet sugar in the USA is now GMO, don't use it. Also, fructose, xylitol, erythritol and sorbitol are all corn sugars, so watch for them on labels if you are allergic to corn, or even if you are not. It is 90% likely that their source is genetically-modified corn.
- Wholesome Sweeteners Organic Blue Agave (Madhava also makes an organic agave). This item is much cheaper at Costco. There is controversy about using Agave, but I tell my patients that small amounts of organic agave are acceptable.
- Chewing Gum. The only one I know that is free from corn-source xylitol or aspartame is B-Fresh, which has birch source xylitol. Check bfreshgum.com If you are not allergic to corn, you can use Spry gum, which is sweetened with corn-source xylitol.

Pasta and Pizza (Mostly not for classic Paleo)

- Manischewitz makes a grain-free gluten-free pasta made of tapioca starch and potato flakes. It does contain egg white. (This is the closest to a Paleo pasta. It does have white potato flakes, but it is grain-free.)
- Trader Joe's organic rice pasta. My family likes this one the best. Here's the Paleo trick for your rice pasta "cheat." Cook your pasta with olive oil in the water. Drain and cool it, refrigerate for 24 hours. Reheat and enjoy a small serving. This lowers the glycemic index as much as 50% and creates resistant starches, which serve as prebiotics.
- Pizza crust—I make Paleo crusts from a recipe or use rounds of fried eggplant as a crust. I use Daiya dairy-free provolone style cheese. Daiya makes a gluten- and dairy-free margarita pizza that many of my patients like, but it does have rice in the crust.

Jams, Candy, Cookies

- All-Fruit Jams (make sure these do not contain any artificial sweetener)
- Wax Orchards Fruit Sweetened Fudge Sauce
- Go Raw agave sweetened dark chocolate squares or chocolate-covered coconut
- For cookies, I make my own almond flour, honey-sweetened Paleo cookies. See the Elana's Pantry recipe in the recipe section.

Alternative Dairy Products

Dairy- and sugar-free ice creams

- So Delicious Ice Cream (they have a line that is fruit-sweetened, make sure you get those and not the items in their product line that have sugar in them, if you are allergic to cane sugar).

- Luna and Larry's coconut milk ice cream is agave-sweetened, and is good if you are allergic to gluten, dairy, egg and sugar.

Milks

- So Delicious unsweetened coconut milk
- Kirkland Organic Almond Milk (no carrageenan)
- Westsoy Unsweetened Organic or Unsweetened Vanilla Soy Milk, (don't use the vanilla if you need to be corn free); Trader Joe's Unsweetened Organic Soy Milk
- Note: A cup of unsweetened almond milk or coconut milk has only 45 calories.

Yoghurts

- So Delicious makes an unsweetened coconut milk yoghurt.

Butter and Cheese

- Purity Farms makes organic ghee (clarified butter) that is obviously not dairy-free, but is casein free, and many people who otherwise react to dairy can tolerate it;
- Earth Balance makes a good coconut butter in a blue-and-white tub, and two other butters, one that has soy and one that is soy-free.
- Melt makes a good organic coconut oil-based butter that is soy-free.
- Daiya cheese has a good flavor and melts well but some of their types of cheese contain corn. The Daiya cream cheese is corn free.
- Leaf Cuisine, Treeline, and Kite Hill are all good brands of dairy-free cheese.
- Go Veggie makes a Vegan dairy-free cheese, the Mexican cheese shreds, which has a good taste and melts well.

However, beware of the other Go Veggie cheeses. They make a whole line of "lactose free" cheeses that actually contain CASEIN, the dairy protein, as a main ingredient. Do not use them if you react to casein!

Condiments, Dressings, Sauces

- Sanji Wheat Free Tamari Sauce
- Annie's Natural Salad Dressings: Cilantro and Lime Vinaigrette, Honey Dijon Vinaigrette are both sugar-free.
- Organicville Salad Dressings: Olive Oil and Wine Vinegar, Sesame Tamari Dressing, Miso Dressing, French Dressing, Pomegranate Vinaigrette, many others—all sweetened with agave nectar.
- Ketchup Organicville also makes a good, agave nectar sweetened ketchup. All the other organic ketchups have sugar in them.
- Organicville and Kirkland also make prepared spaghetti sauces that are organic and corn-free (no citric acid)

Baking

- Wellbee or Honeyville both make good superfine almond flour, available online at Amazon
- Fearn egg replacer (in a box, made from potato starch)
- Hain Featherweight Baking Powder is corn- and aluminum-free
- Wholesome organic coconut sugar works well for baking, and so does honey.
- If you need to be corn-free, use powdered vanilla bean (called "bourbon vanilla") instead of vanilla extract. A teaspoon of the powdered bean equals a teaspoon of the extract in a recipe.
- Almost all chocolate chips contain cane sugar. The ones that do not, Lily's, contain corn sugar. You can make good dark chocolate chunks that work in cookies by cutting Go Raw

agave sweetened chocolate squares into small pieces. Look at Elana's Pantry cookbooks for good dessert recipes.

That's it for the good guys for now. What about the bad guys?

What Not to Eat: The Longer List

- **Cereal grains**: wheat, rye, barley, oats, spelt, kamut, triticale, farro, sorghum, millet, corn, buckwheat, and white or brown rice (see "Eat Occasionally" above)
- **Legumes**. All beans, peas, and peanuts. (One "cheat" on this that is acceptable is pea protein. The problem with legumes is their starch content. The pea protein removes the starch. Yes, it's processed, but the organic versions are acceptable.)
- **All dairy products** from cows, goats, and sheep, including milk, yogurt, cheese, cottage cheese, sour cream, ice cream. Also avoid foods that contain dairy in any form such as cake with milk in the batter or a cream filling.
- **Refined or raw sugars**, including cane and corn sugars, and refined maple sugar.
- **Refined oils**, hydrogenated or partially hydrogenated oils, trans fats, and any foods made with these unhealthy fats, including grain, bean, or seed oils such as soybean, cottonseed, sunflower, grapeseed, corn, safflower, and canola. (Re canola oil, I avoid it almost completely, but you may notice that on the Paleo-friendly prepared foods list below, I have included a non-dairy butter that is primarily made of coconut and flax oils but has organic canola oil as a minor ingredient.) [237]
- **Processed foods**, food additives, artificial sweeteners and flavorings, food dyes, and excess salt.
- **All fast and junk foods.** [238, 239]

Food Additives, Artificial Sugars, Food Dyes and Artificial Flavorings

According to the Asthma and Allergy Foundation of America, seven common food additives are known to cause allergic reactions in some people: Aspartame, Benzoates, BHT, MSG, nitrates and nitrites, sulfites, tartrazine (FD&C Yellow #5 food dye). [240]

The book, *Badditives*, also has a list of what they consider to be the most harmful additives: Aluminum, artificial colors, aspartame, BHA and BHT, carrageenan, fluoride, GMOs, high fructose corn syrup, meat glue (that's right, meat glue!) MSG, Bovine growth hormone. [241]

The main function of additives, preservatives, artificial colors and flavors is to increase the shelf life and marketability of the foods, not to increase your health. The possible exception to that is added vitamins, but they are generally added to refined foods, such as flour or processed cereals, to replace the vitamins that are present in whole grains. We are beginning to know how these additives affect people and none of it is good news. Food additive categories include:

Artificial Sweeteners. I will pause right here and put in an extra paragraph about these "sweet poisons" because they deserve it. They are added to so many "diet" foods. Here's just one of the problems with them: *Diet sodas sweetened with artificial sweeteners have been shown to be associated with* **weight gain, not weight loss**. In a study published in the journal Obesity in 2008, involving more than 3500 people, drinking more than 21 artificially-sweetened beverages a week (three a day) was associated with almost double the risk of being overweight or obese. A partial list of sweeteners to avoid: Aspartame, (also known as Nutrasweet, Equal, and most recently AminoSweet; Acesulfame; Saccharin, Sorbitol, Splenda, and Truvia (sold as a "healthy" stevia sweetener, but not made with pure stevia. They have added erythritol, a processed corn sugar, to the stevia.) [242]

Emulsifiers, stabilizers, gelling agents, and thickeners keep foods from separating, enable foods to gel, and help add body and thickness. However, many of them fall into the category of "modified food starch" and contain wheat and/or corn, both common food allergens.

Flavor enhancers bring out the flavor of foods without imparting one of their own. One of the most controversial of these is monosodium glutamate, or MSG, which is a known migraine trigger. It also does not change the taste of the food, it alters your sense of taste, and affects your nervous system.

Food colors and dyes enhance the way a food looks and make it conform better to consumer expectations but are in the process of being banned in the UK because of their known association with hyperactivity in children.

Preservatives allow foods to be kept safely for a longer time. Using them is the only method of preservation aside from freezing, canning, or drying that can make a food shelf-stable. Sometimes, preservatives can be simple compounds such as salt, sugar, or vinegar. Common chemical preservatives include sulfur dioxide, which stops mold and bacteria growth on dried fruit; sodium sulfite and sodium benzoate. (See below, under the heading "The Connection Between Food Chemicals and Obesity, why those two chemicals contribute to weight gain.") Bacon, ham, corned beef, and other cured meats rely on nitrates and nitrites, which are thought to form carcinogens when heated.

This is only a very bare-bones outline of additives. Mainly, I am saying that there are powerful reasons to avoid eating any foods that contain them. For more detail, and more reasons why they are so bad for your health, get Ruth Winter's excellent book, *Consumer's Dictionary of Food Additives.* [243]

Why Organic Is Best

The weight of the evidence is in: Organically grown and raised fruits, vegetables, meats, and fish are better for us than those sprayed with pesticides or fed pesticide-laced grain. To me, this issue has always been a no-brainer—how could spraying poison on food, and then eating it, be a good thing for the human body? And as far as genetically modified (GMO) produce is concerned, I'm firmly on the side of something called the precautionary principle.

I firmly believe that the proliferation of poisonous chemicals such as pesticides in our environment is linked to the rise in numbers of people whose immune systems are overreacting to once harmless foods. When so many foreign chemicals bombard us, it puts our immune systems on "overdrive" and makes our bodies more likely to react unpredictably. And another thing: As far as I'm concerned, the industry of making and transporting toxic chemicals poses knowable and unknowable risks to our public health and safety. Going organic on a massive scale would lessen our dependence on these poisons— and that, I believe, could have an enormous and positive impact on our health and that of our planet.

Here's what we know about the health impacts of pesticides.

- Exposures to pesticides (more than 17,000 are currently on the market) have been linked to brain and central nervous system disruption, infertility, a multitude of cancers, and even changes to our DNA.
- Children born to mothers who lived near pesticide-treated fields are six times more likely to be autistic.
- Switching to an organic diet for just 5 days virtually eliminates any signs of exposure to organophosphate pesticides among school-age children.
- A nationwide study found elevated risk for several types of childhood cancers for children living near fields treated with pesticides.

- More than 80,000 synthetic chemicals are used in this country, but only a few hundred have been tested for safety. [244]

Look for the green and white USDA Organic label on all the foods you buy. Right now, that label stands for farmers, ranchers, and food processors who sell products following a defined set of standards to produce organic foods. According to the USDA, these standards cover the product from farm to table, including soil and water quality, pest control, livestock practices, and rules for food additives. [245]

The Connection Between Food Chemicals and Obesity

If you're still looking for motivation to choose foods free of chemical food additives (no organic food can contain these potentially toxic substances, by the way), here's some information. In 2012, researchers from the Innsbruck Medical University in Austria discovered a potential link between two food additives and weight gain. In their test-tube study, they learned that sodium sulfite and sodium benzoate appear to delay the release of the hormone leptin. The hormone's job is to tell you that you're full. Based on this study, it's entirely conceivable that eating these additives in processed foods could make feeling full an elusive sensation—thus making overeating (and becoming overweight) more likely. [246]

Researchers are also studying the question as to whether synthetic environmental contaminants could be contributing to the global obesity epidemic, according to a 2014 report in the journal *Current Obesity Reports*. Though the evidence isn't yet solid, the authors suggest that many contaminants do interfere with our endocrine function, insulin signaling, and the way our fat cells behave. But the fact is, we still haven't studied the effects of intentional food additives (such as artificial sweeteners, colors, and emulsifiers) and unintentional compounds (think pesticides, for example) on human metabolism. We don't know what the health consequences of combining these compounds might be, especially years down the road. [214]

And that's another excellent reason to live by the precautionary principle. Until we know for a fact that these additives don't impact us in a negative way, why not go organic and avoid them? I also go by the precautionary principle when it comes to GMO (genetically modified) foods. We do not yet have any convincing evidence that these foods are safe, and until we do, I will advise my patients not to eat them.

Why Avoid Some Traditionally "Staff of Life" Foods?

It is reasonably obvious that additives and dyes are harmful and should be kept out of our foods. But it can be challenging to avoid foods that are traditional "basics" like bread and milk. Why do it? Because they are known common allergens, and they are most often contaminated by food additives, processing chemicals and agricultural chemicals. These foods were common allergens 70 years ago, even before the chemical explosion of the last 50 years. Today, common allergens are even more allergenic and inflammatory. More people are reacting to foods, and it is not a "fad," it is a reality. An article in the Health section of NBC News online, documents the rise of adult food allergies in the United States. Here are the statistics quoted:

> "According to data from FAIR Health, an independent, nonprofit organization focused on transparency in health care costs and health insurance information, private insurance claim lines with diagnoses of anaphylactic food reactions rose 377 percent from 2007 to 2016. And half of adults with food allergies developed them after the age of 18." [247]

In other words, allergic reactions to food have tripled in 9 years. The article says that we don't know why, but I think I may have at least a good educated guess. There are certain substances that increase the allergic or immune response. These are known as *haptens* or *adjuvants*. One of the most common adjuvants added to vaccinations is aluminum, in order to increase the immune response to the vaccination and create more antibodies, and therefore more immunity to the flu virus, or the whooping cough, tetanus, or diptheria bacteria. (The wisdom of injecting children with any item that contains aluminum or mercury (in the case of the multi-dose vials of the flu vaccine) is a story for another day. In the meantime, we know that aluminum increases the immune response. We also know that wheat itself, and the gluten in wheat, are common allergens. And it is obvious that most commercial bakery items are made with baking powder, which contains aluminum. It is possible that one of the factors in increased wheat/gluten allergies is the combination of wheat and the aluminum in baking powder.

In addition to the known adjuvant, aluminum, there are many additives in commercial bread and baked goods that could also function as adjuvants—agricultural pesticides not removed from wheat before it is made into flour, bleaching agents, and the many additives in commercial bread and baked goods. If you want to know more about the potential hazards of wheat and other grains, read at least these two books:

William Davis, M.D.'s book, *Wheat Belly: Lose the Wheat, Lose the Weight, and Find Your Way Back to Health*. You will see how and why avoiding wheat can help your metabolism, your weight, and your whole state of health. [248]

David Perlmutter, M.D.'s book, *Grain Brain*. Dr. Perlmutter has the distinction of being the only doctor in the United States to be board certified in both neurology and nutrition. If you did not understand the connection between food and neurological/psychological illness before, you will, after you read the book. [249]

Another gluten issue is non-celiac gluten hypersensitivity—the delayed-type reaction to gluten that I am discussing in this book. Until 2008, most physicians considered only one response to gluten to be worth consideration—the very serious health problem known as celiac disease. Celiac disease is caused by a gluten allergy that causes lesions and other intestinal damage. A study by Amy C.

Brown, PhD, a registered dietitian and researcher at John A. Burns School of Medicine showed that people with irritable bowel syndrome who did *not* have celiac disease experienced IBS symptom relief after following a gluten-free diet. I am happy that more research is being done. Some of us in the medical profession have already realized that there are people who do not have a diagnosis of celiac disease but do react to gluten. A few doctors already recognize the disease entity known as non-celiac gluten hypersensitivity. [250]

Another traditional food that the Paleo diet avoids is dairy. The best scientific evidence that avoiding dairy may be a good idea comes from a Swedish study published in the prestigious British Medical Journal in 2014. The study followed 61,433 women for 20 years, and 45,339 men for 11 years. They found that during the study period, the more milk people drank, the more likely they were to die or suffer a bone fracture. The risks were greater for women. Women who drank three or more glasses of milk per day had nearly double the risk of dying during the period of the study as those who said they drank only one glass daily. In addition, they had a 16% higher risk of having a bone fracture. [251]

This is a large study of more than a hundred thousand people, conducted over a long period of time. Women were studied for 20 years, men for 11 years. More milk brought about a worse state of health, and people who consumed the most milk had greater risk of fracture and died sooner. This information is so contrary to what we have heard from the U.S. dairy industry all these years, that the blowback has already begun. You can already find material on the Internet that denies the results of this important, large, and longitudinal study. However, the contrary material is generally based on opinion, and some of it appears to fall into the category of disinformation. The study is based on long-term, large-study medical evidence.

Let's do some more myth-busting about dairy. When I discuss dairy products with my patients and suggest that, for most of them, it's best to remove it from their diets, the first reaction is usually, "But what about my calcium and bone strength? Isn't milk essential for that?"

Dairy is not essential for giving you enough calcium intake, according to some scientific studies. While of course it's true that calcium is a key bone-building mineral, dairy products may not be as useful a calcium source as we've been led to believe. "Clinical research shows that dairy products have little or no benefit for bones," states the Physicians Committee for Responsible Medicine [252], a nonprofit organization that supports bringing nutrition into medical education and practice. The organization cites the famous Harvard Nurses' Health Study, which followed 72,000 women for 18 years. It showed "no protective effect of increased milk consumption on fracture risk."

And though we think of milk as a key part of our children's diets, the PCRM points to two studies—one, published in *Pediatrics* in 2005, showing that milk consumption doesn't improve bone integrity in children; and a 2012 paper in the *Archives of Pediatric Adolescent Medicine* that suggested consuming dairy products didn't prevent stress fractures in adolescent girls, after tracking their diets, activity, and incidence of stress fractures over 7 years. [252-251]

Further, it's clear that many people are allergic to dairy products. A bowl of ice cream or a glass of milk might suddenly experience some very uncomfortable digestive complaints.

Two separate issues are involved when we're talking about the problems dairy products cause. One is lactose intolerance; another is an allergy to casein, which is a protein found in dairy products.

One of the worst doctor abuse stories I've heard from my patients concerns lactose intolerance versus casein allergy. One of my patients came in—in tears—to tell me her experience. She'd complained about her digestive problems to her doctor, telling him it happened mostly when she ate dairy. The doc asked, gruffly, "Don't you know about lactose intolerance?" Then he went stalking out of the room, only to return in a minute with packets of Lactaid. He slapped them down in front of her and ordered her to take them.

Now, understand that Dr. Abusive didn't bother to take any additional medical history, nor did he attempt to test whether this woman was reacting to casein, lactose—or both.

And here's the punch line—**if your reaction to dairy involves a delayed-type allergy to casein—the milk protein--then Lactaid, a product intended to break down lactose—the milk sugar--will do you no good at all.**

Here's the difference. When we eat or drink dairy products, they contain lactose, a sugar found in all dairy products. To digest it, the small intestine secretes an enzyme called lactase. It breaks lactose into the sugars glucose and galactose, which are then absorbed into the bloodstream.

If you have "lactose intolerance," you'll experience uncomfortable diarrhea, cramps, bloating, and gas after you drink a glass of milk or eat ice cream. And if you take the lactase enzyme, it will solve the problem. [253]

But what if you weren't "lactose intolerant" in the first place? What if your real problem is the milk protein casein?

The answer is, casein can cause a delayed-type allergic reaction. When your immune system mistakes casein for a harmful invader, it will produce the IgG antibodies we talked about earlier, which are present in the delayed-type response. Your symptoms could appear as digestive symptoms, like diarrhea, gas, or bloating. They could also be congestive symptoms, such as sinus congestion, headaches, and coughing. Whatever reaction you experience, your doctor could mistakenly medicate you for whatever he thinks is wrong with you and be oblivious to the fact that dairy foods are the culprit. Over time, the damage a casein allergy causes to your gut can hurt your digestive system and leave you prone to many of the chronic illnesses with inflammatory components that we discussed in Part II. How can you be sure? Try an elimination diet or ask to be tested for delayed-type reactivity to the milk protein casein.

Even if you're not allergic or intolerant, milk is a pro-inflammatory food, and you will probably feel better if your basic diet is Paleo-style, which does not include dairy.

If you are worried about getting enough calcium, here is a list of non-dairy foods that will give you plenty of calcium.

- *Tofu* - Calcium content: 434 milligrams per half cup
- *Sardines* - Calcium content: 351 milligrams in one 3.75-ounce can
- *Collard Greens* - Calcium content: 268 milligrams per 1 cup cooked
- *Canned Salmon* - Calcium content: 232 milligrams in half a can
- *Figs* - Calcium content: 121 milligrams per 1/2 cup dried
- *Broccoli rabe - Calcium content: 100 milligrams in one 2/3-cup serving*
- *Edamame - Calcium content: 98 milligrams in 1 cup cooked. Also contains all nine* essential amino acids and 8 grams of fiber.
- *Broccoli* - Calcium content: 86 milligrams in 2 cups raw. This amount of broccoli also contains more vitamin C than an orange.
- *Okra* - Calcium content: 82 milligrams in 1 cup. Okra also contains soluble fiber, which is good for lowering cholesterol
- *Almonds* - 75 milligrams per ounce
- *Bok Choy* - Calcium content: 74 milligrams per 1 cup shredded, and only 9 calories.

Eating Out

Of course, you will want to eat out, and you will need to check out what you are eating! I have found that it's easiest to find grain, sugar and dairy-free menu choices at Greek, Middle Eastern, Mexican and farm-to-table restaurants. It's hardest at French restaurants or franchises. When I eat out, sometimes my "cheat" is beans at a Mexican restaurant or rice at a Chinese or Japanese restaurant. (Be sure to ask for no MSG.) One happy thought is that in some major cities, there are at least two restaurant chains that purposely deal in high quality, organic foods—Lyfe Kitchen, and True Food Kitchen. Even some franchises have moved to better quality meats. You won't be eating at franchises often, but there are some that do much better than others. Here is your antibiotic-free franchise survival list from Consumer Reports. They gave A through F grades as follows:

A	Chipotle, Panera Bread
B+	Subway
B	Chick-fil-A
C+	McDonalds
C	Wendy's
D+	Pizza Hut, Starbucks
D	Dunkin Donuts, Jack-in-the-Box, Burger King, Papa John's
F	Dairy Queen, Little Caesars, Sonic, Olive Garden, IHop, Applebee's, Domino's Pizza, Chili's Cracker Barrel, Buffalo Wild Wings [254]

What and What Not to Drink
What to Drink

Now that you've gotten an excellent foundation about how to eat your way to better health (and, hopefully, to a life dominated by fewer pills), let's turn our attention to the liquid portion of the Alive and Well plan. Drinking the right kinds of fluids will be essential to your success, and, as you'll discover, some drinks are clearly superior to others.

Water—Our Watery Bodies [255]

It's easy to understand why drinking enough water is essential for good health, once you realize how much water our organs contain.

Adult human body	60 percent water
Lungs	83 percent water
Bones	31 percent water
Brain and heart	73 percent water
Muscles and kidneys	79 percent water

How much water you need to drink every day has been debated, but I believe that 48 ounces of water or other fluids (from the list that follows) is a good amount to aim for.

I have concerns about chemicals in our water system, which is why I recommend that you use a water filter in your home to make sure you're drinking water that's free of harmful toxins. It is easy to find affordable and effective brands online.

If water's just too boring for you, you can add citrus slices, crushed fresh herbs (I love mint), or even slices of cucumber. If you add lemon, lime, or cucumber slices, be sure to scrub the outside of the lemons or limes with an eco-friendly detergent and rinse them well, and to wash and peel the cucumber. You can also enjoy any of the sparkling waters (not sweetened or artificially sweetened) that come in so many flavors. [256]

Green Tea

Green tea is one of the most health-giving beverages on the planet. Made from the unfermented leaves of the tea plant (*Camellia sinensis*), it's packed with potent antioxidants called polyphenols. Tea's polyphenols are classed as catechins, and green tea contains six different catechin compounds, the most studied and active of which is epigallocatechin gallate (EGCG). Green tea also contains stimulants, including caffeine, theobromine, and theophylline. And, in one of those wonders of nature in which a plant's medicinal compounds balance each other out, green tea also contains L-theanine, an amino acid that has been studied for its calming effects. Green tea has the potential to help balance blood sugar. Several Chinese studies have shown that drinking green tea decreases fasting glucose and lowers A1C numbers, which is why I suggest that my patients who have diabetes drink it regularly. [257]

Black Tea

Like its green cousin, black tea is made from the leaves of the *Camellia sinensis* plant. But green tea is brewed from fresh tea leaves; black tea leaves are aged. In addition to its 2 to 4 percent caffeine content, black tea also contains antioxidants and other compounds that appear to protect the heart and blood vessels. Among black tea's benefits are:

Improved alertness. Like any other beverage containing caffeine, black tea helps keep you alert and sharp.

Reduced stroke risk. Researchers who investigated the relationship between stroke and green or black tea drinking discovered that people who drank more than three cups of either tea a day lowered their risk for stroke by 21 percent. [258]

Reduced ovarian cancer risk. Women who are regular tea drinkers—both green and black—have a significantly lower risk for developing ovarian cancer compared to women who rarely or never drink tea. [259]

Green tea vs. black. Winner: A tie. Both green and black teas delivered high antioxidant levels. Which should you drink? We vote for drinking several cups a day of both kinds of tea for maximum antioxidant power. No matter which type of tea you choose, please make it organic, and again, make sure the bags are unbleached. [260]

Coffee

You may not think of coffee as a health drink, but the research that's been consistently piling up in its favor should convince you otherwise. First, here's a fact that may have escaped your attention: Coffee turns out to be the number one source of antioxidants in the American diet, say researchers at the University of Scranton in Pennsylvania. Sipping just a cup or two a day is enough to deliver coffee's antioxidant benefits. Plus, decaf is as antioxidant-rich as caffeinated coffee. When it comes to decaf, however, read the labels and buy only water-processed decaf. Most commercially decaffeinated coffee is made using a process that employs potentially harmful chemicals.

Studies on coffee have turned up promising evidence for some key health benefits.

Heart Disease and Type 2 diabetes. Researchers investigating cancer and nutrition in a huge (43,659 participants) 2012 European study discovered, after nearly 9 years of follow-up, that coffee drinkers (decaf or regular) had a lower risk for type 2 diabetes than non-coffee drinkers. [261]

Additionally, researchers studying 3,837 Finnish patients with type 2 diabetes in 2006 discovered that the more coffee a patient drank, the lower his risk of dying from heart disease. [262]

Liver problems. Your favorite eye-opener also seems to be particularly liver-friendly. Italian researchers showed that drinking coffee can lower liver cancer risk by about 40 percent; drinking three cups a day slashes risk to about 50 percent. And a study from Kaiser Permanente in Oakland, California, points to coffee's ability to lower the incidence of liver cirrhosis in alcohol drinkers by 22 percent. Finally, a 2014 study published in the journal *Hepatology* suggests that drinking two or more cups of coffee daily reduces the risk of death from liver cirrhosis by 66 percent. [263]

A Word on Wine

Information about wine can be confusing—you might hear that a drink or two is good for your heart, or that it can lessen the risk for type 2 diabetes, or even protect you against Alzheimer's disease. Or you'll hear that drinking raises the risks for those very diseases, and that you're at higher risk for breast cancer if you're a woman who drinks. Where's the truth? [266] [267]

It's all about moderation—and moderation, for most people, involves much less alcohol than you'd think: just two glasses of wine a day, with food, for men, and only one for women. One nightly glass of wine can raise levels of good HDL cholesterol. It can lower blood pressure, prevent artery damage caused by bad LDL cholesterol, and reduce your risk for blood clots, says the American Heart Association. I recommend to my patients that if they want to drink wine, they limit it to one small glass of organic, unsulfited wine, with dinner, a day, and not every day—generally at most three to four times a week.

For some people—such as those who have heart failure, high blood pressure, diabetes, or, for that matter, any chronic illness— drinking even one glass a night is something to discuss with your health care practitioner—especially if you're taking any medications. [268]

What Not to Drink: "Diet" Drinks

Sugary sodas and overly sweetened fruity drinks are absolutely out of our food plan. Sugary drinks are a major player in our obesity and diabetes crises. I won't reiterate all the reasons why you should not drink them because the evidence against them is already overwhelming.

What about diet drinks? It's safe to say this: never drink them!! I do think it's important to let you know how devious these sweeteners are, on the chance that you're not committed to breaking up with your beloved diet drinks quite yet.

Artificial sweeteners are a historically controversial product. They have stirred up concerns ever since they came to market in the 1800s. First, researchers worried that these sweeteners could cause cancer, which, decades later, seemed to become a self-fulfilling prophecy. Headlines went national in the 1960s when the FDA first banned cyclamates and then saccharin due to research findings that they caused cancer in lab animals. Later, we learned that in those studies, the poor lab rats were fed more artificial sweeteners than a normal human could possibly encounter in real life—and that, said the researchers, did not translate to a cancer risk in humans. The ban on saccharine was later lifted. NOTE [264]

Then along came aspartame, another artificial sweetener made from naturally occurring amino acids, aspartic acid, and phenylalanine. It ran into trouble when users complained about experiencing headaches, depression, increased hunger, and even seizures.

Studies on aspartame weren't as clear as we might wish. But one medical authority, neurologist Russell Blaylock, M.D., has written extensively about harm to the brain from aspartame (and MSG) in his excellent book, *Excitotoxins: The Taste That Kills.* I follow his recommendations and make sure that all my patients avoid both these items. I've seen it for myself: Many of my patients have had adverse reactions to aspartame. I tell all my patients to avoid completely any artificially sweetened beverage (or food). And one group of people must be extremely careful to avoid the fake stuff: People who have the rare genetic metabolism disorder phenylketonuria (PKU) can't break down its amino acid, phenylalanine. Taking in any form of phenylalanine causes them serious health problems.

To me, the most fascinating aspect of the artificial sugar controversy is that researchers have started implicating these sweeteners in America's obesity epidemic. Talk about unintended consequences! After all, artificial sweeteners were invented to help people stop drinking sugar-sweetened beverages and to make their weight loss and anti-diabetes efforts easier to accomplish.

A landmark research study in the fall of 2014 showed directly that "diet drinks" can cause weight gain, not weight loss. Conducted in Israel at several leading medical and research facilities, the study looked at the way sweeteners affect beneficial gut bacteria in both lab animals and humans. Here's what the researchers learned: *Artificial sweeteners alter gut bacteria in a way that triggers glucose intolerance.*

In their study, the researchers made a remarkable (and in my opinion, shocking) statement:

> "Artificial sweeteners were extensively introduced into our diets with the intention of reducing caloric intake and normalizing blood glucose levels without compromising the human 'sweet tooth.' This increase in non-caloric artificial sweeteners coincides with the dramatic increase in the obesity and diabetes epidemics."

The researchers connected the dots between the sweeteners and the obesity and diabetes epidemics, adding,

"Artificial sweeteners may have directly contributed to enhancing the epidemic they were intended to fight."[265]

Unsweetened is the way to go when it comes to your beverages. It is best to drink beverages that contain no sugars—no cane sugar, no fruit sugars, no artificial sugars. Watch out for "health drinks" like fruit juices, green juices or kombucha teas. I recently picked up a green juice that contained 34 grams of sugars per serving.

What About Supplements?

When you are already eating a healthy diet, you will generally still need a few supplements. I call myself a minimalist when it comes to dietary supplements. I recommend only those that I believe everyone needs to take, even if you eat an excellent, perfectly balanced diet. Nobody needs to take handfuls of supplements to stay well. Beware any doctor, chiropractor, or nutritionist who wants to send you off with a shoebox full of pill bottles that you are required to buy (from them) every month. The supplements I recommend are truly necessary for health, are made by good companies, are reasonably priced, and can be purchased easily from a store or online. These are my top seven.

Probiotics. I recommend that my patients take a probiotic supplement every day. They improve digestion, immunity, and brain function. Your gut is a microbiome that only stays in balance if it has plenty of good bacteria, and these days, we simply don't get enough in our diets. Yogurt contains probiotics, but to be useful, the person who eats it must be nonreactive to dairy, and the yoghurt must be the plain, organic, unsweetened real thing. Even for people who are not reactive to dairy, I still recommend a daily probiotic supplement. Because many of the people I see are sensitive to dairy, I recommend a dairy-free probiotic supplement. As you know by now, my favorite is Renew Life Ultimate Flora—it is widely available, isn't expensive, and contains a good blend of active bacteria. And you don't have to refrigerate it as you do with other probiotic supplements. That means you can travel with it, and better yet, it's easy to remember to take it because it can be on your table instead of in your refrigerator. I recommend that my patients take one a day with food. Other good dairy-free brands that do not require refrigeration are LiveWell Labs Pro45 and 1MD Complete Probiotics Platinum. Another brand which does need refrigeration is Natren Vegan Probiotic.

Fish oil (omega-3 fatty acids). Almost nobody gets enough omega-3s in their American diet—we eat too little fish, and we don't eat enough of the healthiest fats, such as walnuts, for example. That's bad news for our brains and our cell membranes, because omega-3s are critical to the way your cell membranes function. Surrounding each cell is a membrane that allows the nutrients to enter and the waste to go out. Unhealthy membranes lead to poor food absorption and inefficient waste removal. And manufactured fats (trans fats, hydrogenated and partially hydrogenated fats) can penetrate these membranes. Those bad fats stick around (and I do mean stick, including sticking to the linings of your coronary arteries) for 120 days—4 months!

The fish oil brands I recommend to my patients are NOW Foods Ultra Omega-3, Nordic Naturals, or Carlson. And I recommend that any fish oil supplement they take contain at least 600 milligrams of the EPA/DHA combination. The dosage I recommend to them of the NOW Foods Ultra Omega-3 is one a day, with food.

Vitamin D. If you think that this has become the "wonder vitamin," you're right. Most people in the Northern Hemisphere have deficient levels of this vitamin—and because we're careful to use sunscreen when we're in the sun, we no longer get enough vitamin D from being outside. Vitamin D deficiencies are now being linked to a host of chronic illnesses, including diabetes and even depression. A 2014 study links chronic inflammation to low vitamin D levels. I recommend that my patients over age 60 take 2,000 IU of vitamin

D3 a day; those younger than 60 generally need at least 1,000 IU a day. NOW Foods makes a good, inexpensive vitamin D. I recommend that my patients take one a day, with food. [269]

Vitamin C. Ever since Linus Pauling did his brilliant scientific research on the benefits of vitamin C, it seems that "medical science" has been trying to discredit it. The "minimum daily requirement" of vitamin C is 60 milligrams. As far as I'm concerned, this is a pitifully inadequate amount—maybe it's just enough to prevent "scurvy," or vitamin C deficiency, but certainly not enough to build your collagen and your bones, or to keep your immune system functioning at peak levels. There is even some new evidence that a big part of osteoporosis could be vitamin C deficiency.

I believe that it is helpful to take at least 500 milligrams a day, and according to Linus Pauling's recommendations, it is helpful to take 500 milligrams three to four times a day, with at least 6 to 8 ounces of water. I use NOW Foods Tru-C because it is corn-free.

Multivitamin (and B 12 if necessary.)

There are hundreds, if not thousands of multivitamins on the market. I believe that it is helpful to take a multivitamin, as "insurance" against any possible dietary deficiencies. One of my favorites is Pure Encapsulations "One". A good, corn-free multivitamin is Perque 2, which recommends that you take two a day. Make sure your multi is free of dyes and all other common allergens.

Calcium and Magnesium

Calcium and magnesium work best taken together. It is also important to get the right form, so that they are absorbable and do not irritate the digestive system, and to get the right dose. Doctors have been recommending overdoses of calcium, especially to women in menopause, for a long time. There is now good evidence that humans do not absorb more than 500 mg. of calcium per day, and that if you take more than that, it winds up as unwanted calcification on your bones and in your arteries. This happens more in men than in women, but I believe it is still not a good idea to take more of a mineral per day than your body can absorb. I recommend that my patients use calcium and magnesium glycinate, and that they take no more than 500 milligrams of each per day. I ask them to take it at night, because both minerals can make you feel more tired or sleepy. This is a great thing at night, not so much during the day!

That's it for what and what not to eat and drink. But it is still important to learn about why, when and how you eat. Why? Because if you are an "anxiety eater" or a "binge eater" or you eat a breakfast bar in the car (even a healthy one,) an at-the-desk lunch (even a great salad) and even a Paleo-style dinner at 10 PM in front of the bad news on TV, that can be a problem.

Why You Eat

2.5 million adults in the United States suffer from compulsive overeating. We are barraged with food ads, and food is a giant cultural phenomenon, and a social juggernaut. It is a major part of family celebrations, tailgate and super bowl parties, weddings and funerals. It is associated with love and satisfaction. How to avoid drowning in this flood of associations and expectations about food?

Eat according to nutritional, not emotional needs

If you eat healthy food, and eat only when you are hungry, that's great. But how many of us do that? We have become a nation of snackers and emotional eaters. Getting out of these habits may be challenging but it is crucial for your health.

Be aware of emotional triggers for eating, and disconnect them

If you are an emotional eater, you may want to get help making a change. It could be helpful to try some sessions of Cognitive Behavioral Therapy or EFT. If you feel addicted to food, it may be useful to work with an addictions program. There is a free 12-Step program, Overeaters Anonymous, that will help you stick to a food plan.

Emotional triggers can be powerful and deep-seated, which is why I suggest getting help. In my view, many people, who were bullied about food as children or suffered from CEN (childhood emotional neglect) or suffer from ACE (Adverse Childhood Experiences) have what I call food-related PTSD. In this case, food is tied to trauma. If you believe you have any of these conditions, you might need to get professional help, and you will need emotional support for making changes in what, why, when, or how you eat. If you have anorexia or bulimia, it will be necessary to find professional help.

Avoid trigger foods and addictive foods

If you know that when you open a bag of potato chips and eat one, you won't stop until you eat the whole bag, then you probably want to keep potato chips out of the house. In my experience, work with EFT around food is one of the best ways to let go of underlying issues about trigger foods. It is one of the few methods that can help you break the trigger so that you can enjoy a reasonable serving of potato chips or any other food that was previously a trigger, rather than having to avoid the food completely.

Make your own decisions about food; Don't let others "weigh in" (pun intended).

Food doubters, guilt-trippers and bullies can be everywhere! Many of my patients have family or friends who either subtly or openly try to get them to eat the foods they react to, saying "you ate this when you were a kid" or "you can just have one" or "this can't possibly hurt you." Here's my story. I had a friend who was a doubter. It was clear that she didn't believe I was "really" allergic to wheat. One night she, another friend, and I got together for dinner and made chicken mole. About an hour after dinner (remember, I have delayed-type allergies) welts started to appear on my ankles and climb up my legs. I thought we had made a gluten-free dinner, but remembered we had bought prepared mole sauce, and I hadn't thought to look at the label. I ran to the trash can, grabbed out the label, and there it was—wheat in the mole sauce! My friend stopped being a doubter that very day! In fact, when we went out to eat together after that, she was very supportive in making sure there was no gluten or dairy in what we ordered.

When You Eat

For a long time, "conventional wisdom" has advised us to eat small meals often. A Czech study has shown that eating six small meals is not the best for Type 2 diabetes patients, and it may not be the best for you. Eating two larger meals per day, breakfast and lunch, increased oral insulin sensitivity and lowered fasting glucose, Hemoglobin A1C, and liver fat for the diabetes patients in the study. In general, eating more of your calories at breakfast and lunch, not snacking between meals, and not eating after 7 PM is a good plan. It is important to have at least a 3-hour gap between dinner and bedtime. Remember the eating pattern that helped to reverse Alzheimer's? Check it out in Part II and do your best to follow it.

I'm not saying that you never get to go out for a late dinner or have a snack. That said, binge eating in the evening is something to stay away from. If you find that you are unable to stop evening bingeing, consider trying one of the behavioral change methods I have suggested in Part III. [270]

How You Eat—Mindful Eating

I was first introduced to mindfulness and mindful eating by the wonderful Buddhist teacher, Thich Nhat Hanh. I had been listening to his books on tape in my long commute to the medical center to keep myself from overreacting in the crazy traffic. It seemed like a wonderful idea. However, rush of everyday life sometimes appears to make mindful eating almost impossible. Even sitting down and putting food on a plate becomes a challenge. Too many people gulp down a breakfast bar, coffee, and juice on the run or in the car, eat a sandwich at their desk for lunch, and crash on the couch with today's version of a TV dinner. I understand this. I was a medical resident and worked 36-hour shifts in the hospital. We wolfed down our food and ran. I remember one time when I left my tray to answer my beeper. When I came back to finish it, they had taken it away. Later, in the National Health Service Corps. I clearly remember racing in the car from the office to the hospital, stethoscope in the seat beside me, munching a salted nut roll for my lunch. But the idea of mindful eating had gotten through to me from the Thich Nhat Hanh tapes I was listening to in the car. I went to hear him in person, and he talked about mindful eating.

After that, I set a boundary at work. I began to go out to lunch at the wonderful Mexican restaurant down the block from the clinic. It was full of kind people, beautiful pictures of Mexican scenes, fresh vegetable juices, and great food. Soon, everyone at the medical center knew that I took an hour off for lunch, and either went to the restaurant, or down to the Calumet Harbor beach near the medical center for a picnic. Of course, there were days when I was too busy to do this, but I managed to go at least three or four days a week. Pretty soon everyone accepted this. No one minded. Not a single person said I wasn't doing my job (because I was!). In fact, I was doing my job even better because of my mindful lunches. I believe that these lunches saved me from being overworked and exhausted during my time in the National Health Service Corps.

My favorite definition of mindful eating comes from the Lexicon of Food site:

> "Mindful eating is the practice of cultivating an open-minded awareness of how the food we choose to eat affects one's body, feelings, mind, and all that is around us. The practice enhances our understanding of what to eat, how to eat, how much to eat, and why we eat what we eat. When eating mindfully, we are fully present and savor every bite—engaging all our senses to truly appreciate the food. Beyond just taste,

we notice the appearance, sounds, smells, and textures of our food, as well as our mind's response to these observations. When we eat with this understanding and insight, gratitude and compassion will arise within us. Thus, mindful eating is essential to ensure food sustainability for future generations, as we are motivated to choose foods that are not only good for our health, but also good for our planet." [271]

It is easy to see, just from the definition, that it takes more time to eat mindfully, but there can be big rewards. For more about mindful eating, read Dr. Lynn Rossy's book, *The Mindfulness Eating Solution: proven strategies to end overeating, satisfy your hunger & savor your life.* [272]

Your Weekly Sample Meal Plan

The best thing about the Paleo-type food plan is how delicious the food can be, and how satisfied you'll feel from eating this way. Though I haven't designed this as a weight loss diet, chances are, if you're overweight, you'll probably shed several pounds (or more) without even trying, because you won't be eating fast or junk food or sugary desserts on this plan.

Here's what a week of meals might look like—just follow the dos and don'ts above and you can easily create tasty dishes like these. The recipes are included at the end of Part III.

Monday	
Breakfast	3-egg omelet with chopped peppers and onions
Snack	Nut and Seed Clusters
Lunch	Pork Chops and Sweet Potatoes
Dinner	Roast chicken salad or stir-fry with veggies and mushrooms
Snack	Roasted Kale Chips
Dessert	Peach Melba

Tuesday	
Breakfast	Super Strawberry Smoothie
Snack	Baked Apple
Lunch	Noodle Bowl
Dinner	Tuna, avocado, and broccoli lettuce wrap
Snack	Spiced Pecans
Dessert	Crustless Apple Crumb Pie

Wednesday	
Breakfast	2-egg omelet with chopped peppers and onions
Snack	Avocado Salsa with carrot and celery sticks
Lunch	Hearty Chicken Vegetable Soup
Dinner	Szechuan Chicken
Snack	Roasted Kale Chips
Dessert	Frothy Hot Chocolate

Thursday	
Breakfast	Poached eggs on spinach
Snack	Roasted Kale Chips
Lunch	Pan-Seared Fish Tacos
Dinner	Shepherd's Pie
Snack	5 celery sticks stuffed with almond or cashew butter
Dessert	Strawberry or Peach Coconut Milk Ice Cream

Friday	
Breakfast	Chocolate-Almond Smoothie
Snack	Snacking Nuts
Lunch	Salmon Avocado Wrap
Dinner	Pistachio-Crusted Chicken Breasts
Snack	Eggplant Dip
Dessert	Marinated Summer Berries

Saturday	
Breakfast	Scrambled eggs with mushrooms
Snack	Frothy Hot Chocolate
Lunch	Roasted Chicken and Spinach Salad
Dinner	Tuscan Tuna Steaks
Snack	Nut and Seed Clusters
Dessert	Crustless Apple Crumb Pie

Sunday	

Breakfast	Poached eggs on spinach
Snack	Baked Pumpkin Pudding
Lunch	Tangy Roast Beef Lettuce Wraps
Dinner	Spaghetti Squash Casserole
Snack	Eggplant Dip
Dessert	Peach Melba

How is the SAD Diet Working for Us?

We've challenged a lot of food myths here and we've presented you with a set of guidelines that go "against the grain" (pun intended) of years of diet recommendations. As Americans, we're used to the low-fat diet, the Food Pyramid, the milk mustache campaigns, the food industry and its insidious use of "mouth feel" (combining trans fats and other health-killing ingredients that feel comforting when we eat them) and its addictive strategies that make us crave unhealthy foods.

Here's my question: So, how's that working for us? Why are we dealing with national obesity and diabetes epidemics? Why are there so many kids with middle-aged shapes and middle-aged diseases? Bottom line: Eating what the food industry tells you to eat is like racing your car on a dead-end road full of land mines. At its end, even if you make it through, you'll slam into the wall of chronic diseases that await people who follow the SAD diet (the Standard American Diet).

PART III SECTION 2:
Exercising to Stay Alive and Well

The perfect exercise program is like a three-legged chair—you need all three legs to hold yourself up. The three legs are: aerobics, muscle strengthening, and stretching. What I have outlined here fulfills all three components with an aerobic walking plan, an easy strength-training program, a relaxing yoga routine that helps keep you flexible, and a DVD program that combines aerobics and strength training.

This is a plan for life that, unlike so many other exercise programs, is not specifically designed to help you lose weight or burn calories (those realities will, however, be your happy by-products of following the plan). You'll feel immediately better just a week or two after starting the program—so good, in fact, that I bet you'll want to stick with the combination you have selected from the plan for a long time. That would be a good thing, because study after study shows that being consistently active over time is the key to warding off chronic disease and living a longer, happier life.

The Sitting Disease

Here's one disease your doctor won't prescribe pills for—in fact, he or she may not even diagnose it. But diagnosing it is a must, because sitting is killing us—it's almost as deadly, over time, as some of our most serious chronic diseases, and disease risk. Recently, many people have begun to call the sedentary lifestyle the new secondhand smoke. In fact, despite studies that show that exercise is as effective as pills for heart disease, for example, only one-third of primary care doctors even mention it, much less prescribe it.

We Can Do Better

When it comes to fitness, sadly, most of us are in underwhelming shape. In fact, according to the latest (2011) statistics from the Centers for Disease Control and Prevention, 52 percent of American adults didn't meet nationally recognized recommendations for aerobic exercise or physical activity. And 76 percent of us didn't meet recommendations for doing muscle-strengthening activities. [273]

Here's the scary truth: A couch potato lifestyle increases your risks for chronic disease. A few years ago, researchers did some digging into the television watching habits of Australians. In 2008, they learned something horrifying: The average amount of TV people viewed in Australia reduced life expectancy by *nearly 2 years for men and 1.5 years for women.* They also discovered that people who watched a more-than-average amount of TV shortened their lives even more—6 hours a day for a lifetime of tube watching translates to a lifetime that's nearly 5 years shorter than the lives of people who don't watch TV. Another grim statistic: *Every single hour of TV you watch after the age of 25 reduces your life expectancy by nearly 22 minutes.* Veerman [274]

It might be time to post this sign on top of your TV: "Is watching another *Law & Order* rerun really worth shaving 22 minutes off my life?"

It's not the brain-numbing aspects of television watching that shorten your life—it's the inactivity. We know for a fact that inactivity contributes to disease. Here are just a few of inactivity's insidious effects.

- The less active you are, the higher your risk for developing high blood pressure.

- Inactive people are more likely to develop heart disease than active people are.

- Inactivity may increase your risk for certain cancers.

What happens once you become active? You start fending off diseases instead of developing them. As an example, in 2007, researchers combed through studies that linked exercise with decreased risk of chronic disease and discovered that people who exercised regularly reaped real benefits. They dropped their risks for breast cancer by 75 percent; for heart disease by 49 percent; for diabetes by 35 percent; and for colorectal cancer by 22 percent. [275]

Here is what an article in the America Academy of Family Physicians journal *American Family Physician* has to say about exercise for older adults:

> "Few older adults in the United States achieve the minimum recommended amount of physical activity. Lack of physical activity contributes to many chronic diseases that occur in older adults, including heart disease, stroke, diabetes mellitus, lung disease, Alzheimer's disease, hypertension, and cancer. Lack of physical activity, combined with poor dietary habits, has also contributed to increased obesity in older persons. Regular exercise and increased aerobic fitness are associated with a decrease in all-cause mortality and morbidity, and are proven to reduce disease and disability, and improve quality of life in older persons. In 2008, the U.S. Department of Health and Human Services released guidelines to provide information and guidance on the amount of physical activity recommended to maintain health and fitness. For substantial health benefits, the **guidelines recommend that most older adults participate in at least 150 minutes of moderate-intensity aerobic activity, 75 minutes of vigorous-intensity aerobic activity, or an equivalent combination of each per week. Older adults should also engage in strengthening activities that involve all major muscle groups at least two days a week.** Those at risk of falling should add exercises that help maintain or improve

balance. Generally, healthy adults without chronic health conditions do not need to consult with a physician before starting an exercise regimen." (emphasis mine) [276]

It doesn't take as much activity as you might think to turn your health around. In fact, *overdoing* exercise is as unhealthy as being inactive. In their 2014 *Heart* study that examined exercise and its benefits for people with heart disease, German researchers revealed a bit of a surprise. As you'd expect, people with heart disease who rarely or never exercise have a much worse prognosis than people who engage in strenuous activity (defined as "sweat-inducing activities such as cycling, speedy hiking, gardening, or a sport") two to four times a week. What surprised the researchers, however, was this: They learned that people who performed strenuous exercise five to six times a week had the same number of major cardiovascular events as did people who rarely or never exercised. [277]

The results of that study confirm what I've been telling my patients. I want them to be active three to four times a week, for a total weekly minimum of 90 minutes to a maximum of 160 minutes.

Alive and Well Exercise, Leg 1, Aerobics: Walking Is Your Best Medicine

It's unlikely that you remember that earthshaking day when you took your very first steps. But whoever was lucky enough to be watching you probably would, and it's likely that your audience burst into cheers of joy back then when you first put one little foot in front of the other and teetered across the floor. Too bad you don't hear cheers of joy every time you go walking as an adult—maybe if you did, it would be motivation enough for you to do some walking every day!

Walking is among the best things you can do to prevent the kinds of illnesses that prompt your doctor to prescribe pills. Let's look at the science—it offers many compelling reasons to make walking a part of your life. Here's what walking can do for you.

Lower cholesterol. In their 2014 study, Chinese researchers assigned 330 people with high cholesterol to one of three groups—one group did nothing; the other two groups walked for 30 minutes on at least 5 days a week. One group walked in the morning; the other group walked in the evening. The researchers measured all participants' cholesterol and checked them for signs of system-wide inflammation at the start and finish of the 12-week study. The result? Walking lowered participants' cholesterol in both groups, and it also lowered their inflammation markers. Interestingly, the evening walkers posted better results than did the morning walkers. NOTE: So, the bottom line here is that walking puts you on a path to lowering, or maybe even stopping, your cholesterol drugs. What's more, when you lower your markers for body-wide inflammation, you also lower your chances of developing inflammation-driven diseases such as heart disease, diabetes, and arthritis, to name just a few. [76]

Improve metabolic syndrome. In 2013, Italian researchers studied the effects of a walking program on 176 people with metabolic syndrome—a diagnosis that includes borderline high cholesterol, blood glucose, and waist circumference measurements. Participants were asked to walk at a brisk pace for an hour a day, 5 days a week, for 24 weeks. When participants were tested at the end of the study, their A1C levels (a marker for blood glucose over time) had dropped, their good cholesterol levels had risen, and their total cholesterol and triglyceride levels also had dropped. They also lost about 2 inches off their waist circumference. [278]

Help prevent heart attacks and strokes. In a study of 72,488 nurses, those who walked at least 3 hours a week had a 35 percent lower risk of heart attacks and cardiac death and a 34 percent lower risk of stroke. In another study of 44,452 male health professionals, walking at least 30 minutes a day lowered their risk for coronary artery disease by 18 percent. [279]

Help keep you alive. Now there's a great reason to walk, right? Researchers who looked at the health records of 10,269 male graduates of Harvard College reported that those who walked at least 9 miles a week had a 22 percent lower death rate than did non-walkers. [279]

I encourage my patients to walk 30 to 40 minutes a day, at least three to four times a week. It doesn't matter if you walk outdoors (which is wonderful if you have a safe, scenic route available and the weather isn't treacherous) or indoors on a track, a treadmill, or an elliptical machine. For that matter, if you prefer, you can also ride a bike or a stationary exercise bike.

If you haven't been active for months or years, please start slowly and go at a pace that feels comfortable for you. Personally, I like to walk on my lunch break, and if the weather isn't welcoming, then I just hop on my stationary bike.

I like to add interval work to my walks to increase the aerobic element. This means that for 20 to 30 seconds or so, you walk at your absolute fastest pace. Then you slow down and walk at a slow to normal pace for 2 minutes as your heart rate goes down. Then you speed it up again for another 20 to 30 seconds. Repeat for a total of three times. You can also do your intervals on a stationary bike, a treadmill, an elliptical machine—you get the idea. The goal is to work at your maximum capacity for a very short time, recover, and then repeat. Once you've done this for a while, you'll find that you're probably able to go a little faster and stretch it out a little longer during your "speed" intervals. And I like the fact that during your workout, you're only really pushing yourself for a minute or so, while you're cruising for the rest of the time. Doing intervals seems to make my exercise time fly by.

What's more, there's one incredibly important reason why interval work is an important feature of our exercise and that's the way it helps melt "belly fat." NOTE: You may think of belly fat simply as excess flab that makes your jeans hard to button, but it is far more insidious than that. [280]

Unlike fat deposits on your thighs, butt, or upper arms, the belly fat that lies deep within your abdomen acts in a very similar way to an organ—an evil organ. Unlike the "good" organs—your stomach, intestines, and liver, for example—that keep you alive, the fat that surrounds them produces toxic, inflammatory compounds. When your internal fat secretes these chemicals, it sparks cascades of intricate interactions that (among many other damaging effects) weaken your heart, damage your blood vessels, and dampen your immunity. Belly fat is part of metabolic syndrome, which includes high blood sugar, high blood fats, and belly fat!

If you have diabetes, having excess belly fat is an even bigger danger because it makes your body less sensitive to insulin. It increases insulin resistance, meaning that it takes more and more insulin to take glucose into the cells. Carrying too much fat around your middle puts you on the fast track to beta cell failure. These are the cells in the pancreas that produce insulin; when they burn out completely or partially, you end up taking drugs for the rest of your life. And you'll also be more likely to experience diabetic complications, including heart problems, cognitive difficulties, vision problems, and problems with your feet. NOTE: Bottom line: Losing belly fat is a key to success when it comes to diabetes prevention. And doing interval work is a great way to accomplish that. [281]

Walking Tips

Walking is a simple way to get yourself up and moving regularly. It gently eases you into an activity routine, so it's excellent for people who've been sedentary for a while. If walking for 15 minutes at first is too much for you, no worries. Start with a 5-minute or 10-minute walk and progress from there. These strategies can help you turn into a person who walks regularly—and likes it.

Find your path. Pick a place to walk that's both visually appealing and convenient. This might mean the fresh air and nature you'll find at a nearby park or walking path. Or you may prefer heading to your local gym and using a treadmill or elliptical machine. For some, it's the local mall—just be sure to avoid the food court! Some treadmills have screens with beautiful moving scenery, and you can also download a scenic "walking app" on your phone.

Walk tall. Walking with poor posture or technique can leave you vulnerable to unnecessary pain or injuries. Make sure you're standing straight with your shoulders down and chin parallel to the ground. Keep your lower back straight and bend your arms at a 90-degree angle. Make sure the heel of your foot meets the ground first before your foot rolls forward and push off from your toes. Tip: Walk lightly with a spring in your step and wear good shoes. Too heavy a heel "strike" or poorly padded, ill-fitting shoes can bring on heel pain and plantar fasciitis.

Find a friend. Sometimes a walking friend can provide the extra support you need to maintain your walking program. Consider asking your spouse, co-worker, or neighbor to join you on your walks. Studies have shown that those new to fitness plans are more likely to stick to their routines if they have a partner.

Make it fun. Whether you're starting off with a walk of 5 minutes or 15 minutes, it's important to challenge yourself during each walk. Try to increase your pace or your time, or both—but don't push yourself so hard that you risk an injury. Something as simple as listening to music can make your walks more enjoyable. You can change the song when you change your intensity level to aid in increasing or decreasing your pace. Or you might find it fun to try one of the fitness trackers that monitor your distance and heart rate and provide motivation.

As you progress, be sure to add 30-second intervals into the moderate-pace phase.

Additional Aerobic Exercise, with Added Strength Training

Al Sears, M.D. has a DVD with a set of exercises called the PACE program. I like it so well, I use it myself! It is a scientifically designed interval exercise program with three different levels for every exercise. Doing it takes less than 15 minutes. When you are looking at each exercise, you will see four different people doing it—the trainer, doing the moderate impact version, with three people behind him: one, doing the moderate impact version of each exercise that the trainer is doing; one, doing a high impact "extra" version of each exercise; and one doing a NO impact version of the exercise. Dr. Sears had me at no impact! I have a previous injury that makes no-impact the best for me, and good versions of that can be hard to find! This is an easy-to-follow program that can take care of both your aerobic and strength training needs in about an hour and fifteen minutes a week!

Alive and Well Exercise, Leg Two—Strength Training

Keeping muscles strong is a key to beating the frailty that can accompany aging. The truth is that as we get older, it's all about "use it or lose it." That's because unless you work your muscles, your overall strength will decline significantly after age 50—at the rate of something like 15 percent per decade. That's why I want you to include a gentle weight-training program, using light weights, and I want you to work at a very comfortable pace. Over time, you can increase the weight and repetitions as your muscles get stronger. All it takes is 15 minutes per session 2 days a week. Or, you can use stretch bands or other isometric exercises. It is good to do a session or two with a trainer to get an individualized strength training program. And look for a person who knows how to work with people who are beginners, or who have had injuries or illnesses. I generally advise my patients to stay away from the "no-pain-no-gain" trainers.

Don't worry about looking like a muscle-bound weight lifter. Doing strength exercises regularly will increase your muscle strength, improve your metabolism and bone density, decrease your insulin resistance, and help you sleep better. Be sure to include exercises for your core muscles, those that support your lower back and abdomen. Working these muscles helps improve your balance and stability, lessening your risk of falls.

Bottom line is, you can always start with the strength exercises described below.

Just starting out? Over 55? Begin with these.

These beginning strength training exercises were developed for the American Academy of Family Practitioners. Do 8 to 10 repetitions of each exercise for 2 sets. After 4 weeks, you should be able to move on to a more demanding strength training program that is individually tailored for you. For this, I would try a few sessions with a personal trainer, or if you have previous injuries or other health challenges, with a physical therapist.

For all strength-training exercises:

- Complete all movements in a slow, controlled fashion.
- Don't hold your breath.
- Stop if you feel pain.
- Stretch each muscle after your workout.

Wall Pushups. Place your hands flat against a wall. Slowly lower your body to the wall. Push your body away from the wall to return to the starting position.

Chair Squats. Begin by sitting in a chair. Lean slightly forward and stand up from the chair. Try not to favor one side or use your hands to help you.

Biceps Curls. Hold a weight (start with 1- to 2-pound weights) in each hand with your arms at your sides. Bending your arms at the elbows, lift the weights to your shoulders and then lower them to your sides.

Shoulder Shrugs. Hold a weight in each hand with your arms at your sides. Shrug your shoulders up toward your ears and then lower them back down. [282]

Alive and Well Exercise Leg 3-Stretching

Yoga

My number one preferred stretching exercise is yoga. It was important enough to me that I spent more than a year going back and forth to Canada to get certified to teach Tibetan Yoga. I think it is also useful to begin with a good teacher and go either to individual sessions or a class. There are now many good classes and teachers available. Make sure, if you take a class, that the teacher is qualified. The good ones won't mind you asking about their qualifications and will be happy to tell you who taught them, and how long they have studied. It can also be helpful to look up online reviews. Simple Hatha Yoga is a good place to start. I would not jump into anything strenuous like hot yoga, unless you are in your teens or 20s and already an athlete.

If you have a chronic illness, or more than one, or previous injuries, or even if you just sit in a desk chair all day, chair yoga may be the best for you. An excellent book and guide to chair yoga is nationally recognized celebrity yoga and Pilates teacher Kristin McGee's *Chair Yoga: Sit, Stretch, and Strengthen Your Way to a Happier, Healthier You* New York: Harper Collins, 2017.

Pilates

Pilates system of physical fitness invented by Joseph Pilates, has an interesting history. Pilates had asthma and other illnesses as a child. He studied and did exercise to make himself stronger, and got strong enough to dive, ski, and work as a gymnast and a boxer. When the German army asked him to teach his methods of exercise to its soldiers, he left Germany and moved to England. When World War I began, he was put in an internment camp, and began teaching the people who were interned with him. In 1926, he moved to New York, and opened a studio right next to the New York City ballet. The rest is history. Pilates began to teach dancers, taught George Balanchine, and the method became popular throughout the United States.

Pilates is a series of controlled exercises done both with equipment and on a mat. It includes both strengthening and stretching, toning up the body core, and the whole body. It is appropriate for a wide range of people—those who have previous injuries, are recovering from an injury, pregnant women, as well as people who want to get fit, and athletes, all the way up to professional and Olympic levels. If you are planning to start Pilates, be sure to look at reviews and talk to people who have taken it, so that you get a good teacher.

Simple Stretches

There are many good, simple stretching programs online. Mayo Clinic's stretching video is available at:

http://www.mayoclinic.org/healthy-lifestyle/fitness/multimedia/stretching/sls-20076840

Tai Chi and Qigong

These two forms of exercise are part of Traditional Chinese Medicine. Both are based on whole-body movement and are especially good for the muscles of balance. Your ability to balance is more and more important as you age and prevents you from falling. You will need to find a good teacher to learn both Tai Chi and Qigong. Look them up online, and check for reviews. One of my favorite forms of Qigong is Spring Forest Qigong. The founder, Master Chunyi Lin, holds periodic workshops. He also has a DVD series for home use. For more information, check https://www.springforestqigong.com/

PART III SECTION 3:

Alive and Well Strategies for Reducing Stress and Building Emotional Intelligence, Resilience, and Community Support

Reducing Stress

Of course, stress is a part of life. It can be that happy, tingly anticipation you feel when you're waiting for something wonderful to happen—the trip to the airport to embark on your vacation, for example. Who'd want to live without that? On the other hand, stress can also be getting stuck in traffic on your way to a job interview. Just picturing that scenario is enough to make your heart start pounding. But, when stressful moments become chronic, stress becomes dangerous. Unfortunately, for many of us, unrelenting chronic stress is a fact of life. Surveys commissioned by the American Psychological Association have concluded that about 25 percent of us live with high levels of stress—that's 8 on a 10-point scale! Another 50 percent of us report having moderate levels of daily stress. It's no wonder. In 21st-century America, we're subject to a 24/7 news cycle that focuses on one horrifying calamity after another. It's certainly easy to see how we all absorb way more than our share of worrisome messages. NOTE: And in these still shaky economic times, many of us have burdensome worries about our job security and finances. [283]

The Stress Response

You're familiar with the fight-or-flight response. That's what nature gave our Paleo ancestors as a survival mechanism. It begins in the brain. When you confront danger (these days, the terrible driver instead of the saber-toothed tiger), your eyes and ears send the information to your brain's processing center, called the amygdala. When the amygdala registers danger, it shoots an SOS to the hypothalamus, your brain's central command. Its job is to send signals, via the autonomic nervous system, to trigger responses that help you deal with whatever crisis confronts you.

The command center also signals the adrenal glands to start pumping adrenaline throughout your system. This ramps up your heartbeat so that blood—and energy—can flow into your muscles, heart, and other vital organs. Up go your pulse and blood pressure. Your blood vessels widen or narrow, depending on your need (if you've been wounded, for example, your vessels would constrict to stem blood loss). Your breathing speeds up so your lungs and brain get more oxygen. Now, you're in a state of heightened alertness. You can hear and see more sharply, and you're better equipped to manage whatever challenge you're facing.

And, by the way, you're probably unaware that this miracle of nature is occurring, because it happens nearly instantaneously. That's why you're able to swerve and slam on the brakes almost before you even perceive that there is a car coming at you head on. NOTE: This is an amazing system we're blessed with—miraculous, even. You can probably recall a time or two when your stress response saved your life or helped you avoid danger.

But when your stress response gets stuck in the "on" position and continually pumps adrenaline and other stress hormones throughout your body, it begins to feel like a burden instead of a miracle. [283]

Sara's Stress Story

Sara, a writer I have worked with off and on for more than 25 years, experienced what happens when stress spirals out of control, and stress, illness and pain get tied into a knot that stops life as you know it. Sara shared her story with me. Within months of each other, death claimed two beloved sisters-in-law. Then, budget cuts vaporized her husband's teaching position. A magazine job she loved came to a sudden end, and some other writing projects dried up.

Out of the blue, Sara's left knee started to hurt, but she ignored the pain—so much else was going on that needed her attention. Then she developed a nasty case of shingles. Now, in addition to her knee pain, she felt as if sharp, hot needles were tattooing her right flank.

Nothing good ever comes from ignoring your body when it's desperately trying to tell you something important. Pain is one way your body gets your attention.

Sara finally learned she had a torn meniscus (the cushion that surrounds the knee), complicated by a bone shard. The answer was arthroscopic surgery to mend the meniscus and remove the fragment. She had the procedure, but a few days later, the pain was fiercer than ever. It was eye-popping! Then she acquired *another* case of shingles—this bout even more painful than the first.

Her doctors were sympathetic and prescribed opioids to help her cope with the pain. What an imperfect solution that was! All she got was mushiness where her brain used to be, and her attention-getting sharp pains didn't disappear—they simply became dull, throbbing aches.

Finally, she'd had it. She asked me what else she could do. I advised that she try water exercise and acupuncture. Sara signed up for a 4-day-a-week aqua aerobics and aqua Zumba program at the Y. She also found a great acupuncturist and began weekly treatments. Additionally, I recommended that she take curcumin and fish oil supplements to deal with the inflammation. Then, a near-miracle happened. The pain started easing after just one week. I'm convinced the pool work and the acupuncture blunted her stress response. Stress has been shown to increase pain levels, and when the stress goes down, the pain generally goes down too. The acupuncture, a proven pain-reliever, and extensively studied for knee pain relief, also took effect. The supplements eased the inflammation. What's more, those gentle water exercises were also great for strengthening her knee muscles, she was able to stop taking narcotic pain pills.

Of course, Sara's stress didn't completely disappear—but now that she was in less pain, she felt more hopeful about dealing with the causes of her stress.

Stress—Bad for the Mind, Bad for the Body

Scientists have been scrutinizing the connections between stress and disease for at least 80 years. Back in 1936, Hans Selye, the pioneering stress researcher, defined stress as a "general adaptation syndrome" and believed that people experience physical reactions to various "noxious environmental agents." By the mid-1970s, the notion that stress could trigger chronic illness was gaining serious traction. That's when scientists began to identify the key stressors that they believed could heighten a person's susceptibility to disease. (Among them, two major stressors are clearly illustrated in Sara's story—bereavement and job loss.) Rabkin [284]

Today, it is pretty much common knowledge that stress plays a role in disease. Two recent studies shed light on two different ways stress influences disease and health. These studies are fascinating.

The Direct Link Between Stress and Inflammation

There's a direct link between stress and inflammation, say researchers at Carnegie Mellon University in Pittsburgh. In their 2012 study, they learned that when you're under chronic psychological stress, your body seems to lose its ability to control the inflammatory response. "Inflammation is partly regulated by the hormone cortisol," says Sheldon Cohen, PhD, the Robert E. Doherty Professor of Psychology at CMU's Dietrich College of Humanities and Social Sciences. Dr. Cohen goes on to explain that when you're under chronic stress, cortisol pumps out continually. Cells consistently subjected to this "cortisol waterfall" begin to lose their sensitivity to the hormone. Among the cells that become insensitive to cortisol are the immune cells, which are supposed to keep disease-causing elements away. Since insensitive immune cells are ineffective immune cells, that's how runaway inflammation can promote the development and progression of many diseases. Cohen [285]

Dr. Cohen is no stranger to studying the effects of stress on the human body. Back in 1991, in his landmark *New England Journal of Medicine* study, he gave 394 healthy adults questionnaires to measure their stress levels. His team then administered nose drops to them that contained various common cold viruses. He quarantined them all for 5 days and monitored them for signs of infection. And guess what? The participants developed colds at rates that matched their stress levels. Nearly half of the most stressed-out people developed colds, while only 27 percent of people experiencing less stress got sick. [286]

Epigenetics and Stress

Over the years, studies have shown that chronic psychological stress alters DNA, which could explain why stress makes some people more susceptible to chronic disease. But in a 2012 study, researchers discovered that even *fleeting* stress (as you might experience during a job interview, for example) could change DNA in a way that might promote chronic disease. "Epigenetic changes may well be an important link between stress and chronic diseases," says lead author, Gunther Meinlschmidt, professor and head of the research department of psychobiology, psychosomatics, and psychotherapy at the LWL University Hospital of Ruhr University in Bochum, Germany. He and his team of European researchers noted that complex epigenetic stress patterns would be the target of future study. [191]

Molecules of Emotion, the Biology of Belief and the Biology of Intention

And speaking of the science of epigenetics in relationship to stress and illness, this is where we need a change, and are suffering from the old "clockwork" aspects of our medical system. This paragraph could as easily be titled "Why are we ignoring cellular biology and epigenetics in clinical medicine?" But the title I have used is catchier, and besides, it is a combination of the titles of two dazzlingly brilliant books by two different cellular biologists, Candace Pert, and Bruce Lipton. Reading them is enough to make you understand how desperately we need to bring the discoveries of cellular biology into clinical medicine. And reading Robert O. Becker, M.D. will help you understand that the body has its own electrical network. Reading the work of Dawson Church, Ph.D. will introduce you to the science of epigenetics and make you want to see a practitioner who understands it, has a practice based on it, and can help you resolve your intergenerational PTSD from the generations of alcoholism in your family.

For decades, scientific research has examined, at a cellular level, the chain of events that happens when the mind produces chemicals that bring about illness in the body. All the disease burden of unresolved core emotional issues, adverse childhood experience, childhood emotional neglect and intergenerational stress (for example, children of holocaust survivors) has most often been poorly addressed in the medical industry. The industry is still grudgingly accepting the idea that stress is related to illness, while scientists are examining the epigenetics of stress, the molecules of emotion, and the biology of belief. They are still saying, "Do you have to believe in acupuncture for it to work?" when scientists have already defined the acupuncture network as a microvolt, nanoamp DC current system.

I am looking forward to a time when all these internal environmental factors are considered in addressing health and illness. More examination of the findings of cellular biologists and other advanced scientists and their application to human health is well beyond the scope of this book. If you are interested in more information, I recommend four books, by the people I mentioned above: Dr. Robert O. Becker's *The Body Electric*, Candace Pert's *The Molecules of Emotion*, Dr. Bruce Lipton's The Biology of Belief, and Dr. Dawson Church's *The Genie in Your Genes*. [287-290]

Alive and Well Stress-Relieving Strategies

Dealing with the two kinds of stress we encounter—chronic and acute—means you will need to set aside time to practice one or more of the methods known to keep stress at bay. Just as you're bringing a new way of eating into your life, and learning how to become more active, I believe it is important to make conscious stress relief part of your daily plan. In this section of Part III, we'll outline some of the most tested and trusted stress-relieving methods available. When you add these to your Alive and Well eating and exercise programs, you'll be helping to chase away chronic disease. Community support, friendship, time in nature, music, are also wonderful stress relievers, along with the methods I will describe here.

Mindfulness Meditation

Mindfulness meditation is one of the oldest ways of gaining awareness and reducing stress. This classic method of meditation centers on the breath. You sit on a chair or a cushion with your back straight, hands in your lap or on your legs, and simply focus your attention on your breath, breathing in, and breathing out naturally. You never force your breath, just observe your own natural breathing. If your mind wanders away from focusing on your breath, you simply make a mental note "thinking" and gently bring your mind back to focusing on your breath.

There many books that teach meditation. I have three favorites—two books and an audiobook. They are Pema Chodron's book, *How to Meditate,* Jack Kornfield's book, *Meditation for Beginners,* and Jon Kabat-Zinn's audiobook, *Guided Mindfulness Meditation: A Complete Guided Mindfulness Meditation Program from Jon Kabat-Zinn.* [291-293]

One precautionary note about meditation is that it is best to start with very short periods of meditation. The Dalai Lama recommends that at the beginning, you meditate for only three minutes at a time.

Another is that meditation may not be for you. For some people, sitting still and trying to meditate can cause more restlessness or anxiety and not relaxation. If that is true for you, try an activity that is relaxing for you, like walking in nature, or listening to music.

Guided Imagery

Guided Imagery is a method that not only reduces stress, it enhances healing & wellness, reduces side effects of medications, and the pain of medical procedures. It can also help to achieve goals, aid peak performance and motivate behavior change. Guided imagery can carry you off to the sights and sounds of your favorite beach or mountain when the reality of your situation couldn't be more different—when you are in the middle of work stress, family stress, pain, anxiety, or even in the middle of surgery!

Guided imagery has been fortunate to have a guiding star here in the United States, Belleruth Naparstek. She has been tireless in producing guided imagery CDs and downloads for everything from anxiety to surgical recovery, making sure scientific studies got done to prove the efficacy of guided imagery, and distributing guided imagery CDs free to veterans and other people who need them.

Guided imagery can be effective for daily stress and anxiety, test anxiety or other performance anxiety, relationship stress, and stress around major life events—a birth or death in the family, a new marriage, or a new job. It can also help you cope better with one of the most stressful places you can go—the hospital! Here is a definition of guided imagery and information about its use in medical settings from Belleruth Naparstek herself. She defines guided imagery as:

> "An immersive, hypnotic, self-administered audio intervention made up of a guided narrative scored to music, designed to drive attention inward, to experience a desired outcome of healing, wellness or behavioral change... It promotes relaxation, healing and wellness, while requiring very little training or prep from the listener." [294]

Who is guided imagery good for in the hospital? Ms. Naparstek's list:

1. Patients facing anxiety-inducing medical procedures, such as surgery, dialysis, chemo, radiation, MRIs, cardiac caths, biopsies, proctological or gynecological procedures, ventilator weaning, etc.

2. Those with emotional challenges, i.e., anxiety, depression, PTS, panic attacks, phobias, acute or chronic stress, anger & impulse management, compulsive or addictive behaviors—supports other treatments and does not compete.

3. People seeking tools to support a healthier lifestyle, wanting help with losing weight, sleeping better, smoking cessation, stress reduction, chemical dependency.

4. Patients in pain. Increases comfort. Reduces need for and use of opioids. Applies to post-surgical pain, headache, functional pain conditions, injuries, etc.

5. Soothing and calming for most Alzheimer's, dementia patients & family caregivers.

6. Cardiac, hypertensive, diabetes patients found to benefit thru impact of stress relief on biochemistry.

7. Helps with breathing in asthma, COPD and hospice patients. Assists and enhances rehab and physical therapy results for stroke, TBI recovery, Parkinson's.

8. Reduces pain, aids in range of motion in osteoarthritis patients.

9. Increases feelings of efficacy, well-being, empowerment in those seeking to be proactive in their own medical care. [294]

Are there contraindications for using guided imagery? Of course:

1. Should not be imposed on anyone who is made more anxious or distressed by having to sit still, "relax" and listen to someone else's guidance.

2. A minority of people with posttraumatic stress can become triggered or flooded with anxiety when introduced to guided imagery. For them, simple breath work, progressive relaxation, yoga or biofeedback can be preferred.

3. Not recommended for those with paranoid schizophrenia, active bipolar illness or other serious mental disorders. [294]

For more information, visit www.HealthJourneys.com.

EFT—Emotional Freedom Technique

EFT is based on doing acupressure by tapping on specific points while talking about aspects of situations that have caused emotional responses and stress. EFT has been available for anyone to use for a long time. A manual that describes in detail how to do it is downloadable for free, at www.eft-universe.com. EFT is considered in general to be something that you can learn to do pretty easily and do safely for yourself. For the last 15 years, more and more good studies have been accumulating showing its safety and effectiveness, including studies of near-miraculous results with veterans who have suffered from PTSD, sometimes for decades. That said, if you have known PTSD, or a background now called ACE (adverse childhood experience) or CEN (childhood emotional neglect, or any other psychological or psychiatric diagnosis, I recommend that you do EFT with a qualified practitioner. For a list of these (people who have gone through a rigorous certification program that includes 50 supervised by a certified mentor, thousands of pages of reading followed by a very comprehensive final exam, and an ethics exam) see either Association for Comprehensive Energy Psychology site www.energypsych.org, or the EFT Universe site, www.eft-universe.com.

EFT evolved from a practice called Thought Field Therapy, which was developed in the early 1980s by a clinical psychologist named Roger Callahan. I was fortunate to hear him talk about the method and see a film showing him free a woman from her phobia of water in one session. Thought Field Therapy was simplified a decade later by Dr. Callahan's student, Gary Craig, a Stanford graduate engineer.

To do EFT, you tap with fingertip pressure on a set pattern of acupressure points. As you tap, you murmur a phrase—an intention—that focuses you and helps you counter your current stress in a positive way. Though it sounds fairly incredible, this exercise lowers your body's stress response and even makes changes in old neurologic patterns, notably in severe post-traumatic stress disorder (PTSD). There are now many good studies, including a number of studies done with veterans suffering from PTSD, documenting the effectiveness of EFT. [295, 296]

According to Mark Hyman, M.D., who recently opened the Center for Functional Medicine at the Cleveland Clinic, EFT's "tapping interrupts the body's stress response quickly and effectively." In his foreword to *The Tapping Solution,* a book by renowned EFT expert Nick Ortner, Dr. Hyman writes that tapping is a "fast-acting, noninvasive way to proactively manage the stress that so often leaves our bodies vulnerable to disease." [296]

The standards of EFT research are rigorous and adhere to American Psychological Association guidelines. There are more than 100 qualified studies listed on the www.eft-universe.com. Here is a quote from the research section of the site regarding research standards:

> "There are over 5,000 stories on this web site written by people who have recovered from a wide variety of physical and psychological challenges using EFT. This anecdotal evidence is consistent with rigorous scientific research showing that EFT is an 'evidence-based' method. Studies show that EFT is effective as a self-help tool, while it is also used in many healthcare settings by medical and mental health professionals."

This EFT research bibliography lists more than 100 papers published in peer-reviewed professional journals. To provide a context for this research, which has been shaped by the criteria for evidence-based treatments defined by the American Psychological Association's Division 12 Task Force on Empirically Validated Treatments, we begin with on overview of the criteria.

The abstracts are organized into a number of categories. These include Outcome Studies, Clinical Reports, Mechanisms Papers, Review Articles and Meta-Analyses, and Skeptical and Opposing Viewpoints. Outcome studies are further divided by condition, such as anxiety, depression, and post-traumatic stress disorder (PTSD). From the given links, you can jump to any of these sections immediately.

APA Standards for Empirically Validated Treatments

EFT Universe supports the evidence-based standards defined by the American Psychological Association (APA) Division 12 (Clinical Psychology) Task Force ("APA standards" for short). These define an "empirically validated treatment" as one for which there are two different controlled trials conducted by independent research teams.

For a treatment to be designated as "efficacious," the studies must demonstrate that the treatment is better than a wait list, placebo, or established efficacious treatment.

To be designated as "probably efficacious," a treatment must have been shown to be better than a wait list in two studies that meet these criteria or are conducted by the same research team rather than two independent teams.

The APA standards advocate that studies contain sufficient subjects to achieve a level of statistical significance of $p < .05$ or greater, which means that there is only one possibility in 20 that the results are due to chance. The status of EFT as an evidence-based practice is summarized in this statement published in the APA journal *Review of General Psychology:*

> "A literature search identified 51 peer-reviewed papers that report or investigate clinical outcomes following the tapping of acupuncture points to address psychological issues. The 18 randomized controlled trials in this sample were critically evaluated for design quality, leading to the conclusion that they consistently demonstrated strong effect sizes and other positive statistical results that far exceed chance after relatively

few treatment sessions. Criteria for evidence-based treatments proposed by Division 12 of the American Psychological Association were also applied and found to be met for a number of conditions, including PTSD."

If you think you would like to do EFT, I recommend that you download the free EFT mini-manual from www.eftuniverse.com, and do at least a few coaching sessions with a certified EFT practitioner.

Don's Story

I've used EFT successfully to help many people overcome stress-linked problems, but one patient I learned about in my EFT studies is particularly unforgettable. This story comes from EFT coach, Ingrid Dinter.

"Don" is a 61-year-old Vietnam War veteran who has Parkinson's disease.

He worked with therapist Dinter for a total of six EFT session hours. Since returning from Vietnam, Don hadn't experienced a single night of uninterrupted sleep—he never slept more than a couple of hours at a stretch, and never more than 4 or 5 hours a night. Even worse, horrific nightmares woke him at least twice a night.

His first session took only minutes—it was all Don could handle that day. Before starting with EFT, he told Dinter his thoughts were like bumper cars, bouncing all over, but the tapping helped him relax and release the tension in his mind. It also stopped the Parkinson's tremors and shaking. The therapist helped him tap on finding peace with the war and peace with Vietnam. After this brief first session, his sleep greatly improved: He now slept 6 to 7 hours, woke up twice briefly, and felt rested instead of fatigued.

In each of the subsequent sessions, Dinter worked through several traumatic war-related memories with Don. She released his sadness and guilt using the gentle EFT techniques and tapped on deserving forgiveness.

By the end of his therapy, Don was going to bed between 9:45 and 10:15, was sleeping 7 to 8 hours, and had no more nightmares. Reviewing his progress, Don said, "I still think about Vietnam, but it doesn't seem to bother me." He continues to tap on his Parkinson's symptoms to keep the shaking under control. His wife has noticed that he seems happier and more relaxed, Dinter reported. He feels comfortable socializing now and is a true believer in EFT. [297]

Laughter

One of the best summaries on the benefits of laughter comes from www.helpguide.org. They outline a list of the physical, mental, and social benefits of laughter.

Physical Benefits: Boosts immunity, lowers stress hormones, decreases pain, relaxes your muscles, prevents heart disease

Mental Benefits: Adds joy and zest to life, eases anxiety and tension, relieves stress, improves mood, strengthens resilience

Social Benefits: Strengthens relationships, attracts others to us, enhances teamwork, helps defuse conflict, promotes group bonding

And they have a list of ways to create opportunities to laugh. Here they are:

- Watch a funny movie, TV show, or YouTube video
- Invite friends or co-workers to go to a comedy club
- Read the funny pages
- Seek out funny people
- Share a good joke or a funny story

- Check out your bookstore's humor section
- Host game night with friends
- Play with a pet
- Go to a "laughter yoga" class
- Goof around with children
- Do something silly
- Make time for fun activities (e.g., bowling, miniature golfing, karaoke)

https://www.helpguide.org/articles/mental-health/laughter-is-the-best-medicine.htm

It's clear that we all need to laugh more. One of my favorite people who has promoted humor to reduce stress for many years, is Loretta LaRoche. You might want to try her DVD, "The Joy of Stress."

HeartMath—Refocusing emotion to reduce stress

A while back, I learned about a wonderful system called HeartMath, whose mission is to help people reduce stress and increase their emotional balance. The rationale behind the program's techniques is that you can "learn how to neutralize and counter the effects of stress by actively adding a positive feeling such as appreciation, care, and compassion to the process," say the HeartMath experts. They believe that you can experience positive emotions by generating feelings of appreciation, care, or compassion—and that doing so can help you manage your stress.

I use and recommend one of their techniques, called Freeze-Frame.

There are five steps to Freeze-Frame.

1. **Recognize** that you're feeling stress and take a time out so you can put your feelings and thoughts on hold.

2. **Shift** your focus to the area of your heart. Now, breathe in as if your breath is flowing in through the center of your chest and out through your stomach area. Practice breathing this way to ease into the technique. Breathe in for 4 to 5 seconds and then breathe out for 4 to 5 seconds. Breathe quietly and naturally. Continue this rhythmic breathing as you do the rest of the steps.

3. **Activate** make a sincere effort to activate a positive feeling. This can be a genuine feeling of appreciation or caring for someone, some place (your favorite beach or hiking trail, for example), or something wonderful in your life. It's important to feel the feeling this thought engenders.

4. **Ask** yourself: What would be a better way to handle this situation, or what action would reduce your stress? Try to select a less stressful perspective, even if you can't feel it yet.

5. **Notice** any change in the way you think and feel about the situation. Try to remember any new thoughts and feelings for as long as you can.

The HeartMath organization has many stress-reducing resources. For more, check out www.heartmath.org. [298]

How Mindfulness and Compassion Calm You Down

In a similar vein to the HeartMath approach is the much more ancient technique called self-compassion. Its kindred concept is practicing compassion for everyone—including compassion toward people who actively get your goat or do you wrong, deliberately or not. Although compassion has its roots in Buddhist tradition, its practice is nondenominational; I view it as mindfulness. I've found one practice, called *metta bhavana,* to be especially helpful for relieving stressful feelings, especially after a long day of caring for patients. You might also find it helpful after a full day at work.

Proving the point that compassion can lead to calmer feelings, a 2014 study investigated the health benefits of self-compassion. The study looked at 3,252 records that linked compassion with a set of health-promoting behaviors. The researchers concluded that self-compassion could help promote healthy behaviors. The study was published in the journal *Health Psychology* by Jameson K. Hirsch, PhD, associate professor in the department of psychology at East Tennessee State University in Johnson City, Tennessee. [299]

What does this mean for you? We asked Dr. Hirsch to explain. First, he says, being mindful is key to reaping the health benefits of compassion. "Understanding that others are in similar or even worse situations than you are, and then being mindful of your pain, discomfort, stress, or fears, rather than ignoring them or worrying about them, is an important outcome of practicing mindfulness," he says.

In his studies, Dr. Hirsch and his team learned that self-compassion was linked to healthy behaviors, such as exercising and eating—and they also learned that the more people practice self-compassion, the more they also practiced these beneficial behaviors. What's more, the researchers learned that self-compassion improves your mood—and the better your mood, the more likely you'll be "kind" to yourself by exercising more or eating healthier foods, says Dr. Hirsch. "It may also be the case that self-compassion allows you to effectively cope with the setbacks that often accompany working toward your health goals, so that if you mess up on your diet, or miss a workout, it will be easier for you to get back on track," says Dr. Hirsch. That's because practicing self-compassion means you're not so hard on yourself, and so it's easier to forgive yourself when you slip, and to get back to your program the next day.

The word *metta* means nonromantic love, which translates to friendliness or kindness. That's why the Buddhists refer to it as loving-kindness. You feel loving-kindness in your heart, says the Buddhist tradition. The word *bhavana* refers to the practice part of this exercise: It means cultivation. I learned to practice *metta bhavana* in six stages.

Here's how to get started. The entire exercise should take you about five minutes.

1. Focus on yourself. Start by becoming aware of yourself, and focus on feelings of peace, calm, and tranquility.

2. Feel confidence and love. Let yourself feel strength and confidence, and then develop that into a feeling of love within your heart. You can use an image, like golden light flooding your body, or a phrase such as "may I be well and happy," which you can repeat to yourself. These are ways of stimulating the feeling of metta for yourself.

3. Think of a good friend. Bring them to mind as vividly as you can and think of their good qualities. Feel your connection with your friend, and your liking for him or her, and encourage these to grow by repeating "may she be well; may she be happy" quietly to yourself.

4. Think of someone neutral. This may be someone you do not know well but see around. You reflect on their humanity and include them in your feelings of metta.

5. Think of someone you actually dislike. Here's the challenging part: Don't get caught up in your feelings of hatred; instead, think of them positively and send your metta to them as well.

6. Finally, think of all four people together. Think of yourself, your friend, your neutral person, and your enemy. Then extend your feelings further, to everyone around you—to everyone in your neighborhood, in your town, your country, and so on throughout the world. Have a sense of waves of loving-kindness spreading out from you.

For almost everyone, this practice can be helpful in reducing stress. [300]

Breathing Stress Away

Rhythmic breathing, or "breath work," is a stress-relieving practice used in many complementary healing practices, including Traditional Chinese Medicine and Ayurveda, the traditional medicine of India. According to Andrew Weil, M.D., the father of integrative medicine, "Practicing regular, mindful breathing can be calming and energizing, and can even help with stress-related health problems ranging from panic attacks to digestive disorders." Among the stress-relieving breathing techniques Dr. Weil recommends frequently is one called the 4-7-8 (or Relaxing Breath) Exercise.

You can practice this exercise anywhere, and it takes just a few minutes to learn. Commit it to memory and you'll have a tool to calm you down even in the heat of the most stressful times.

You can do 4-7-8 in any position, but while you're learning, Dr. Weil recommends that you sit down, keeping your back nice and straight. Place the tip of your tongue against the ridge of tissue behind your upper front teeth and keep it there throughout the exercise. You will exhale through your mouth around your tongue. If it's easier for you, purse your lips slightly.

1. Exhale completely through your mouth, making a whooshing sound.

2. Close your mouth and inhale quietly through your nose to a mental count of four.

3. Hold your breath while silently counting to seven.

4. Exhale completely through your mouth, making a whooshing sound to a silent count of eight.

5. This is one breath. Now, inhale again and repeat the cycle three more times for a total of four breaths. [301]

There Is an App for That

There are many meditation apps. Two of my favorites are Calm, and Breethe. Either one will give you short periods of guided meditation. I especially like Breethe—it follows the principles of simple breath meditation and encourages you to meditate every day. You can also download guided meditations. My favorites are from www.healthjourneys.com. Just be sure you are out of your car, or that it is parked when you are using the apps or the downloads!

Discover What Works for You

Some of these strategies are likely to resonate better with you than others, so pick the ones that feel most natural. Set aside some time each day to practice—5 to 20 minutes once or twice a day is ideal. Put your stress relief time in your calendar, and don't let anything get in the way of your practice. In just a few weeks, if not sooner, you'll notice that you feel calmer and more centered, and that the little things that once made you tense aren't quite so alarming anymore. That's the whole point! Just remember that some people might have difficulty with some—even all—of these methods. Sometimes, if you have unresolved trauma, or are just a very high-energy person, sitting and trying to relax may end up being too much "trying" and not relaxing at all. In fact, if you're this kind of person, sitting quietly may even make you feel more anxious. If that's true for you, pick some other activity that feels relaxing. For you, it may be running, yoga, listening to music, or even reading a book.

Developing Emotional Intelligence, Resilience and Community Support

Emotional Intelligence

It's becoming clear today, in our increasingly divided society, that we all could use more emotional intelligence! A good place start is Daniel Goleman's book, *Emotional Intelligence: Why It Can Matter More Than IQ*. Since the book was written, more than 20 years ago, we have adopted the term emotional intelligence into our language, and many of us have accepted it with our minds, but most of us could still use more help in living our lives with greater emotional intelligence. [302]

A highly skillful explanation of emotional intelligence, with illustrations and examples, comes from a brilliant review of studies of emotions and emotional regulation in breast cancer survivors. They point to emotional distress as the "sixth vital sign" in cancer care, and document that emotional distress can cause poor treatment compliance, and higher risk of disease progression and death. In my opinion, their findings are equally applicable to chronic illness and life stressors.

One of the most informative and useful items in the study is a table they constructed about emotional regulation. They noted that not all emotional regulation is helpful, and divided it into two types: engagement strategies, and disengagement strategies. They stated that engagement strategies can improve health outcomes, but disengagement strategies can make them worse.

The engagement strategies, descriptions and examples are these:

1. Acceptance: Assent to the reality of the situation without attempting to change it. Examples: "I've been accepting the reality of it; I've been learning to live with it

2. Active coping: Taking active steps to remove/circumvent the emotional stimulus or minimize its effects. Examples: "I've been trying to do something about it; I've been taking action to improve the situation."

3. Cognitive reappraisal: Construing an emotional stimulus in different terms, also known as reframing. Examples: "I've

been trying to see it in a different light; I've been looking for the good in the situation."

4. Problem solving: Discovering, analyzing and finding a solution that best resolves the issue (does NOT include taking active steps toward a solution). Examples: "I've been thinking about a strategy for action. I've been thinking about what steps to take."

5. Seeking instrumental support: Seeking advice, assistance, or information from others. Example: "I've been seeking help and advice from others."

The disengagement strategies, descriptions and examples are these:

1. Behavioral Avoidance: Reducing one's effort to deal with the emotional stimulus or attain related goals. Examples: "I've been giving up trying to deal with it. I've been giving up the attempt to cope."

2. Cognitive avoidance: Using distraction to prevent oneself from thinking about the emotional stimulus and/or related goals. Examples: "I've been trying to take my mind off things. I've been doing something to think about it less."

3. Denial: The refusal to accept reality or fact, acting as if an emotional stimulus did not exist. Examples: "I've been thinking this can't be real. I refuse to believe that this has happened."

4. Substance use: Using drugs or alcohol to disengage from or numb an emotional stimulus. Example: "I've been using alcohol or other drugs to make me feel better."

5. Suppression: Actively trying to put thoughts or feelings about the emotional stimulus out of one's mind (does NOT include replacing those thoughts with a distraction). Examples: "I tried to put it out of my mind. I tried to avoid thoughts about it." [303]

This list can be used to check whether you are handling a stressful life event or illness with engagement strategies—that is, emotional intelligence, or disengagement strategies. If you find that you are stuck in disengagement strategies, it is well worth your while to get help. Cognitive behavioral therapy, (see the Depression and Anxiety section of Part II) or EFT (see the description above in Part III). The wonderful thing about emotional intelligence is that it is a teachable, learnable skill that can help you make big improvements in the way you manage stressful situations.

Building Resilience

Building resilience works the same way as building emotional intelligence. It is a skill that can be taught and learned. Martin Seligman, the founding father of positive psychology, has probably studied and written more about the development of positive qualities like resilience than anyone else, ever. He began by studying learned helplessness, but soon realized that if people could learn helplessness, they could probably learn optimism too. He began to study people who "bounced back" from some adverse circumstances and had successful lives, so that he could identify positive qualities in people and teach them. He has written 25 books and many scholarly articles. My favorite book of his is *Flourish*, for its dynamic advocacy of individual, community, and global well-being as a standard of managing human affairs that we all need to adopt. His website, www.authentichappiness.org is full of resources and information and is a great contribution to the field of positive psychology. For a practical, beginning handbook, I like Christian Moore's *The Resilience Breakthrough: 27 Tools for Turning Adversity into Action.* [304-305]

You can learn a lot about the qualities of resilience and well-being just from two of Seligman's concepts: The 3 Ps and PERMA.

Seligman's "3 Ps" are Personalization, Pervasiveness, and Permanence, and are a good litmus test for the kinds of responses you may be making after a stressor shows up in your life. Let's say there's a death in the family. At a time like that, it is all too easy to get into the three Ps. The first one, personalization, is the idea that somehow you are at fault for the situation. The second one, pervasiveness, is the thought that this affects every level of your life. The third, permanence, is the belief this after-the-loss feeling will go on forever and will never go away. The first step in taking down the fortress walls of the 3 Ps to notice that they are there. You recognize that this is how you are thinking about the situation and then begin to see whether there are any chinks developing in the fortress walls.

For example, you might be bogged down in personalization, and be blaming yourself for not knowing about an illness your loved one had. Then one day you think about it again and you realize that his doctors hadn't even diagnosed it. How could you? This could be the first chink in the wall.

If you are stuck in pervasiveness, the belief that no parts of your life can ever be happy again because of the stressful event, maybe one day you go to work and find that you are so absorbed in what you are doing that you have forgotten the stress for a moment. That could be a second chink.

And permanence? Again, as you are living along, you may step into a different part of your life that reveals to you that your emotional state has changed, and you are no longer feeling the way you did right after the event. You have a direct experience that your emotional state is not permanent. This realization may be even bigger than a chink in the wall and look more like the beginning of the light at the end of the tunnel.

The other one of Seligman's concepts I will discuss here is a set of qualities that, together, according to Seligman, constitute well-being, and can be applied to individuals, families, schools, companies, communities, and the whole world. It is an outline of the qualities of well-being, represented by the letters PERMA, which stand for: Positive emotion, Engagement, Relationships (positive), Meaning, Achievement.

For any individual, Seligman's point is to "keep your eyes on the prize"—and work toward building a life or an organization that makes the development of these qualities of well-being a priority. Seligman is working to advise businesses, cities (Adelaide, in Australia) and even countries (the U.K.) about the skills needed to make well-being a value and a practice for management and public policy.

The bottom line is, when it comes to building resilience, if you feel you need more than self-help, get someone to help you! I believe that one of the best ways to start learning is with another human being. It could be a friend. Or if you need more than a friend, then it could be a professional who knows how teach you to turn the 3P fortresses into sand castles and sweep them away, and to recognize your strengths and help you to build on them. A good cognitive behavioral therapist or EFT practitioner can most likely help you. (See the CBT information in the Depression and Anxiety section of Part II, and the EFT information here in Part III.)

Building Family and Community Support

Finding support with family, friends and community is the last preventive health strategy I will discuss here. There is a city in Roseto, Pennsylvania, that in the early 1960s used to be one of the healthiest places to live, had fewer deaths from heart attacks and no crime. Why? Because the Italian-Americans who lived there had strong family ties and community relationships. They drank wine, and ate sausages, meatballs, and cheese. Some of them smoked cigars, and many of the men worked in slate quarries. But they had a family-centered life. In general, three generations of a family lived in the same household, so no one was isolated. And the community had a value on modesty when it came to money. People who had more wealth didn't flaunt it, so people in Roseto were not pressured to "keep up with the Joneses." Many people pointed out that if the family and community values and structure failed, their health would fail too. Unfortunately, the community started to develop suburbs, and a suburban lifestyle in the 1970s and people began to live in single-family homes. By the 1990s, their health statistics matched those of the surrounding communities.

People might respond to this story by saying, "oh, too bad." But my response is, "this is still important information, and we can do something with it. Since we know how much harm social isolation and "keeping up with the Joneses" can do to human health, and how much good family/community ties, and a modest approach to income level can do, we can move toward putting these elements into effect in our current communities. There are already hopeful signs. In the Netherlands, day care is being integrated into elder care facilities. Many communities have care centers for dementia patients that provide support and socialization that wasn't available before.

There is a movement in American public education toward community building in the classroom. One of the largest groups of teachers and mentors of classroom community skills is Ojai Foundation's Council in Schools. Council is a practice of sitting together in community and talking and listening from the heart, so that true understanding and connection are fostered between everyone in the school community, both children and adults. Imagine if we all learned to do that and practiced it in our homes, schools, and workplaces! One of the largest Council in Schools programs serves more than 12,000 students in southern California schools. If you look back at the story about Roseto, you can see that this kind of education directly addresses the two social practices that kept Roseto healthy—it promotes community connection and cooperation, rather than isolation and competition. And if you look back at Dr. Martin Seligman's PERMA qualities of well-being, Council in Schools helps people to create school communities that foster all the qualities—positive emotion, engagement, relationships, meaning and achievement. Council in Schools also teaches another community skill—restorative justice, a method of non-violent conflict resolution. Imagine if we all had those skills too—and what it would do for all the health problems connected with violence in this country. For more information, check out either www.ojaifoundation.org, or www.councilinschools.org.

And there are smaller, but important changes among families and friends. Families are keeping in closer touch with each other, even if they live in distant cities by "Face-timing" on phones and sending pictures. Many people are already insisting—at dinners out with friends or during family time at home--that people put their phones away, or in a basket in the middle of the table, and spend the time talking to each other about what is going on in their lives.

On that hopeful note, I will say good-bye, with the wish that you stay alive and well; that we will see the profit-driven disease management system, the Five Horsemen, and the health care apocalypse itself, gradually fade away; and that we will witness the rising growth of a system that practices and values health and prevention.

RECIPIES

In the spirit of "life is short, eat dessert first," I am going to start with desserts, and then add recipes for Breakfasts, Lunches, Dinners and Sides, Snacks, and lastly, one for a Vegetarian Paleo-style diet.

Desserts

I think it is completely fitting for me to begin the dessert and snack section with a recipe from Elana Amsterdam, fabulous cook, and author of one of the best paleo cookbooks I have found, *Paleo Cooking from Elana's Pantry*. See the end of this section for more information about the book!

In writing about the development of this recipe, Elana said she tried 14 different versions to get it right. When I read that I knew that she was a real cook, and every one of her recipes that I have tried have turned out well for me. I have made her cookie recipe hundreds of times by now. My children and grandchildren love them and eat them 4 or 5 at a time. I make them smaller, so they are "cookie bites." No worries. One of them contains only 2 grams of sugars from honey, and no cane sugar, wheat or other grains, dairy or egg. My family especially loves it when I make a whole batch and give it to them as a present! I have added pecan halves to the recipe and have substituted Go Raw agave sweetened chocolate chunks instead of chocolate chips.

Elana's Pantry Paleo Chocolate Chip Cookies
Makes 24

2 cups blanched and finely ground almond flour
(such as Honeyville)
1/2 teaspoon baking soda
1/4 teaspoon fine sea salt
1/4 cup Spectrum organic all-vegetable shortening
1 tablespoon vanilla extract

1⁄2 cup chocolate chunks made from organic, agave-sweetened Go Raw chocolate squares. Cut each square into 16 chunks
24 pecan halves

1. Preheat the oven to 350°F. Line 2 large baking sheets with parchment paper.
2. In a food processor, combine the almond flour, baking soda, and salt. Pulse to
3. thoroughly combine. Add the shortening and vanilla and pulse until thoroughly
4. combined. Remove the blade from the food processor and stir in the chocolate
5. chips. Scoop the dough a tablespoon at a time onto the baking sheets, pressing
6. down to flatten, leaving at least 1" between each cookie. Place a pecan half
7. on top of each cookie.
8. Bake for 8 to 11 minutes, or until golden. Let cool on the baking sheets for 5 minutes.
9. Transfer the cookies to racks to cool completely.

Per serving: 98 calories, 3 g protein, 4 g carbohydrates, 1 g fiber, 8 g total fat, 2 g saturated fat, 54 mg sodium

Baked Pumpkin Pudding

Makes 8 servings

1 can (15 ounces) organic pumpkin
1 can (13.66 ounces) unsweetened coconut milk
1⁄4 cup maple syrup
2 eggs, lightly beaten
1 teaspoon ground cinnamon
1⁄4 teaspoon ground nutmeg
1⁄4 teaspoon ground ginger
1 teaspoon vanilla extract
3⁄4 cup unsweetened almond milk

1. Preheat the oven to 350oF. Lightly coat eight 6-ounce custard cups with cooking spray.

2. In a medium bowl, whisk together the pumpkin, coconut milk, maple syrup, eggs, cinnamon, nutmeg, ginger, vanilla, and almond milk.
3. Divide the mixture among the custard cups. Place the cups in a large baking
4. dish. Fill the dish with water 1" up the sides.
5. Bake for 20 minutes, or until the centers are just barely set.

Per serving: 164 calories, 3 g protein, 13 g carbohydrates, 2 g fiber, 12 g total fat, 10 g saturated fat, 45 mg sodium

Frothy Hot Chocolate
Makes 1 serving

1 cup Almond Breeze unsweetened chocolate almond milk
1 teaspoon unsweetened cocoa powder
4–7 drops (to taste) Sweet Leaf
Liquid Stevia chocolate sweetener drops

In a small saucepan over medium heat, whisk the almond milk, cocoa, and stevia to combine. Bring to a slow boil, reduce the heat to a simmer, and heat for 2 minutes, whisking constantly until hot and frothy.

Per serving: 52 calories, 2 g protein, 4 g carbohydrates, 1 g fiber, 4 g total fat, 0 g saturated fat, 180 mg sodium

Marinated Berries
You can use frozen organic berries for this recipe, but it works a lot better with fresh berries
Makes 6 servings

2 cups raspberries
2 cups blueberries
2 cups blackberries
1 cup sliced peaches
4 cups sparkling seltzer or white wine

In a medium bowl, combine the raspberries, blueberries, blackberries, and peaches. Pour the seltzer or wine over the fruit and let stand for 1 hour before serving.

Per serving: 80 calories, 2 g protein, 19 g carbohydrates, 7 g fiber, 1 g total fat, 0 g saturated fat, 1 mg sodium

Baked Apples
Makes 1 serving

1 Granny Smith apple, cored and cut into 6 wedges
1 teaspoon coconut oil
1/2 teaspoon ground cinnamon

1. Preheat the oven to 425°F.
2. Arrange the apple wedges peel side down on a baking sheet. Drizzle with the oil. Sprinkle with the cinnamon.
3. Bake for 10 to 15 minutes, or until the apple wedges are tender and lightly browned.

Per serving: 151 calories, 1 g protein, 20 g carbohydrates, 4 g fiber, 9 g total fat, 8 g saturated fat, 2 mg sodium

Strawberry or Peach Coconut Milk Ice Cream
Makes 4 servings

2 cups fresh or frozen strawberries or peach slices
1 can full-fat unsweetened coconut milk
1/4 cup maple syrup

In a blender or food processor, combine the fruit, coconut milk, and maple syrup. Blend or process until combined. Enjoy immediately!

NOTE: The ingredients can be processed in an ice cream maker for 15 to 20 minutes for a creamier version.

Per serving: 241 calories, 2 g protein, 15 g carbohydrates, 3 g fiber, 21 g total fat, 18 g saturated fat, 15 mg sodium

Crustless Apple Crumb Pie

Makes 6 servings

5 Granny Smith apples, peeled, cored, and sliced
2 tablespoons maple syrup, divided
1 tablespoon lemon juice
1 1/2 teaspoons ground cinnamon, divided
1 1/4 cups ground pecans
1/4 teaspoon ground ginger
3 tablespoons Spectrum organic all-vegetable shortening, softened

1. Preheat the oven to 375°F. Lightly oil a 9" pie plate and set aside.
2. In a large bowl, combine the apples, 1 tablespoon of the maple syrup, the lemon juice, and 1 teaspoon of the cinnamon. Mix gently. Transfer to the pie plate and set aside.
3. In a small bowl, combine the pecans, the remaining 1/2 teaspoon cinnamon, the ginger, the remaining 1 tablespoon maple syrup, and the shortening. With clean hands, mix to thoroughly combine. Sprinkle the topping over the apple
4. mixture. Bake for 40 to 45 minutes, or until the fruit is cooked and the topping is browned.
5. Variation: Use 5 cups of peeled and sliced peaches instead of apples and replace the pecans with almonds.

Per serving: 314 calories, 3 g protein, 25 g carbohydrates, 5 g fiber, 25 g total fat,5 g saturated fat, 2 mg sodium

Peach Melba

Makes 8 servings

4 ripe peaches
2 teaspoons honey
2 tablespoons Spectrum organic all-vegetable shortening, melted
4 teaspoons raspberry no-sugar spread
8 mint springs, for garnish (optional)

1. Preheat the oven to 450°F.
2. Cut each peach in half and remove the pits. Place the halves cut side up in an 11" x 7" glass baking dish.

3. Brush each peach half with the honey and then with the shortening. Bake for25 to 30 minutes, or until glazed and very tender. Remove from the oven and let cool for a few minutes.
4. To serve, spoon 1/2 teaspoon of the raspberry spread into each peach half.
5. Place a peach half on each of 8 dessert plates and garnish each with a mint sprig, if using.

Per serving: 74 calories, 1 g protein, 11 g carbohydrates, 1 g fiber, 4 g total fat,2 g saturated fat, 0 mg sodium

For more recipes, a good book to start with is Elana Amsterdam's wonderful paleo cookbook I mentioned at the beginning of this section: Amsterdam, Elana Paleo Cooking from Elana's Pantry Berkeley: Ten Speed Press, 2013. Also, try this book: Michail, Deb et. al. Paleo Treats: 55 Decadent Desserts for Your Paleo Sweet Tooth Paleo Secret, 2017.

Greens and Fruit Smoothie

Makes 2 servings

1 cup water
31/2 cups chopped organic spinach
1/2 cup chopped parsley
1 banana, frozen
1 pear, cored and chopped
1/2 cup unsweetened frozen blueberries
2 tablespoons ground golden flaxseed

In a blender, combine the water and spinach. Blend on high speed for 30 seconds to 1 minute, or until smooth. Add the parsley, banana, pear, blueberries, and flaxseed and blend on high speed for 1 minute, or until all ingredients are thoroughly blended.

Per serving: 173 calories, 4 g protein, 36 g carbohydrates, 8 g fiber, 4 g total fat,0.5 g saturated fat, 49 mg sodium

Chocolate-Almond Smoothie

Makes 2 servings

11/2 cups unsweetened almond milk
1 tablespoon maple syrup
1 teaspoon ground flaxseed or white chia seeds
1 tablespoon almond butter
11/2 teaspoons unsweetened cocoa powder
Ice cubes (optional)

1. In a blender, combine the almond milk, maple syrup, flaxseed or chia seeds,
2. almond butter, and cocoa. Blend on high speed for 30 seconds. Let stand for5 minutes.
3. Blend again on high speed for 30 seconds, or until smooth and frothy. Pour into glasses over ice (if using) and serve.

Per serving: 114 calories, 3 g protein, 11 g carbohydrates, 2 g fiber, 7 g total fat,1 g saturated fat, 154 mg sodium

Blueberry Cardamom Flaxseed Muffins

Makes 6

3/4 cup almond meal or almond flour
1/3 cup ground flaxseed
1/2 teaspoon ground cardamom or 1 teaspoon ground cinnamon
1 teaspoon baking powder
2 eggs
1/4 cup honey
1/4 cup unsweetened almond milk
1 tablespoon olive oil
1 tablespoon vanilla extract
1/2 cup fresh blueberries

1. Preheat the oven to 350ºF. Coat a nonstick 6-cup muffin pan with cooking spray or line with paper or foil liners.
2. In a medium bowl, whisk together the almond meal or flour, flaxseed, cardamom or cinnamon, and baking powder.
3. In another medium bowl, whisk together the eggs, honey, milk, oil, and vanilla. Stir in the blueberries and the flour mixture.
4. Divide the batter among the muffin cups.
5. Bake for 18 minutes, or until a wooden pick inserted into the center of a muffin comes out clean.

Per muffin: 219 calories, 7 g protein, 19 g carbohydrates, 3 g fiber, 14 g total fat, 1 g saturated fat, 129 mg sodium

Turkey and Fennel Breakfast Sausage

Makes 10 servings

1 small carrot
1 rib celery
1 small onion
1/2 teaspoon black peppercorns, freshly ground
1/2 teaspoon dried basil
1 teaspoon coconut oil
1/4 teaspoon Himalayan salt
1 clove garlic
1 teaspoon fennel seeds
1/2 teaspoon fenugreek seeds or ground fenugreek
1/2 teaspoon dried thyme

1/2 cup ground walnuts
1-pound lean, organic ground turkey
1 egg, beaten

1. Preheat the oven to 350ºF. Finely chop the carrot, celery, and half of the onion (reserve the other half). In a medium skillet over medium heat, heat the oil. Cook the chopped vegetables until lightly browned. Be sure not to let the oil smoke. Allow the vegetables to cool.
2. In a food processor, combine the remaining onion and the garlic. Process until finely chopped. Add the cooked vegetables and pulse. Transfer the vegetable mixture to a large bowl and add the fennel, fenugreek, pepper, basil, salt, thyme, and walnuts. Combine until mixed. Add the turkey and egg and mix together until the vegetables and seasonings are evenly distributed.
3. Cut parchment paper into 1 piece approximately 10" long. Place the turkey mixture in the center of the parchment and shape into a large log. Tightly wrap the parchment around the log and place in a baking pan.
4. Bake for 1 hour. Allow to cool and then refrigerate for at least 1 hour. Remove the parchment from the turkey log and slice into 1" disks. If freezing, lay the disks out on a baking sheet and place in the freezer. Once frozen, place the sausage patties into freezer bags and keep frozen until using.
5. In a skillet, fry the sausage patties until lightly browned on both sides.

Per serving: 125 calories, 11 g protein, 7 g carbohydrates, 1 g fiber, 7 g total fat, 2 g saturated fat, 66 mg sodium

Eggs Florentine

Makes 2 servings

4 eggs
2 teaspoons olive oil
1 bag (6 ounces) fresh baby spinach
1/8 teaspoon salt
1/8 teaspoon ground black pepper

1. Preheat the oven to 350°F.
2. Coat four 1-cup custard cups with cooking spray and add 1 tablespoon of water to each cup. Break 1 egg into each cup. Bake for 15 to 20 minutes.

3. Meanwhile, in a small nonstick skillet over medium heat, heat the oil. Cook the spinach, stirring constantly, until wilted. Season with the salt and pepper.
4. Divide the spinach between 2 plates. Place 2 baked eggs on top of each serving of spinach.

Per serving: 273 calories, 15 g protein, 6 g carbohydrates, 2 g fiber, 14 g total fat, 4 g saturated fat, 378 mg sodium

Western Scramble

Makes 4 servings

1 sweet potato (6–8 ounces total weight), peeled and cut into 1/2" chunks
1 tablespoon sunflower oil
1 onion, coarsely chopped
1/2 cup chopped extra-lean organic cooked ham
6 large eggs
1/2 teaspoon coarsely ground black pepper
1 red bell pepper, coarsely chopped
1 green bell pepper, coarsely chopped
Pinch of salt

1. Place the potato chunks in a saucepan. Add cold water to just cover. Bring to a boil over high heat. Reduce the heat to a simmer, partially cover, and cook for 10 minutes, or until tender. Drain and set aside.
2. In a large nonstick skillet over medium-high heat, heat the oil. Cook the onion and bell peppers, stirring often, for 8 minutes, or until tender and lightly golden. Stir in the ham and potato chunks and cook, stirring often, for 2 minutes, or until just starting to brown.
3. Meanwhile, in a medium bowl, beat the eggs. Add the black pepper and salt.
4. Pour the egg mixture into the skillet. Reduce the heat and cook, turning often with a nylon spatula, for 3 to 5 minutes, or until just set.

Per serving: 214 calories, 14 g protein, 14 g carbohydrates, 3 g fiber, 11 g total fat, 3 g saturated fat, 263 mg sodium

Honey-Sweet Broiled Grapefruit Halves

Makes 4 servings

2 medium red or pink grapefruit (about 1 pound each), halved and sectioned
4 teaspoons honey
1/4 teaspoon ground cinnamon
1/4 teaspoon ground cardamom

1. Preheat the broiler. Line the bottom of a broiler pan with foil.
2. Place the grapefruit halves in the pan. Drizzle 1 teaspoon of the honey over each half, spreading it evenly. Sprinkle each grapefruit half with a tiny bit of cinnamon and cardamom.
3. Broil 4 to 5" from the heat for 5 to 7 minutes, or until glazed and heated through.

Per serving: 75 calories, 1 g protein, 19 g carbohydrates, 2 g fiber, 0 g total fat, 0 g saturated fat, 0 mg sodium

Omelet Italian Style

Makes 1 serving

2 tablespoons chopped onion
2 tablespoons chopped green bell pepper
2 tablespoons chopped tomato + additional for garnish
3 eggs, beaten
1/2 teaspoon dried oregano
1 teaspoon chopped fresh parsley

1. Coat a medium skillet with cooking spray. Place over medium heat. Cook the onion and pepper, stirring occasionally, for 2 minutes, or until sizzling. Add the tomato.
2. Cook for 1 minute, or until just starting to soften. Add the eggs and sprinkle with the oregano. Cook, lifting the cooked edges of the egg mixture with a fork so the uncooked egg can run underneath, for 5 minutes, or until the bottom is set. Cook undisturbed for 1 to 2 minutes, or until the eggs are completely set. Sprinkle with the parsley and fold the omelet in half. Slide onto a plate and garnish with additional tomato.

Per serving: 232 calories, 20 g protein, 5 g carbohydrates, 1 g fiber, 14 g total fat, 5 g saturated fat, 507 mg sodium

Peachy Quinoa Breakfast

Makes 1 serving

2/3 cup water
1/4 cup quinoa
1 teaspoon honey
1/4 cup sliced fresh or frozen, thawed peaches
2 tablespoons sliced almonds
1 tablespoon unsweetened coconut
Pinch of ground cinnamon
Pinch of ground ginger

> In a heavy saucepan, combine the water, quinoa, and honey. Stir to mix well. Simmer, stirring frequently until thickened and the liquid is absorbed. Stir in the peaches and top with the almonds and coconut. Sprinkle with the cinnamon and ginger.

Per serving: 294 calories, 9 g protein, 41 g carbohydrates, 6 g fiber, 12 g total fat, 4 g saturated fat, 11 mg sodium

Super Strawberry Smoothie

Makes 1 serving

1 cup sliced strawberries
1/4 cup coconut milk
1/2 cup vanilla almond milk
1/4 cup unsweetened pomegranate juice

> In a blender or food processor, combine the strawberries, coconut milk, almond milk, and juice. Blend or process until thick and smooth. Spoon into a glass and serve.

Per serving: 218 calories, 3 g protein, 24 g carbohydrates, 5 g fiber, 14 g total fat, 11 g saturated fat, 105 mg sodium

Sweet Potato Pancakes

Makes 2 servings

1 large sweet potato, peeled and cubed
2 scallions, chopped
2 egg whites
1/8 teaspoon ground black pepper
Pinch of grated nutmeg
Pinch of ground ginger
1 tablespoon sunflower oil, divided
1 cup unsweetened applesauce
teaspoons maple syrup

1. In a steamer set in a pan of boiling water, steam the potato for 12 to 15 minutes, or until very tender. Transfer to a large bowl and mash until almost smooth. Add the scallions, egg whites, pepper, nutmeg, and ginger and mash to combine.
2. In a nonstick skillet coated with cooking spray, heat 11/2 teaspoons of the oil over medium heat. Drop half of the potato mixture by 1/4 cupful into the skillet
3. Flatten into 3" rounds. Cook, turning once, for 6 to 8 minutes, or until golden brown. Transfer to a plate and cover to keep warm. Repeat with the remaining 11/2 teaspoons of oil and potato mixture to make 6 pancakes total. Serve the pancakes with the applesauce. Drizzle each serving with maple syrup.

Per serving: 207 calories, 5 g protein, 32 g carbohydrates, 4 g fiber, 7 g total fat, 1 g saturated fat, 99 mg sodium

Noodle Bowls
Makes 4 servings

1/4 cup almond butter
2 tablespoons honey
2 teaspoons less-sodium soy sauce
2 teaspoons rice vinegar
2 tablespoons water
2 packages (7 ounces each) shirataki noodles, drained
2 cups shredded cooked chicken breast
3/4 cup grated carrots
1/2 yellow bell pepper, very thinly sliced (about 2/3 cup)
1/4 cup sliced almonds, toasted
2–3 radishes, very thinly sliced (about 1/3 cup)
8 scallions, white and some green, thinly sliced (about 1/2 cup)
2 tablespoons chopped cilantro

1. In a small bowl, combine the almond butter, honey, soy sauce, vinegar, and water.
2. Prepare the noodles according to package directions. Drain, rinse with cold water, and drain thoroughly.
3. In a large bowl, combine the noodles and almond butter mixture, stirring well to coat. Stir in the chicken, carrots, pepper, almonds, radishes, scallions, and cilantro. Divide among 4 bowls and serve.

Per serving:332 calories, 29 g protein, 23 g carbohydrates, 7 g fiber, 15 g total fat,2 g saturated fat, 182 mg sodium

Salmon Avocado Wrap
Makes 2 servings

1 can (6 ounces) wild-caught Alaskan salmon
1/2 cup chopped scallions
2 tablespoons chopped fresh parsley
1 tablespoon extra-virgin olive oil
Juice of 1/2 lime
1/4 cup chopped avocado
1/2 cup cherry tomatoes, halved
Salt and pepper to taste

4 large bok choy or Chinese cabbage leaves

1. In a large mixing bowl, combine the salmon, scallions, parsley, oil, lime juice, avocado, tomatoes, salt, and pepper. Divide the mixture among the bok choy or
2. Chinese cabbage leaves and fold into a wrap. Place 2 wraps on each of 2 plates and serve.

Per serving: 242 calories, 19 g protein, 7 g carbohydrates, 3 g fiber, 16 g total fat,3 g saturated fat, 326 mg sodium

Hearty Chicken or Beef Vegetable Soup
Makes 6 servings

1 tablespoon coconut oil
1 pound organic, grass-fed, lean ground beef or shredded cooked chicken
1 onion, chopped
2 cloves garlic, chopped
8 ounces mushrooms, chopped
2 carrots, sliced
2 zucchini, sliced
2 quarts organic chicken or vegetable broth
1 can (14.5 ounces) organic crushed tomatoes
1 can (28 ounces) organic diced tomatoes
1 tablespoon fresh lemon juice (optional)
2 teaspoons dried basil
1/8 teaspoon crushed red pepper flakes, or to taste
2 cups chopped kale leaves
1/4 cup cilantro, chopped
1/4 cup fresh parsley, chopped

1. In a stockpot over medium-high heat, heat the oil. Cook the beef or chicken, stirring frequently, for 5 minutes, or until cooked or heated through. Drain and transfer to a plate.
2. In the same pot, cook the onion, garlic, and mushrooms for 5 minutes, or until soft.
3. Stir in the carrots, zucchini, broth, crushed and diced tomatoes, lemon juice (if using), basil, pepper flakes, and kale. Cover and simmer for 20 minutes.
4. Add the cilantro and parsley and cover. Simmer for 20 minutes.

Per serving: 287 calories, 23 g protein, 21 g carbohydrates, 5 g fiber, 13 g total fat,6 g saturated fat, 640 mg sodium

Roasted Chicken and Spinach Salad

Makes 2 servings

2 tablespoons red wine vinegar
2 teaspoons extra virgin olive oil
1 teaspoon Dijon mustard
1/4 teaspoon salt
1/8 teaspoon ground black pepper
1 bag (6 ounces) baby spinach
1 boneless, skinless organic chicken breast (about 6 ounces), roasted or grilled and thinly sliced
2 red-skinned pears, cored and thinly sliced
1/2 red onion, thinly sliced
1/4 cup pecans, toasted

1. In a large serving bowl, whisk together the vinegar, oil, mustard, salt, and pepper.
2. Add the spinach, chicken, pears, and onion. Toss to coat well.
3. Divide among 2 plates and top each serving with the pecans.

Per serving: 419 calories, 30 g protein, 41 g carbohydrates, 11 g fiber, 17 g total fat, 2 g saturated fat, 553 mg sodium

Chicken Noodle Soup with Spinach and Basil

Makes 4 servings

1 package (7 ounces) shirataki spaghetti noodles, rinsed and drained
2 tablespoons olive oil
11/2 pounds boneless, skinless chicken breasts, cut into bite-size pieces
2 scallions, thinly sliced 1 carton (32 ounces)
low-sodium organic chicken broth
4 cups spinach leaves, shredded
1 cup basil leaves, shredded
1 tablespoon fresh lemon juice

1. Prepare the noodles according to package directions. Drain and set aside.
2. Meanwhile, in a large saucepan over medium-high heat, heat the oil. Cook the chicken and scallions for 5 minutes, or until lightly browned. Add the broth, reduce the heat to medium, and bring to a simmer. Add the spinach, basil, and lemon juice. Simmer for 4 minutes, or until the spinach is wilted and the chicken is cooked through.
3. Add the noodles to the soup and stir.

Per serving: 288 calories, 29 g protein, 6 g carbohydrates, 2 g fiber, 11 g total fat, 2 g saturated fat, 307 mg sodium

Warm Sweet Potato and Onion Salad with Toasted Walnuts

Makes 4 servings

2 large sweet potatoes (about 2 pounds), peeled and cut into 1" pieces
2 large red onions, cut into wedges
1/2 teaspoon dried rosemary
1/2 teaspoon dried oregano
1/4 teaspoon salt
1/4 teaspoon ground black pepper
1 tablespoon balsamic vinegar
1 teaspoon honey
1/2 teaspoon Dijon mustard
2 tablespoons sunflower oil
5 ounces baby arugula (5 cups)
6 tablespoons walnut halves, toasted

1. Preheat the oven to 400°F. Coat a baking sheet with cooking spray.
2. Place the potatoes and onions on the baking sheet and toss with the rosemary, oregano, salt, and pepper. Roast for 30 minutes, turning once, or until tender and browned.
3. In a large bowl, whisk together the vinegar, honey, and mustard. Whisk in the oil. Add the arugula and toss to coat. Toss in the vegetables.
4. Divide the salad among 4 plates and top each serving with the walnuts.

Per serving: 361 calories, 12 g protein, 33 g carbohydrates, 6 g fiber, 22 g total fat, 7 g saturated fat, 377 mg sodium

Fish and Chips

Makes 4 servings

2 sweet potatoes, peeled and cut lengthwise into wedges
11/2 teaspoons olive oil
1/2 teaspoon smoked paprika
1/8 teaspoon salt
1/4 teaspoon ground black

pepper, divided
1 egg, lightly beaten
1 teaspoon Dijon mustard
1/8 teaspoon ground red pepper
1 cup finely ground almonds or pecans
1/2 teaspoon dried thyme
4 skinless halibut fillets (6 ounces each)
Lemon wedges or malt vinegar, for serving (optional)

1. Preheat the oven to 425°F. Line 2 large baking sheets with parchment paper.
2. In a large bowl, combine the sweet potatoes, oil, paprika, salt, and 1/8 teaspoon of the black pepper, tossing well to coat. Arrange on 1 of the baking sheets in a single layer. Bake for 15 minutes.
3. Meanwhile, in a shallow dish, whisk the egg, mustard, red pepper, and remaining 1/8 teaspoon black pepper. In another shallow dish, combine the nuts and thyme. Working with 1 fillet at a time, dip the halibut in the mustard mixture, shake off the excess, and then roll in the nut mixture to coat. Place on the second baking sheet. Repeat with the remaining fillets.
4. Remove the vegetables from the oven and toss. Return to the oven with the halibut fillets. Bake for 12 to 15 minutes, or until the halibut is golden and flakes easily.
5. Divide the fish and sweet potatoes among 4 plates. Serve with the lemon wedges or malt vinegar, if using.

Per serving: 278 calories, 35 g protein, 20 g carbohydrates, 2 g fiber, 6 g total fat, 1 g saturated fat, 312 mg sodium

Tangy Chicken Lettuce Wraps

Makes 4 servings

1/4 cup vegan sour cream
2 teaspoons prepared horseradish, drained
4 large leaves green leafy lettuce
6 ounces thinly sliced grilled chicken
1 apple, cut into 16 slices

1. In a small bowl, combine the sour cream and horseradish until blended.
2. Place the lettuce leaves on a work surface. Spread each leaf with the sour cream mixture. Evenly layer the beef and apple slices down the center of each lettuce leaf. Fold each leaf around the filling and serve.

Per serving: 106 calories, 12 g protein, 8 g carbohydrates, 1 g fiber, 4 g total fat, 1 g saturated fat, 88 mg sodium

Pan-Seared Fish Tacos
Makes 4 servings

1 Hass avocado, halved, pitted, peeled, and cubed
3 tablespoons finely chopped red onion
2 tablespoons chopped cilantro
1/2 jalapeño Chile pepper, finely chopped (wear plastic gloves when handling)
1 tablespoon lime juice
1/2 teaspoon salt, divided
1-pound cod fillet, cut into 1" pieces
1 teaspoon cumin
1/2 teaspoon chili powder
1 tablespoon olive oil
8 gluten-free or gluten and corn free tortillas
(6" diameter)
1 cup shredded romaine lettuce

1. In a small bowl, combine the avocado, onion, cilantro, jalapeño pepper, lime juice, and 1/4 teaspoon of the salt until blended. Set aside. In a medium bowl, toss the cod with the cumin, chili powder, and remaining 1/4 teaspoon salt.
2. In a large nonstick skillet over medium-high heat, heat the oil. Cook the cod for 8 minutes, turning occasionally, or until opaque in the center. Transfer to a plate and keep warm.
3. Wipe out the skillet. Heat the tortillas in the skillet for 30 seconds per side, or according to package directions, until hot and lightly toasted. Dividing evenly, top each tortilla with the romaine, reserved avocado mixture, and cod. Place 2 tacos on each of 4 plates and serve hot.

Per serving: 370 calories, 23 g protein, 39 g carbohydrates, 13 g fiber, 15 g total fat, 1 g saturated fat, 737 mg sodium

Sweet Potatoes Stuffed with Picadillo
Makes 4 servings

4 orange-fleshed sweet potatoes (yams), 6 ounces each
8 ounces organic, grass-fed, extra-lean ground beef

1 medium onion, chopped

2 cloves garlic, minced

1/2 teaspoon dried oregano

1/4 teaspoon ground cinnamon

1 can (14.5 ounces) no-salt added petite diced tomatoes

1/3 cup packed golden raisins (optional)

2 tablespoons no-salt-added tomato paste

1/4 teaspoon salt

1/8 teaspoon ground black pepper

1. Preheat the oven to 425°F.
2. Place the sweet potatoes on a baking sheet and roast for 35 minutes, or until easily pierced with a knife.
3. Meanwhile, heat a medium nonstick skillet over medium-high heat. Add the beef, onion, garlic, oregano, and cinnamon. Cook, breaking the beef into smaller pieces with a wooden spoon, for 4 minutes, or until no longer pink. Stir in the diced tomatoes, raisins (if using), and tomato paste. Cook, stirring occasionally, for 5 to 6 minutes, or until slightly thickened. Stir in the salt and pepper.
4. Cut the sweet potatoes in half lengthwise and set 2 halves on each of 4 plates. Top each potato half with 1/4 cup of the beef mixture.

Per serving: 307 calories, 16 g protein, 45 g carbohydrates, 7 g fiber, 8 g total fat, 3 g saturated fat, 263 mg sodium

Moroccan Quinoa
Makes 6 servings

1 cup quinoa
1 tablespoon coconut oil
1 small onion, finely chopped
1 clove garlic, minced
1/2 teaspoon ground coriander
1/2 teaspoon ground cinnamon
1/4 teaspoon ground turmeric
Pinch of saffron threads (optional)
1 cup low-sodium vegetable broth
2/3 cup water
1 tomato, chopped
1/3 cup golden raisins
1 /2 teaspoon salt
3 tablespoons finely chopped fresh parsley

1. In a fine sieve, rinse the quinoa under cold water for 1 minute. Drain well and set aside.
2. In a large saucepan over medium heat, heat the oil. Cook the onion and garlic, stirring, until softened. Add the coriander, cinnamon, turmeric, and saffron (if using). Cook, stirring constantly, for 30 seconds.
3. Add the reserved quinoa and stir for 1 minute, or until the quinoa is coated with the spices.
4. Add the broth, water, tomato, raisins, and salt and stir to combine. Simmer, covered, for 15 minutes, or until the liquid is absorbed.
5. Remove the pan from the heat. Let the mixture stand, covered, for 5 minutes. Stir in the parsley and serve.

Per serving: 167 calories, 5 g protein, 28 g carbohydrates, 3 g fiber, 4 g total fat, 2 g saturated fat, 224 mg sodium

Veggie "Soufflé"
Makes 6 servings

1-pound cauliflower florets (about 4 cups)
1-pound broccoli florets (about 6 cups)

2 teaspoons olive oil
1/2 cup chopped onion
1 large shallot, finely chopped
11/2 cups sliced mushrooms
2 large eggs, divided
4 egg whites, divided
2/3 cup ground pecans, divided
1 teaspoon salt, divided
1 teaspoon ground black pepper, divided
Ground red pepper

1. Preheat the oven to 350°F. Coat an 8" x 4" loaf pan with cooking spray or use a nonstick loaf pan.
2. Place the cauliflower and 3-4 tablespoons of water in a heavy saucepan and cook until softened (to taste) and drain the liquid.
3. Do the same with the broccoli.
4. In a skillet, heat the oil. Cook the onion, shallot, and mushrooms, stirring frequently, for 5 minutes, or until soft. Set aside.
5. In a food processor, combine the reserved cauliflower, 1 egg, 2 egg whites, 1/3 cup of the pecan crumbs, 1/2 teaspoon of the salt, and 1/2 teaspoon of the black pepper. Pulse until almost smooth. Scrape into the loaf pan.
6. In the food processor, combine the reserved broccoli and the remaining 1 egg, 2 egg whites, 1/3 cup pecan crumbs, 1/2 teaspoon salt, 1/2 teaspoon black pepper, and a pinch of red pepper (no need to rinse the bowl after the cauliflower). Pulse until almost smooth.
7. Arrange the reserved mushroom mixture over the cauliflower layer. Gently spread the broccoli mixture over the top. Sprinkle with a pinch of red pepper.
8. Bake for 45 to 50 minutes, or until a wooden pick inserted into the center comes out clean.

Per serving: 193 calories, 10 g protein, 12 g carbohydrates, 6 g fiber, 13 g total fat, 2 g saturated fat, 493 mg sodium

Shepherd's Pie

Makes 4 servings

11/4 pounds sweet potatoes, peeled and cut into 1" pieces
1/2 cup almond milk
11/2 tablespoons coconut oil, divided
3/4 teaspoon salt, divided

1/4 teaspoon ground black pepper, divided
1-pound organic, grass-fed, lean ground beef
1 medium leek, white part only, washed and chopped (about 1/2 cup)
1 onion, chopped
2 cups chopped carrots
1/2 teaspoon dried oregano
1/2 cup low-sodium, fat-free beef broth
1/4 cup red wine
1/4 cup tomato paste
Ground paprika

1. Preheat the oven to 350°F.
2. Coat a 6-cup (1-1/2 quart) baking dish with cooking spray and set aside.
3. Place the sweet potatoes in a small pot with enough water to cover by 3". Bring to a boil and cook for 10 to 12 minutes, or until tender. Drain the potatoes, return to the pot, and add the almond milk, 1 tablespoon of the oil, 1/4 teaspoon of the salt, and 1/8 teaspoon of the pepper. Mash until smooth. Set aside.
4. In a nonstick skillet over medium-high heat, heat the remaining 1/2 tablespoon oil. Cook the beef, stirring occasionally, for 5 to 6 minutes, or until browned.
   Drain the fat from the pan and transfer the beef to a bowl.
5. Return the skillet to the heat and add the leek, onion, carrots, and oregano. Cook, stirring occasionally, for 5 to 7 minutes, or until the vegetables are soft.
6. Return the beef to the skillet and stir in the broth, wine, and tomato paste. Cook for 2 to 3 minutes, or until the liquid is almost evaporated. Stir in the remaining 1/2 teaspoon salt and 1/8 teaspoon pepper.
7. Transfer the beef mixture to the baking dish. Spread the reserved mashed sweet potatoes evenly over the top of the beef. Sprinkle with paprika. Bake for 25 to 30 minutes, or until the potatoes are lightly browned.

Per serving: 363 calories, 29 g protein, 37 g carbohydrates, 7 g fiber, 10 g total fat, 6 g saturated fat, 782 mg sodium

Coconut Vegetable Curry

Makes 4 servings

2 tablespoons extra virgin olive oil
1 tablespoon chopped fresh ginger
1 1/2 teaspoons cumin seeds

3 cups peeled and cubed butternut squash
3 carrots, chopped
1/2 teaspoon ground turmeric
2 teaspoons ground coriander
1 teaspoon curry powder
1 tablespoon tomato paste
1 can (13.66 ounces) full fat coconut milk
1/4 cup water
2 cups frozen peas
1 teaspoon salt
1/2 cup chopped cilantro

1. In a large pot over medium heat, heat the oil. Cook the ginger and cumin seeds for 1 to 2 minutes, or until the seeds begin to "pop."
2. Add the squash, carrots, turmeric, coriander, and curry powder. Stir well and cook for 1 minute. Add the tomato paste, coconut milk, and water. Stir well.
3. Simmer, covered, for 5 to 10 minutes, or until the squash and carrots are almost done but still a little firm. Add the peas and salt, cover the pot, and simmer for 6 to 7 minutes, or until the vegetables are tender. Remove from the heat and stir in the cilantro.

Per serving: 356 calories, 6 g protein, 26 g carbohydrates, 7 g fiber, 28 g total fat, 19 g saturated fat, 672 mg sodium

Tuscan Tuna Cakes

Makes 4 servings

1-pound yellowfin tuna, cut into 1/4" cubes
1 large egg
1 large egg white
1/4 cup finely chopped fennel (about 1/4 of a medium bulb)
1 small onion, finely chopped
1 tablespoon drained capers
1 tablespoon lemon juice
2 teaspoons grated lemon peel
1 teaspoon chopped fresh oregano
1 cup pine nuts, finely ground
1/2 teaspoon salt
1/4 teaspoon ground black pepper
2 tablespoons olive oil, divided
4 lemon wedges

1. In a large bowl, combine the tuna, egg, egg white, fennel, onion, capers, lemon juice, lemon peel, and oregano. Mix well. Gently fold in the pine nuts, salt, and pepper until just combined.
2. Divide the tuna mixture into 8 equal portions. Shape each into a disk approximately 31/2" in diameter and about 1/2" thick.
3. In a large nonstick skillet over medium heat, heat 1 tablespoon of the oil. Add 4 tuna cakes and cook for 3 to 4 minutes per side, or until the cakes are golden and cooked through. Repeat with the remaining 1 tablespoon oil and tuna cakes. Serve with the lemon wedges.

Per serving: 448 calories, 34 g protein, 9 g carbohydrates, 2 g fiber, 32 g total fat, 3 g saturated fat, 432 mg sodium

Hearty Winter Harvest Stew

Makes 8-10 servings

2 tablespoons olive oil
4 boneless, skinless chicken breast halves (about 6 ounces each), cut into 1/2" pieces
1 onion, chopped
1/2 cup sliced leek
3 cloves garlic, minced
10 cups peeled and cubed harvest vegetables, such as sweet potatoes, butternut squash, or parsnips
8 cups low-sodium organic chicken broth
2 tablespoons finely chopped fresh ginger
1 tablespoon ground cumin
2 teaspoons sweet paprika
1 teaspoon ground black pepper
1/2 teaspoon salt
1/2 teaspoon ground cardamom
3 strips orange peel, white pith removed
2 bay leaves
3 cups winter greens, such as spinach or kale (ribs removed), chopped
1/2 cup snipped fresh Italian parsley
1/2 cup chopped pistachios, toasted

1. In a large pot over medium-high heat, heat the oil. Cook the chicken, onion, leek, and garlic until lightly browned. Stir in the vegetables, broth,

ginger, cumin, paprika, pepper, salt, cardamom, orange peel, and bay leaves. Bring to a boil.
2. Reduce the heat and simmer, uncovered, for 45 to 50 minutes, or until the vegetables are tender. Remove from the heat and discard the bay leaves. Stir in the greens and let wilt. Just before serving, stir in the parsley and pistachios.

Per serving: 254 calories, 23 g protein, 19 g carbohydrates, 4 g fiber, 9 g total fat, 1 g saturated fat, 365 mg sodium

Mock Mashed Potatoes
Makes 4 servings

2 pounds rutabagas, peeled and cubed (approximately 5–6 cups)
2 tablespoons coconut oil
1/2 cup coconut milk
1/8 teaspoon salt
1/8 teaspoon ground black pepper

1. In a large saucepan over medium-high heat, cook the rutabagas in boiling water for 10 minutes, or until fork-tender. Drain.
2. In a small saucepan over medium-low heat, combine the coconut oil and coconut milk and bring to a slow simmer.
3. Using an electric mixer or food processor, puree the rutabagas until smooth.
4. Add the warmed milk mixture. Blend for 30 seconds, or until creamy. Season with the salt and pepper.

Per serving: 356 calories, 3 g protein, 16 g carbohydrates, 4 g fiber, 13 g total fat, 11 g saturated fat, 97 mg sodium

Grilled Salmon with Citrus Salsa
Makes 4 servings

Salsa
2 tablespoons sherry vinegar
3 tablespoons extra virgin olive oil
1 navel orange, peeled and cut into 1/4" pieces
1/2 cup pitted and chopped
Kalamata olives

1/3 cup finely chopped red onion
1/3 cup chopped fennel
1 tablespoon chopped fresh oregano
1 tablespoon chopped flat-leaf parsley
Salmon
4 wild-caught salmon fillets (6 ounces each)
2 teaspoons extra virgin olive oil

1. To make the salsa: Pour the vinegar into a large bowl and whisk in the oil. Stir in the orange, olives, onion, and fennel. Let sit at room temperature while preparing the salmon.
2. To make the salmon: Heat a ridged grill pan over medium-high heat. Brush both sides of the salmon lightly with the oil. Grill the salmon, shaking the pan occasionally to keep the fish from sticking and turning once, for 6 to 8 minutes, or until it is opaque.
3. Transfer the salmon to a serving platter. Add the oregano and parsley to the salsa and spoon evenly over the salmon.

Per serving: 499 calories, 35 g protein, 12 g carbohydrates, 2 g fiber, 34 g total fat, 5 g saturated fat, 135 mg sodium

Pistachio-Crusted Chicken Breasts

Makes 4 servings

2 tablespoons ground flaxseed
3/4 cup pistachios, crushed to very fine crumbs
1 tablespoon sliced almonds, crushed
1 teaspoon dried basil
1 teaspoon dried oregano
1 teaspoon smoked paprika
2 eggs, beaten
4 boneless, skinless chicken breasts (5–6 ounces each)
1 tablespoon sunflower oil

1. On a large flat plate, combine the flaxseed, pistachios, almonds, basil, oregano, and paprika and mix well. Pour the beaten eggs in a shallow dish. Dip each chicken breast in the beaten egg and then press both sides of the chicken breasts into the crumb mixture. Make sure the chicken breasts are completely covered in the crumbs.
2. In a 10" skillet over medium heat, heat the oil. Cook the chicken for 8 to 12 minutes, turning once, or until golden brown, a thermometer inserted in the thickest portion registers 165°F, and the juices run clear.

Per serving: 387 calories, 39 g protein, 8 g carbohydrates, 3 g fiber, 22 g total fat, 3 g saturated fat, 208 mg sodium

Beef and Cabbage Stir-Fry

Makes 4 servings

2 tablespoons wheat free tamari
2 cloves garlic, minced
1 tablespoon honey
2 teaspoons toasted sesame oil
1 teaspoon hot-pepper sauce
1 teaspoon arrowroot
1-pound organic, grass-fed top sirloin or round steak, sliced across the grain into thin strips
1/4 cup unsweetened apple juice
1/2 cup low-sodium organic beef broth
1 cup chopped onions
3 cups shredded Napa cabbage
1 cup sliced carrots

1. In a shallow glass dish, combine the soy sauce, garlic, honey, oil, hot-pepper sauce, and arrowroot. Add the beef strips and stir. Cover and refrigerate for 30 minutes, stirring occasionally.
2. Coat a large nonstick skillet with cooking spray and heat over medium-high heat until hot. Add the beef, reserving the marinade. Cook, stirring, for 5 minutes, or until browned and just slightly pink in the center. Transfer to a plate and cover to keep warm.
3. Add the apple juice and broth to the skillet. Bring to a brisk simmer, scraping the bottom to loosen any browned bits.
4. Add the onions. Cook, stirring, for 1 to 2 minutes, or until the onions are tender. Add the cabbage and carrots. Cook, stirring, for 3 to 4 minutes, or until the vegetables are tender. Return the beef and the reserved marinade to the skillet. Bring to a boil. Cook, stirring, for 1 to 2 minutes, or until the sauce thickens slightly.

Per serving: 237 calories, 27 g protein, 14 g carbohydrates, 2 g fiber, 8 g total fat, 2 g saturated fat, 402 mg sodium

Spaghetti Squash with Stir-Fry Vegetables

Makes TK servings

1 medium spaghetti squash (about 2 1/2 to 3 pounds)
3 tablespoons sunflower oil
2 cups sliced red bell peppers
2 cups broccoli florets
1/4 cup Asian garlic chili paste
1/4 teaspoon crushed red pepper
1 toasted sesame oil

1. Preheat Oven to 375°F.
2. Carefully cut the squash in half lengthwise
3. Oil the surface of the squash with olive oil and place on parchment paper on a sheet pan
4. Bake for 45 minutes, or until the squash flesh becomes tender and separates easily into strands with a fork.
5. Using a fork, scrape the squash strands into a large serving bowl. Set aside.
6. In a large nonstick skillet over medium-high heat, heat the sunflower oil. Cook the bell pepper and broccoli, tossing frequently, for 5 to 7 minutes, or until the vegetables are crisp-tender. Add the chili paste and crushed red pepper and stir to coat the vegetables. Cook for 5 minutes. Add the vegetables to the spaghetti squash, toss, and drizzle with the sesame oil.

Per serving: 241 calories, 5 g protein, 23 g carbohydrates, 5 g fiber, 16 g total fat, 1 g saturated fat, 177 mg sodium

Homestyle Roast Beef

Makes 6 servings

1 organic, grass-fed, boneless beef tri-tip roast (bottom sirloin) (about 2–2 1/2 pounds)
1 cup cippolini onions, peeled
2 cups sliced carrots
2 cloves garlic, minced
1 tablespoon sunflower or olive oil
1 teaspoon dried thyme
1 teaspoon dried oregano
1/2 teaspoon salt

1/4 teaspoon ground black pepper
1 cup low-sodium organic beef broth

1. Preheat the oven to 375°F. Coat the inside of a heavy roasting pan with cooking spray. Place the roast, onions, carrots, and garlic in the pan. Drizzle the oil over the meat and vegetables. Sprinkle on the thyme, oregano, salt, and pepper.
2. With clean hands, toss to coat the vegetables and to rub the seasonings all over the beef.
3. Roast for 50 to 60 minutes, or until a thermometer inserted in the center registers 155°F. Transfer the roast and vegetables to a serving platter. Let stand for 10 minutes.
4. Meanwhile, place the roasting pan over medium heat. Add the broth and cook, scraping the bottom of the pan with a spatula to release the browned particles.
5. Boil for a few minutes to reduce. Slice the roast. Serve the beef and vegetables drizzled with the pan juices.

Per serving: 213 calories, 26 g protein, 8 g carbohydrates, 2 g fiber, 8 g total fat, 2 g saturated fat, 237 mg sodium

Pork Chops and Sweet Potatoes

Makes 4 servings

2 large sweet potatoes, peeled and cut into 8 wedges each
1 large onion, peeled and cut into 8 wedges
1 tablespoon sunflower oil
2 teaspoons finely chopped fresh ginger
1/4 teaspoon salt
1/4 teaspoon ground cinnamon
1/4 teaspoon ground black pepper
4 thin-cut boneless pork chops (about 3 ounces each)
1/4 cup low-sodium vegetable broth or water

1. Preheat the oven to 400°F. Coat a large shallow baking pan with cooking spray.
2. Add the sweet potatoes and onion to the pan.
3. In a small bowl, whisk the oil, ginger, salt, cinnamon, and pepper. Drizzle over the vegetables. With clean hands, rub the seasoning mixture evenly into the vegetables.
4. Bake, tossing occasionally, for 20 to 30 minutes, or until the vegetables start to brown. Reduce the heat to 375°F. Add the pork chops to the pan.

Roast for 10 to 15 minutes, or until a thermometer inserted in the center of a chop registers 160°F and the juices run clear. Transfer the pork and vegetables to a serving platter. Add the broth or water to the pan juices and stir to combine, scraping up any bits left in the pan. Pour the pan juices over the pork and vegetables.

Per serving: 332 calories, 18 g protein, 23 g carbohydrates, 4 g fiber, 19 g total fat, 4 g saturated fat, 505 mg sodium

Spaghetti Squash Casserole

Makes 6 servings

1 spaghetti squash (2 1/2–3 pounds), halved and seeded
1 tablespoon olive oil
1 small onion, chopped
2 cloves garlic, chopped
2 tablespoons chopped fresh basil or 1 teaspoon dried
1 can (14.5 ounces) no-salt added diced tomatoes
1/4 cup chopped fresh parsley
1/4 teaspoon salt
1/4 teaspoon ground black pepper
3/4 cup pine nuts, lightly toasted and chopped

1. Preheat the oven to 400°F. Coat a 13" x 9" baking dish and a baking sheet with cooking spray. Place the squash, cut sides down, on the baking sheet. Pierce the skin with a small paring knife or fork. Bake for 30 minutes, or until tender. With a fork, scrape the squash strands into a large bowl.
2. Meanwhile, in a medium skillet over medium heat, heat the oil. Cook the onion, garlic, and basil for 4 minutes, or until the onion is soft. Add the tomatoes and cook for 5 minutes.
3. Add the parsley, salt, pepper, and the tomato mixture to the bowl with the squash. Toss to coat. Place in the baking dish.
4. Bake for 20 minutes, or until hot and bubbly. Sprinkle with the pine nuts.

Per serving: 201 calories, 4 g protein, 17 g carbohydrates, 4 g fiber, 15 g total fat, 1 g saturated fat, 131 mg sodium

Szechuan Chicken

Makes 4 servings

1 teaspoon minced garlic
1 teaspoon grated fresh ginger
1⁄2 teaspoon salt
1⁄4 teaspoon ground black pepper
1⁄2 teaspoon crushed fennel seeds
Pinch of ground cloves
1-pound chicken tenders, cut into 1⁄2"-thick crosswise slices
1⁄4 cup sunflower oil
12 ounces bok choy, cut into 1⁄2"-thick crosswise slices
1⁄4 cup low-sodium chicken broth
1 tablespoon gluten-free tamari
Crushed red-pepper flakes

1. In a large bowl, combine the garlic, ginger, salt, pepper, fennel seeds, and cloves. Add the chicken. With your hands or a fork, toss well to coat all of the pieces with the seasoning.
2. Place a wok or large skillet over medium-high heat until very hot. Add the oil and swirl to coat the pan. Place the chicken pieces in the pan so they are separated.
3. Cook for 2 to 3 minutes, turning once, or until browned on both sides.
4. Reduce the heat to medium-high. Add the bok choy. Cook, tossing, for 2 minutes, or until the leaves begin to wilt. Add the broth and tamari. Bring to a boil, reduce the heat, and simmer for 2 minutes, or until the chicken is no longer pink and the juices run clear.
5. Serve, garnished with pepper flakes.

Per serving: 272 calories, 26 g protein, 3 g carbohydrates, 1 g fiber, 17 g total fat, 2 g saturated fat, 637 mg sodium

Spiced Pecans

Makes 4 servings

1 cup raw pecans
1 tablespoon honey
1 teaspoon extra virgin olive oil
1/8 teaspoon ground cinnamon
1/8 teaspoon ground ginger
1/8 teaspoon salt
1/4 teaspoon ground black pepper

1. Preheat the oven to 300°F.
2. In a small bowl, combine the pecans, honey, and oil. Add the cinnamon, ginger, salt, and pepper and toss to coat. Spread on a baking sheet and bake for 15 minutes, stirring once. Cool slightly before serving.

Per serving: 215 calories, 3 g protein, 8 g carbohydrates, 3 g fiber, 21 g total fat, 2 g saturated fat, 73 mg sodium

Snacking Nuts

Makes 12 servings

2 teaspoons olive or sesame oil
4 cups mixed raw nuts
1 teaspoon garlic powder
1/2 teaspoon ground cumin
1/4 teaspoon ground turmeric

1. Preheat the oven to 375°F.
2. In a medium bowl, stir together the oil, nuts, garlic powder, cumin, and turmeric.
3. Spread on a rimmed baking sheet and bake for 12 to 15 minutes, or until toasted. Store the nuts in an airtight container. Keeps for 2 weeks.

Per serving: 231 calories, 4 g protein, 5 g carbohydrates, 3 g fiber, 24 g total fat, 2 g saturated fat, 1 mg sodium

Roasted Kale Chips

Makes 4 servings

2 bunches kale (about 2–2½ pounds), hard stems removed, chopped finely
(about 9 cups chopped)
¼ cup coconut or extra virgin olive oil
¼ teaspoon kosher salt
¼ teaspoon ground black pepper
2 tablespoons nutritional yeast flakes

1. Arrange 3 oven racks evenly spaced apart in the oven. Preheat the oven to 375°F.
2. In a large bowl, toss the kale with the oil, salt, and pepper.
3. Arrange on 3 baking pans or roast kale in batches. (It's important to roast kale with lots of space. If kale is too tight on the pan, it will steam rather than roast and will never get crispy.) Roast for 15 minutes, or until crisp. Sprinkle with yeast flakes.

Per serving: 207 calories, 8 g protein, 15 g carbohydrates, 4 g fiber, 16 g total fat, 12 g saturated fat, 179 mg sodium

Avocado Salsa

Makes 4 servings

1 ripe avocado
1 tablespoon finely chopped red onion
2 scallions, minced
1 tablespoon finely chopped jalapeño chili pepper
(wear plastic gloves when handling)
1 Roma tomato, seeded and chopped
1 tablespoon lime juice
1 tablespoon coarsely chopped cilantro
1 clove garlic, minced
¼ teaspoon ground cumin
Pinch of salt
Pinch of ground black pepper
Carrot and celery sticks, for serving

1. In a large bowl, mash the avocado. Add the onion, scallions, jalapeño pepper, tomato, lime juice, cilantro, and garlic and stir to combine. Stir in the cumin, salt, and black pepper.

2.   Serve with carrot and celery sticks.

Per serving: 66 calories, 1 g protein, 5 g carbohydrates, 3 g fiber, 5 g total fat, 1 g saturated fat, 114 mg sodium

Eggplant Dip
Makes 6 servings

2 large eggplants (about 2 pounds total), halved lengthwise
1 large onion (unpeeled), halved
3 tablespoons lemon juice (from 11/2 lemons)
3 cloves garlic, minced
1 tablespoon tahini (sesame paste)
1–2 tablespoons water
1/4 cup olive oil
11/2 teaspoons salt
2 tablespoons chopped fresh parsley

1.   Preheat the oven to 425°F. Line a baking sheet with foil and brush with olive oil.
2.   Place the eggplants and onion cut side down on the baking sheet. Bake for 30 minutes, or until soft and caramelized. Let stand until cool enough to handle.
3.   In a medium bowl, combine the lemon juice, garlic, and tahini. Stir in 1 tablespoon of the water. Scrape the seeds from the eggplant and discard. Scrape out the remaining flesh, put in a strainer, and press out as much liquid as possible with the back of a spoon. Add to the bowl. Peel and chop the onion. Add to the bowl.
4.   Stir in the oil and salt. Add the remaining 1 tablespoon water if needed to reach desired consistency. Sprinkle with the parsley before serving.

Per serving: 139 calories, 2 g protein, 11 g carbohydrates, 4 g fiber, 11 g total fat, 1 g saturated fat, 587 mg sodium

Nut and Seed Clusters
Makes 8 servings

1 tablespoon ground white chia seeds
3 tablespoons water
1 tablespoon honey

1 teaspoon ground cinnamon
1 teaspoon ground ginger
1/4 teaspoon ground cardamom
1/2 cup pecans, chopped
1/2 cup almonds, chopped
1/2 cup raw pumpkin seeds (pepitas)
1/4 cup sesame seeds

1. Preheat the oven to 350°F. Line a baking sheet with parchment paper.
2. In a small bowl, soak the chia seeds in the water for 5 minutes.
3. In a medium bowl, whisk the seed mixture, honey, cinnamon, ginger, and cardamom. Add the pecans, almonds, pumpkin seeds, and sesame seeds and toss to coat well. Spread the mixture onto the parchment paper. Bake for 20 minutes, or until browned.
4. Cool on a rack for 30 minutes, or until cooled. Break into bite-size pieces.

Per serving: 182 calories, 6 g protein, 8 g carbohydrates, 3 g fiber, 16 g total fat, 0 g saturated fat, 3 mg sodium

Vegetarian and Vegan Paleo-type Diet

It is more challenging to put together a low-carb, anti-inflammatory diet as a vegetarian or vegan, but it is possible. Vegetarians and vegans will need to eat legumes to get enough protein, and this is not the "classic Paleo." What is enough protein? Even for the most sedentary person, .36 grams per pound is the current recommended daily amount (RDA). For a more active person, you will need more protein, and there is some evidence that doubling this amount can be beneficial. That said, you can get 60 grams of protein from ¾ cup of mature roasted soy beans. Vegetarians will get their main proteins from eggs, legumes, nuts and seeds, and vegans will use legumes, nuts and seeds. One great thing about this diet for vegans and vegetarians is that fruits and vegetables contribute a greater percentage of daily intake because there is not a "fallback" to grains. And, so-called "pseudocereals"—quinoa, amaranth, buckwheat—can be a great resource. For example, quinoa is more related to spinach and beets than it is to grains, but makes a great hot cereal, stuffing, or base for tabbouleh. Wild rice is also good. It is not a grain, but an aquatic grass. One of my grandnieces is vegan. This thanksgiving, we made a great stuffing with organic vegetable broth, wild rice, mushrooms, almonds and dried cranberries, cooked in a slow cooker. There wasn't much left over because it was so good that everyone else ate it too. Here is the recipe from Erin Clarke, at www.wellplated.com.

Ingredients:

2 tablespoons extra virgin olive oil
1 small yellow onion, diced
2 ribs celery, finely sliced
16 ounces cremini (baby bella) mushrooms, sliced
1/2 teaspoon kosher salt
1/4 teaspoon black pepper
2 1/2 cups uncooked brown and wild rice blend, rinsed and drained
5 1/2 cups low sodium vegetable broth (I use organic)
2/3 cup reduced sugar dried cranberries (I use fruit sweetened dried cranberries)
1 tablespoon chopped fresh sage
1 tablespoon chopped fresh thyme
1/2 cup slivered almonds, toasted

Directions:

1. In a large skillet, heat the olive oil over medium. Add the onions and celery and let cook, stirring occasionally, until the onion is softened and lightly brown, about 8 minutes. Increase the heat to medium high, then add the mushrooms. Let cook, stirring often, until the mushrooms are soft and most of the liquid has evaporated, about 6 minutes. Stir in 1/2 teaspoon salt and 1/4 teaspoon pepper. Remove from heat and set aside.

2. In a 3 or 4-quart slow cooker, stir together the wild rice blend and sautéed vegetables. Carefully pour in the chicken broth (if using a 3-quart slow cooker, it will be full nearly to the top). Gently stir, then cover and cook on low for 5 to 6 hours or high for 2 to 3 hours, until the rice is tender. Turn off the slow cooker, then stir in the cranberries, sage, and thyme. Taste and add additional salt and/or pepper as desired. Cover and let stand 10 minutes. Just before serving, sprinkle the toasted almonds over the top. Serve warm.

Leftover Crock Pot Stuffing with Wild Rice can be stored in an airtight container in the refrigerator for up to four days or frozen for up to two months.

Make it ahead: the celery, mushrooms, and onions can be sautéed up to 2 days in advance and stored in the refrigerator. Add all the ingredients to the crock pot just before cooking.

NUTRITION FACTS
Serving Size: 1 (of 12, about 1 cup)

Amount Per Serving:

Calories: 218
Total Fat: 6g
Saturated Fat: 1g
Cholesterol: 0mg
Sodium: 248mg
Carbohydrates: 38g
Fiber: 7g
Sugar: 3g
Protein: 7g

This is only the beginning of your adventures with paleo recipes. They are widely available online, and there are many good recipe books. Happy eating!

Acknowledgments

Dean Gwynne R. Winsberg, Ph.D. Without her pioneering spirit and belief that there should be more women, and older people with some life experience in medical school, I would not have been accepted to medical school, and would never have written this book.

Robert Carlson, MD for his skill in teaching the value of compassion in medicine, and for being a living example of Dr. William Osler's principle, "Listen to your patient. He is telling you the diagnosis."

Frank R. Murphy, MD for mentoring me in critical thinking, and showing me that reactions to food can be the source of many illnesses.

Gene Arbetter for years of loving kindness, skill, and untold contributions at home and at work.

Sarah Howard for her love, generosity, and encouragement to look at the "upside".

David Howard for his love, sense of humor, and ability to laugh in the face of the apocalypse.

Atyani Howard for her love, encouragement and skill in reading and commenting on the manuscript, and for her suggestions about the Council in Schools program.

Chris Costas, MD for 38 years of friendship, for his laughing, loving support through medical school, and for his generous help in working with Wellness of Chicago.

Laura Lim for her kindness, intelligence, and skill in making contributions to the practice and to the book.

Sara Altshul for her friendship, writing skill, and many contributions to the book.

Rachel Lyon for 50 years of friendship, and her insistence that I must write a book about what I do.

Valerie Mrak for her friendship, and support since the 90's, and for cheering me on during the creation of this book.

Belleruth Naparstek, LCSW, for friendship, support, inspiration, and for her pioneer spirit and tireless work in bringing guided imagery into the mainstream of health care.

Diane Rapaport, MD, for hauling me into medical school, for her view of the health care apocalypse, and for being my friend for more than 40 years.

Alina Frank for her brilliant mentoring in EFT, and her encouragement and support for the publication of the book.

Lisa Bess Kramer for her personal touch in editing.

Victor Popoola for amazing editing skills, understanding, and patience.

Howard Wolinsky for his inspiring medical reporting, and his dedication to keeping the medical profession honest.

About the Author

Martha H. Howard, MD

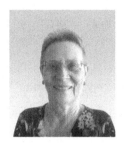 At the age of 30, I was teaching Chinese history and theater, and taking classes in social work. On my way to a class, I was sitting at a stop light with my turn signal on, and a drunk driver plowed into my car at 55 miles an hour! The accident broke my neck. In the process of recovering, I got very little help from the health care industry. Their first action was to misread my x-ray and send me out of the emergency room with a soft cervical collar and a broken neck. I was in constant pain. I went back to get help but was told I just had to "live with it" and take pain pills. Fortunately, in a few years, I did get help from an acupuncturist. After three months of treatment, my constant pain was almost gone, and I was sold on acupuncture! I studied for two years in an apprenticeship with the acupuncturist who had helped me, and then was surprised to learn that although acupuncture and Traditional Chinese Medicine had become board-certified specialties in California in 1974, the practice of acupuncture was in a legal "gray area" in Illinois. It turned out I would have to be an M.D., D.O. or chiropractor to practice acupuncture legally in Illinois in 1978. I decided to become an M.D. (Acupuncture was not officially a licensed specialty in Illinois until 20 year later, so as the years went by, and the fight to get acupuncture licensed here dragged on, I was happy that I had made that decision!) I was lucky enough to get accepted to Loyola University Stritch School of Medicine at the age of 38 and graduated in 1982. After medical school, I did a three-year residency in Family Practice, and then worked for four years in the National Health Service Corps. Then I started an integrative practice, Wellness Associates of Chicago, and I am still working in that practice. Along the way, I have served on the boards of the American Association of Acupuncture and Oriental Medicine (AAAOM) and the National Institute for the Clinical Application of Behavioral Medicine. I have earned national board certification in Acupuncture from the National Commission on Acupuncture and Oriental Medicine [129], have maintained my board-eligible status in Family Practice, and have been certified as a practitioner of EFT. I live in Chicago with my husband Gene. We have five children and eight grandchildren.

Bibliography

PART I NOTES

Brown, T. (2015). "100 Best-Selling, Most Prescribed Branded Drugs Through March." Retrieved Nov 21, 2017, from https://www.medscape.com/viewarticle/844317.

Buttorff, C., et al. (2017). Multiple Chronic Conditions in the United States. Santa Monica, CA, RAND Corporation.

CDC (2017). "Infographic: Antibiotic Resistance The Global Threat." Retrieved Nov 20, 2017, from https://www.cdc.gov/globalhealth/infographics/antibiotic-resistance/antibiotic_resistance_global_threat.htm

CDC (2017). "Opioid Overdose." Retrieved Nov 20, 2017, from https://www.cdc.gov/drugoverdose/.

Center, J. D. (2017). "Oral Diabetes Medications Summary Chart." Retrieved Vov 18, 2017, from joslin.org/info/oral_diabetes_medications_summary_chart.html.

Cha, A. (2016). "Researchers: Medical errors now third leading cause of death in the United States." Washington Post. Retrieved Nov 18, 2017, from https://www.washingtonpost.com/news/to-your-health/wp/2016/05/03/researchers-medical-errors-now-third-leading-cause-of-death-in-united-states/?utm_term=.1e0c1c1bc6ea.

Davis, K., et al. (2014). "Mirror, Mirror on the Wall, 2014 Update: How the U.S. Health Care System Compares Internationally, The Commonwealth Fund, June 2014.". Retrieved Nov 20, 2017, from http://www.commonwealthfund.org/publications/fund-reports/2014/jun/mirror-mirror.

Dueñas-Laita, A., et al. (2009). "Hypersensitivity to Generic Drugs with Soybean Oil." New England Journal of Medicine 361(13): 1317-1318.

Edney, A. (2014). "Drug Quality in China Still Poses Risks for U.S. Market." Retrieved Nov 19, 2017, from www.bloomberg.com/news/print2014-04-03/drug-quality-in-china-still-poses-risks-for-u-s-market.html.

eDrugSearch (2017). "New Chart Exposes the Inhumanity of US Drug Prices Compared to Other Countries." Retrieved Nov 20, 2017, from https://edrugsearch.com/chart-inhumanity-us-drug-prices/.

ewg (2017). "Nation's Pediatricians, EWG Urge EPA to Ban Pesticide that Harms Kids' Brains." Retrieved Nov 23, 2017, from https://www.ewg.org/testimony-official-correspondence/nation-s-pediatricians-ewg-urge-epa-ban-pesticide-harms-kids#.Wf8QZ2hSyyK.

Fluoridation (nd). "Fluoridation status of some countries." Retrieved Nov 21, 2017, from http://www.fluoridation.com/c-country.htm.

Hedlund, B. (2017). "Homepage." Retrieved Nov 23, 2017, from www.baumhedlundlaw.com.

Huen, K., et al. (2012). "Organophosphate pesticide levels in blood and urine of women and newborns living in an agricultural community." Environ Res 117: 8-16.

Johnson, D. A. and E. C. Oldfield (2013). "Reported side effects and complications of long-term proton pump inhibitor use: dissecting the evidence." Clinical gastroenterology and hepatology 11(5): 458-464.

Jones, C. M., et al. (2014). "Alcohol involvement in opioid pain reliever and benzodiazepine drug abuse-related emergency department visits and drug-related deaths-United States, 2010." MMWR Morb Mortal Wkly Rep 63(40): 881-885.

Kantor, E. D., et al. (2015). "Trends in prescription drug use among adults in the United States from 1999-2012." JAMA 314(17): 1818-1830.

Kearns, C., et al. (2016). "Sugar Industry and Coronary Heart Disease Research: A Historical Analysis of Internal Industry Documents." JAMA 176(11): 1680-1685.

Makary, M. and M. Daniel (2016). "Medical Errors—The Third Leading Cause of Death in the US." BMJ 353.

McLean, B. (2015). Everything You Know About Martin Shkreli Is Wrong—Or Is It?" Vanity Fair.

Meier, B. (2007). Narcotics Maker Guilty of Deceit Over Marketing. The New York Times/Business Day. The New York Times/Business Day.

Moss, M. (2013). Salt Sugar Fat: How the Food Giants Hooked Us. , 2013. New York City, NY, Random House Publishing Group.

Network, F. A. (2007, 2007). "Statements from European Health, Water & Environment Authorities on Water Fluoridation." Retrieved Nov 21, 2017.

Network, F. A. (2017). "National Research Council." Retrieved Nov 21, 2017, from fluoridealert.org/researchers/nrc/findings/.

NIDA (2017, Sept 2017). "Overdose Death Rates." Retrieved Nov 20, 2017, from https://www.drugabuse.gov/related-topics/trends-statistics/overdose-death-rates.

NIH (2017). "Understand your risk for high blood pressure." Retrieved Nov 20, 2017, from nhlbi.nih.gov/health-topics/topics/hbp/printall-index.html; heart.org/HEARTORG/Conditions/HighBloodPressure/UnderstandYourRiskForHighBloodPressure/Understand-Your-Risk-For-High-Blood-Pressure_UCM_002052_Article.jsp;.

Potter, K., et al. (2016). "Deprescribing in frail older people: a randomised controlled trial." PLoS one 11(3): e0149984.

Reeve, E., et al. (2015). "A systematic review of the emerging definition of 'deprescribing' with network analysis: implications for future research and clinical practice." British journal of clinical pharmacology 80(6): 1254-1268.

Sarpatwari, A., et al. (2017). "The Opioid Epidemic: Fixing a Broken Pharmaceutical Market"." Harvard Law and Policy Review 11: 463-484.

Spain, E. (2014). "Scientists Find Heart Disease Can Be Reversed by Adopting Healthy Habits." Retrieved Nov 22, 2017, from feinberg.northwestern.edu/news/2014/06/reverse_heart_disease.html.

Sugiyama, T., et al. (2014). "Different time trends of caloric and fat intake between statin users and nonusers among US adults: gluttony in the time of statins?" JAMA internal medicine 174(7): 1038-1045.

Walker, E. R. and B. G. Druss (2017). "Cumulative burden of comorbid mental disorders, substance use disorders, chronic medical conditions, and poverty on health among adults in the USA." Psychology, health & medicine 22(6): 727-735.

Whittaker, B. (2017). Ex-DEA agent: Opioid crisis fueled by drug industry and Congress. CBS News 60 Minutes Politics, CBS News.

Will, M. (2017, Jan13, 2017). "The 16 countries with the world's best healthcare systems." Retrieved Nov 18, 2017, from http://nordic.businessinsider.com/the-16-countries-with-the-worlds-best-healthcare-systems-2017-1/.

Zhong, W., et al. (2013). Age and sex patterns of drug prescribing in a defined American population. Mayo Clinic Proceedings, Elsevier.

PART II NOTES

aafa (2017). "Allergies." Retrieved Nov 21, 2017, from aafa.org/display.cfm?id=9&sub=24&cont=34.

Abas, F., et al. (2006). "Biological evaluation of curcumin and related diarylheptanoids." Zeitschrift für Naturforschung C, **61**(9-10): 625-631.

Abbasi, B., et al. (2012). "The effect of magnesium supplementation on primary insomnia in elderly: A double-blind placebo-controlled clinical trial." Journal of research in medical sciences: the official journal of Isfahan University of Medical Sciences, **17**(12): 1161.

Abramson, J. and R. Redberg (2013). "Don't Give More Patients Statins." Retrieved Nov 22, 2017, from http://www.nytimes.com/2013/11/14/opinion/dont-give-more-patients-statins.html.

ADAA (2016). "Generalized Anxiety Disorder (GAD." Understanding the facts. Retrieved Nov 23, 2017, from adaa.org/understanding-anxiety/generalized-anxiety-disorder-gad.

ADAA (2016). "Medication." Retrieved Nov 23, 2017, from adaa.org/finding-help/treatment/medication.

ADAA (2016). "Symptoms." Retrieved Nov 23, 2017, from https://adaa.org/understanding-anxiety/generalized-anxiety-disorder-gad/symptoms.

AHA (2014, Oct 24, 2016). "Atherosclerosis and Stroke." Retrieved Nov 22, 2017, from strokeassociation.org/STROKEORG/LifeAfterStroke/HealthyLivingAfterStroke/UnderstandingRiskyConditions/Atherosclerosis-and-Stroke_UCM_310426_Article.jsp.

AHA (2014). "High stress, hostility, depression linked with increased stroke risk." Retrieved Nov 23, 2017, from http://newsroom.heart.org/news/high-stress-hostility-depression-linked-with-increased-stroke-risk.

AHA (2017). "The American Heart Association's Diet and Lifestyle Recommendations." Retrieved Nov 25, 2017, from http://www.heart.org/HEARTORG/GettingHealthy/NutritionCenter/HealthyEating/Trans-Fats_UCM_301120_Article.jsp.

AHA (2017). "What is cardiovascular disease?". Retrieved Nov 22, 2017, from heart.org/HEARTORG/Caregiver/Resources/WhatisCardiovascularDisease/ What-is-Cardiovascular-Disease_UCM_301852_Article.jsp.

AHA (nd). "Eating probiotics regularly may improve your blood pressure." Retrieved Nov 25, 2017, from http://newsroom.heart.org/news/eating-probiotics-regularly-may-improve-your-blood-%20pressure.

Akbaraly, T., et al. (2013). "Does overall diet in midlife predict future aging phenotypes? A cohort study." The American journal of medicine, 126(5): 411-419. e413.

Altshul, S. (2013). Get a leg up on diabetes, Prevention.

Altshul, S. (2013). Outsmart diabetes, Prevention.

Altshul, S. (2014). "21 Healing Herbs and Supplements Doctors Prescribe." Retrieved Nov 24, 2017, from https://www.prevention.com/mind-body/herbs-and-supplements-natural-remedies-doctors-prescribe.

Altshul, S. (2014). "Docs gone wild." Retrieved Nov 23, 2017.

AMA (nd). "Human Microbiome." Retrieved Nov 26, 2017, from academy.asm.org/images/stories/documents/FAQ_Human_Microbiome.pdf.

Amsterdam, J. D., et al. (2012). "Chamomile (matricaria recutita) may have antidepressant activity in anxious depressed humans-an exploratory study." Alternative therapies in health and medicine, 18(5): 44.

Anglia, U. o. E. (2011, Jan 15, 2011). "Eating blueberries can guard against high blood pressure, according to new research." Retrieved Nov 23, 2017, from sciencedaily.com/releases/2011/01/110114155241.htm.

Arnadottir, T. S. and A. K. Sigurdardottir (2013). "Is craniosacral therapy effective for migraine? Tested with HIT-6 Questionnaire." Complementary therapies in clinical practice, 19(1): 11-14.

Babyak, M., et al. (2000). "Exercise treatment for major depression: maintenance of therapeutic benefit at 10 months." Psychosomatic medicine, 62(5): 633-638.
Beck (2016). "What is Cognitive Behavior Therapy (CBT)?". Retrieved Nov 25, 2017, from https://beckinstitute.org/get-informed/what-is-cognitive-therapy/.

Bernardy, K., et al. (2012). "Cognitive behavioural therapies for fibromyalgia syndrome." The Cochrane database of systematic reviews, 9.

Bhatt, J. K., et al. (2012). "Resveratrol supplementation improves glycemic control in type 2 diabetes mellitus." Nutrition research, 32(7): 537-541.

Blumenthal, J. A., et al. (2007). "Exercise and pharmacotherapy in the treatment of major depressive disorder." Psychosomatic medicine, 69(7): 587.

Blumenthal, J. A., et al. (1999). "Effects of exercise training on older patients with major depression." Archives of internal medicine, 159(19): 2349-2356.

Blumenthal, J. A., et al. (2003). "Depression as a risk factor for mortality after coronary artery bypass surgery." The Lancet, 362(9384): 604-609.

Blumenthal, J. A., et al. (2012). "Is exercise a viable treatment for depression?" ACSM's health & fitness journal, 16(4): 14.

Bredesen, D. E. (2014). "Reversal of cognitive decline: A novel therapeutic program." Aging (Albany NY), 6(9): 707.

Breus, M. J. (2013). "Kiwi: Super Food for Sleep?". Retrieved Nov 26, 2017, from psychologytoday.com/blog/sleep-newzzz/201311/kiwi-super-food-sleep.

Brooks, M. (2017). "Antidepressants Tied to a Significantly Increased Risk for Death." Retrieved Nov 23, 2017, from https://www.medscape.com/viewarticle/886015.

Castano, G., et al. (2001). "Effects of policosanol 20 versus 40 mg/day in the treatment of patients with type II hypercholesterolemia: a 6-month double-blind study." International journal of clinical pharmacology research, 21(1): 43-57.

Castro-Marrero, J., et al. (2015). Does oral coenzyme Q10 plus NADH supplementation improve fatigue and biochemical parameters in chronic fatigue syndrome?, Mary Ann Liebert, Inc. 140 Huguenot Street, 3rd Floor New Rochelle, NY 10801 USA.

CDC (2017, March 17, 2017). "Leading causes of death." Retrieved Nov 23, 2017, from cdc.gov/nchs/fastats/leading-causes-of-death.htm.

CDC (2017, Nov 7, 2017). "Myalgic Encephalomyelitis/Chronic Fatigue Syndrome." Retrieved Nov 23, 2017, from cdc.gov/cfs/symptoms/.

CDC (nd). "Pennsylvania." Retrieved Nov 25, 2017, from https://www.cdc.gov/diabetes/prevention/recognition/states/Pennsylvania.%20ht m?choice=states%2FPennsylvania.htm.

Chatzi, L., et al. (2007). "Protective effect of fruits, vegetables and the Mediterranean diet on asthma and allergies among children in Crete." Thorax, **62**(8): 677-683.

Chawla, J. (2017). "Migraine Headache Treatment & Management." Retrieved Nov 24, 2017, from emedicine.medscape.com/article/1142556-treatment.

Chiu, H.-Y., et al. (2015). "Effects of acupuncture on menopause-related symptoms and quality of life in women in natural menopause: a meta-analysis of randomized controlled trials." Menopause, **22**(2): 234-244.

Clinic, C. (2015). "Menopause & Osteoporosis." Retrieved Nov 26, 2017, from my.clevelandclinic.org/health/diseases_conditions/hic-what-is-perimenopause-menopause-postmenopause/hic_Menopause_and_Osteoporosis.

Clinic, M. (2017, Oct 5, 2017). "Chronic fatigue syndrome." Retrieved Nov 23, 2017, from mayoclinic.org/diseases-conditions/chronic-fatigue-syndrome/basics/treatment/ con-20022009.

Cohen, H. (2016, July 17, 2016). "Depression versus Anxiety." Retrieved Nov 23, 2017, from https://www.nimh.nih.gov/health/topics/depression/index.shtml.

Connect, N. (nd). "Sinusitis: Dietary and Lifestyle Recommendations to improve symptoms." Retrieved Nov 26, 2017, from naturopathconnect.com/articles/sinusitis-dietary/.

consumerlab.com (2012, Apr 5, 2016). "Product Review: Acetyl-L-Carnitine Supplements Review." Retrieved Nov 23, 2017, from consumerlab.com/reviews/Acetyl-L-Carnitine-Supplements-Review/Acetyl-L-Carnitine/.

consumerlab.com (nd). "Turmeric curcumin supplements spice review." Retrieved Nov 25, 2017, from https://www.consumerlab.com/reviews/turmeric-curcumin-supplements-spice-review/%20turmeric/.

Cordero, M. D., et al. (2013). Can coenzyme q10 improve clinical and molecular parameters in fibromyalgia?, Mary Ann Liebert, Inc. 140 Huguenot Street, 3rd Floor New Rochelle, NY 10801 USA.

Crosta, P. (2017). "What is Lyrica (pregabalin)?: Uses, dosage, and side effects." Retrieved Nov 23, 2017, from medicalnewstoday.com/articles/151139.php.

Dog, T. L. (2013). "3 Ways To Cool Hot Flashes." Retrieved Nov 26, 2017, from https://www.prevention.com/health/health-concerns/natural-remedies-hot-flashes.

Drugs.com (2014). "U.S. Pharmaceutical Sales - Q4 2013." Retrieved Nov 23, 2017, from https://www.drugs.com/stats/top100/sales.

drweil (nd). "Irritable Bowel Syndrome." Retrieved Nov 26, 2017, from https://www.drweil.com/.

eatright (2017). "Understanding the New Nutrition Facts Label." Retrieved Nov 23, 2017, from eatright.org/Public/content.aspx?id=6442472548.

ewg (2016). "Homepage." Retrieved Nov 25, 2016, from https://www.ewg.org/.

Feinman, R. D., et al. (2015). "Dietary carbohydrate restriction as the first approach in diabetes management: critical review and evidence base." Nutrition, **31**(1): 1-13.

fmswaws (2014). "Treatments-Medications." Retrieved Nov 23, 2017, from fmswaws.org/medications.html.

Foundation, A. (2012). "Cause of Osteoarthritis." Retrieved Nov 21, 2017, from arthritistoday.org/about-arthritis/types-of-arthritis/osteoarthritis/who-gets-oa-and-why/cause-of-osteoarthritis.php.

Foundation, A. (2012, 2012). "Snow conference." Retrieved Nov 21, 2017, from arthritistoday.org/about-arthritis/types-of-arthritis/osteoarthritis/treatment-plan/snow-conference-2012.php.

Foundation, A. (nd). "Osteoarthritis." Retrieved Nov 21, 2017, from arthritis.org/arthritis-facts/disease-center/osteoarthritis.php.

Friedman, R. (2012). "A Call for Caution on Antipsychotic Drugs." Retrieved Nov 23, 2017, from http://www.nytimes.com/2012/09/25/health/a-call-for-caution-in-the-use-of-antipsychotic-drugs.html.

Fujimura, K. E., et al. (2010). "Role of the gut microbiota in defining human health." Expert review of anti-infective therapy, **8**(4): 435-454.

Givi, M. (2013). "Durability of effect of massage therapy on blood pressure." International journal of preventive medicine, **4**(5): 511.

Glatthaar-Saalmüller, B., et al. (2011). "Antiviral activity in vitro of two preparations of the herbal medicinal product Sinupret® against viruses causing respiratory infections." Phytomedicine, **19**(1): 1-7.

Gray, S. L., et al. (2015). "Cumulative use of strong anticholinergics and incident dementia: a prospective cohort study." JAMA internal medicine, **175**(3): 401-407.

Grisanti, R. (nd). "Insomnia Solution." Retrieved Nov 26, 2017, from functionalmedicineuniversity.com/public/906.cfm.

Gulati, S., et al. (2014). "Effects of pistachio nuts on body composition, metabolic, inflammatory and oxidative stress parameters in Asian Indians with metabolic syndrome: a 24-wk, randomized control trial." Nutrition, **30**(2): 192-197.

Gulliver, W. P. and H. J. Donsky (2005). "A report on three recent clinical trials using Mahonia aquifolium 10% topical cream and a review of the worldwide clinical experience with Mahonia aquifolium for the treatment of plaque psoriasis." American journal of therapeutics, **12**(5): 398-406.

Gunn, J., et al. (2013). Diabetes and Natural Products. San Diego, CA, Academic Press

Habashy, J., et al. (2017). "Psoriasis." Retrieved Nov 24, 2017, from https://emedicine.medscape.com/article/1943419-overview.

Harrar, S. and S. A. O'Donnell (1999). The Woman's Book of Healing Herbs: healing teas, tonics, supplements, and formulas, Rodale Press.

Hastings, D. (2013, Jan 23, 2013). "The 25 Best Foods for Your Heart." Retrieved Nov 22, 2017, from https://www.prevention.com/health/health-concerns/best-foods-for-heart-health?s=25.

Häuser, W., et al. (2010). "Efficacy of different types of aerobic exercise in fibromyalgia syndrome: a systematic review and meta-analysis of randomised controlled trials." Arthritis research & therapy, **12**(3): R79.

Health, N. L. (2017). "Conditions we treat." Retrieved Nov 21, 2017, from med.nyu.edu/content?ChunkIID=21574.

Herber-Gast, G.-C. M. and G. D. Mishra (2013). "Fruit, Mediterranean-style, and high-fat and-sugar diets are associated with the risk of night sweats and hot flushes in midlife: results from a prospective cohort study." The American journal of clinical nutrition, **97**(5): 1092-1099.

HSPH (2017). "Fats and Cholesterol." Retrieved Nov 22, 2017, from hsph.harvard.edu/nutritionsource/fats-full-story/.

Huth, T., et al. (2016). "Pilot study of natural killer cells in chronic fatigue syndrome/myalgic encephalomyelitis and multiple sclerosis." Scandinavian journal of immunology, **83**(1): 44-51.

Hypertension-cholesterol (nd). "Hypertension." Retrieved Nov 23, 2017, from http://hypertension-cholesterol.com/hypertension-cholesterol/hypertension-1-2557.%20html.

Institute, S. A. (nd). "DSM-5 Definition of Social Anxiety Disorder." Retrieved Nov 24, 2017, from socialanxietyinstitute.org/dsm-definition-social-anxiety-disorder.

Javed, Y. and A. Zagham (2016). "Role of Omega-3 Fatty Acids in Irritable Bowel Syndrome (IBS)." International Journal of Pharmacological Research **6**(8): 1-6.

Jones, C. M., et al. (2014). "Alcohol involvement in opioid pain reliever and benzodiazepine drug abuse-related emergency department visits and drug-related deaths-United States, 2010." MMWR Morb Mortal Wkly Rep, **63**(40): 881-885.

Kaplan, M. (2014). "Worn Out At the Finish Line." Retrieved Nov 22, 2017, from http://anapsid.org/cnd/coping/hillenbrand.html.

Katta, R. and S. P. Desai (2014). "Diet and dermatology: the role of dietary intervention in skin disease." The Journal of clinical and aesthetic dermatology, **7**(7): 46.

Kemps, E., et al. (2014). "Exposure to television food advertising primes food-related cognitions and triggers motivation to eat." Psychology & health, **29**(10): 1192-1205.

Khalsa, S. B. S. (2004). "Treatment of chronic insomnia with yoga: a preliminary study with sleep–wake diaries." Applied psychophysiology and biofeedback, **29**(4): 269-278.

Khanna, S. and P. K. Tosh (2014). A clinician's primer on the role of the microbiome in human health and disease. Mayo Clinic Proceedings, Elsevier.

Kim, J., et al. (2009). "Comparative clinical trial of S-adenosylmethionine versus nabumetone for the treatment of knee osteoarthritis: an 8-week, multicenter, randomized, double-blind, double-dummy, Phase IV study in Korean patients." Clinical therapeutics, **31**(12): 2860-2872.

Kling, J. (2000). "he Strange Case of Premarin." <u>Modern Drug Discovery</u>, **3**(8): 46-52.

Ladabaum, U., et al. (2014). "Obesity, abdominal obesity, physical activity, and caloric intake in US adults: 1988 to 2010." <u>The American journal of medicine</u>, **127**(8): 717-727. e712.

Lashner, B. (2014). "Best and Worst Foods for IBS." Retrieved Nov 23, 2017, from health.clevelandclinic.org/2014/02/take-control-of-ibs-with-low-fodmap-diet/.

Lawler, S. P. and L. D. Cameron (2006). "A randomized, controlled trial of massage therapy as a treatment for migraine." <u>Annals of Behavioral Medicine</u>, **32**(1): 50-59.

Lee, T. (2010). "Ask the doctor: Is no-flush niacin as effective as other types of niacin?." Retrieved Nov 23, 2017, from https://www.health.harvard.edu/newsletter_article/is-no-flush-niacin-as-effective-as-other-kinds-of-niacin.

Lewis, J. E., et al. (2013). "The effect of methylated vitamin B complex on depressive and anxiety symptoms and quality of life in adults with depression." <u>ISRN</u> psychiatry, **2013**.

Lian, X.-Q., et al. (2014). "The influence of regular walking at different times of day on blood lipids and inflammatory markers in sedentary patients with coronary artery disease." <u>Preventive medicine</u>**58**: 64-69.

Lin, H.-H., et al. (2011). "Effect of kiwifruit consumption on sleep quality in adults with sleep problems." <u>Asia Pacific journal of clinical nutrition</u>, **20**(2): 169-174. Lopresti, A. L., et al. (2014). "Curcumin for the treatment of major depression: a randomised, double-blind, placebo controlled study." <u>Journal of affective disorders</u>, **167**: 368-375.

Lv, H. and G. She (2010). "Naturally occurring diarylheptanoids." <u>Natural product communications</u>, **5**(10): 1687-1708.

Maghbooli, M., et al. (2014). "Comparison between the efficacy of ginger and sumatriptan in the ablative treatment of the common migraine." <u>Phytotherapy research</u>, **28**(3): 412-415.

Markham, H. (2013). "4 Ways to Fight Your Night Sweats." Retrieved Nov 26, 2017, from prevention.com/health/health-concerns/activity-linked-fewer-night-sweats-menopause.

Marshall-Gradisnik, S. M., et al. (2015). "Examination of single nucleotide polymorphisms (SNPs) in transient receptor potential (TRP) ion channels in chronic fatigue syndrome patients." Immunology and Immunogenetics Insights7: 1.

Maslej, M. M., et al. (2017). "The Mortality and Myocardial Effects of Antidepressants Are Moderated by Preexisting Cardiovascular Disease: A Meta-Analysis." Psychotherapy and Psychosomatics, **86**(5): 268-282.

Masters, P. A. (2014). "Insomnia." Annals of internal medicine, **161**(7): ITC1-ITC1.

Mauskop, A. and B. Fox (2007). What Your Doctor May Not Tell You About (TM): Migraines: The Breakthrough Program That Can Help End Your Pain, Grand Central Publishing.

McIntosh, J. (2016). "Serotonin: Facts, What Does Serotonin Do?". Retrieved Nov 25, 2017, from medicalnewstoday.com/articles/232248.php.

McIntosh, J. (2017). "What's to know about eczema?". Retrieved Nov 24, 2017, from https://www.medicalnewstoday.com/articles/14417.php.

McVeigh, G. (2011). "Mood Booster: B12." Retrieved Nov 24, 2017, from prevention.com/mind-body/natural-remedies/vitamin-b12-and-depression.

Medicinenet (2017). "Aripiprazole (Abilify, Abilify Maintena, Aristrada)." Retrieved Nov 23, 2017, from medicinenet.com/aripiprazole/article.htm.

Medicinenet (2017). "fexofenadine - oral, Allegra." Retrieved Nov 21, 2017, from medicinenet.com/fexofenadine-oral/page2.htm.

MedlinePlus (2014). "Venlafaxine." Retrieved Nov 23, 2017, from nlm.nih.gov/medlineplus/druginfo/meds/a694020.html.

MedlinePlus (2016). "Duloxetine." Retrieved Nov 23, 2017, from https://medlineplus.gov/druginfo/meds/a604030.html.

MedlinePlus (2016). "Sinusitis." Retrieved Nov 26, 2017, from nlm.nih.gov/medlineplus/sinusitis.html.

MedlinePlus (2017, Nov 6, 2017). "High blood pressure - medicine-related." Retrieved Nov 23, 2017, from https://medlineplus.gov/ency/article/000155.htm.

MedlinePlus (2017). "Triglyceride level." Retrieved Nov 21, 2017, from nlm.nih.gov/medlineplus/ency/article/003493.htm.

MedlinePlus (2017, May 15, 2017). "Zolpidem." Retrieved Nov 26, 2017, from nlm.nih.gov/medlineplus/druginfo/meds/a693025.html.

Millsop, J. W., et al. (2014). "Diet and psoriasis, part III: role of nutritional supplements." Journal of the American Academy of Dermatology, 71(3): 561-569.

Milner, J. (nd, nd). "New Insights into the Mechanism of Action of Antioxidants." Retrieved Nov 23, 2017.

MIRECC/CoE (nd). "Benzodiazepines." Retrieved Nov 26, 2017, from https://www.mirecc.va.gov/visn4/bhl/docs/benzodiazepines.pdf.

Mitrou, P., et al. (2015). "Vinegar consumption increases insulin-stimulated glucose uptake by the forearm muscle in humans with type 2 diabetes." Journal of diabetes research, 2015.

Moore, E. M., et al. (2013). "Increased risk of cognitive impairment in patients with diabetes is associated with metformin." Diabetes care, 36(10): 2981-2987.

Naci, H. and J. P. Ioannidis (2013). "Comparative effectiveness of exercise and drug interventions on mortality outcomes: metaepidemiological study." BMJ, 347: f5577.

nccaom (nd). "Home." Retrieved Nov 24, 2017, from nccaom.org.

Newman, A. M. (2011). "The Essential IBS Book: Understanding and Managing Irritable Bowel Syndrome & Functional Dyspepsia. Robert Rose." Inc. Toronto, Canada.

NHF (2012). "Headache Sufferers' Diet." Retrieved Nov 13, 2017, from http://www.headaches.org/2012/01/13/headache-sufferers-diet/.

NHLBI (2015, Sept 10, 2015). "Description of High Blood Pressure`." Retrieved Nov 23, 2017, from nhlbi.nih.gov/health/health-topics/topics/hbp/#.

NIDDK (nd). "Acid Reflux (GER & GERD) in Adults." Retrieved Nov 25, 2017.

NIDDK (nd). "Diabetes Prevention Program." Retrieved Nov 24, 2017, from diabetes.niddk.nih.gov/dm/pubs/preventionprogram.

NIDDK (nd). "Irritable Bowel Syndrome (IBS)." Retrieved Nov 23, 2017, from digestive.niddk.nih.gov/ddiseases/pubs/ibs/.

NIH (2005, June 2005). "High Blood Cholesterol: What You Need to Know." Retrieved Nov 22, 2017, from nhlbi.nih.gov/health/resources/heart/heart-cholesterol-hbc-what-html.htm.

NIH (2014, March 4, 2014). "Prevalence of allergies the same, regardless of where you live." Retrieved Nov 21, 2017, from nih.gov/news/health/mar2014/niehs-04.htm.

NIMH (2016). "Anxiety Disorders." Retrieved Nov 23, 2017, from https://www.nimh.nih.gov/health/topics/anxiety-disorders/index.shtml.

NIMH (2016). "Depression." Retrieved Nov 23, 2017, from nimh.nih.gov/health/topics/depression/index.shtml.

NIMH (2016). "Post-Traumatic Stress Disorder." Retrieved Nov 23, 2017, from https://www.nimh.nih.gov/health/topics/anxiety-disorders/index.shtml.

NINDS (nd). "Brain Basics: Understanding Sleep." Retrieved Nov 23, 2017, from https://www.ninds.nih.gov/Disorders/Patient-Caregiver-Education/Understanding-Sleep.

NLM (nd). "Migraine." Retrieved Nov 25, 2017, from https://www.ncbi.nlm.nih.gov/pubmedhealth/PMHT0024778/.

Novella, S. (2011). "Statins – The Cochrane Review." Retrieved Nov 19, 2017, from sciencebasedmedicine.org/statins-the-cochrane-.

Osher, Y. and R. Belmaker (2009). "Omega-3 fatty acids in depression: A review of three studies." CNS neuroscience & therapeutics, 15(2): 128-133.

Paddock, C. (2012). "Stress may cause illness by changing genes." Retrieved Nov 28, 2017, from https://www.medicalnewstoday.com/articles/249215.php.

Pareek, A., et al. (2011). "Feverfew (Tanacetum parthenium L.): A systematic review." Pharmacognosy reviews 5(9): 103.

Passos, G. S., et al. (2014). "Exercise improves immune function, antidepressive response, and sleep quality in patients with chronic primary insomnia." BioMed research international, 2014.

PCOM (2017). "Improve Your Sinuses Today: What to Eat to Avoid Inflammation." Retrieved Nov 26, 2017, from pacificcollege.edu/acupuncture-massage-news/articles/1126-improve-your- sinuses-today-what-to-eat-to-avoid-inflammation.html.

Pongdee, T. (2012). "Colds, Allergies and Sinusitis—How to Tell the Difference." Retrieved Nov 21, 2017, from aaaai.org/Aaaai/media/MediaLibrary/PDF%20Documents/Libraries/EL- allergies-colds-allergies-sinusitis-patient.pdf.

Prevention (nd). "Eating pepper helps you eat fewer calories." Retrieved Nov 26, 2017, from prevention .com/food/healthy-eating-tips/eating-pepper-helps-you-eat-fewer-calories.

Prevention (nd). "Natural remedies: Safety herbal supplements." Retrieved Nov 24, 2017, from prevention.com/mind-body/natural-remedies/safety-herbal-supplements?page=3&cm_BULbczB8WctNB879b%24ADD8jS47h=1412283273&cm_BUPYW3B8WctNB879b%24ADD8jS3oh=1413319480.

Prevention, E. o. (2012). The Belly Melt Diet. Emmaus, A, Rodale.

Ramsden, C. E., et al. (2013). "Targeted alteration of dietary n-3 and n-6 fatty acids for the treatment of chronic headaches: a randomized trial." PAIN® **154**(11): 2441-2451.

Rhee, M. K., et al. (2010). "Many Americans have pre-diabetes and should be considered for metformin therapy." Diabetes care, **33**(1): 49-54.

Ried, K., et al. (2010). "Does chocolate reduce blood pressure? A meta-analysis." BMC medicine, **8**(1): 39.

Ritsner, M. S., et al. (2011). "L-theanine relieves positive, activation, and anxiety symptoms in patients with schizophrenia and schizoaffective disorder: an 8-week, randomized, double-blind, placebo-controlled, 2-center study." Journal of Clinical Psychiatry, **72**(1): 34.

Rockett, D. (2017). "'Unrest' puts spotlight on disease that affects millions, including Riverside girl, 12." Retrieved Nov 23, 2017, from http://www.chicagotribune.com/lifestyles/health/ct-life-me-cfs-unrest-film-20170928-story.html.

Rognmo, Ø., et al. (2004). "High intensity aerobic interval exercise is superior to moderate intensity exercise for increasing aerobic capacity in patients with coronary artery disease." European Journal of Cardiovascular Prevention & Rehabilitation, **11**(3): 216-222.

Ross, S. M. (2012). "Menopause: a standardized isopropanolic black cohosh extract (remifemin) is found to be safe and effective for menopausal symptoms." Holistic nursing practice, 26(1): 58-61.

Roundtable, T. M. (2012). "Fibromyalgia: New Clinical Concepts." Retrieved Nov 23, 2017, from themedicalroundtable.com/article/fibromyalgia-new-clinical-concepts.

Salo, P. M., et al. (2014). "Prevalence of allergic sensitization in the United States: results from the National Health and Nutrition Examination Survey (NHANES) 2005-2006." Journal of Allergy and Clinical Immunology, 134(2): 350-359.

Sambrook, J. (nd). "IBS Diet Sheet." Retrieved Nov 23, 2017, from patient.co.uk/health/irritable-bowel-syndrome-diet-sheet.

Schapowal, A. (2005). "Treating intermittent allergic rhinitis: a prospective, randomized, placebo and antihistamine-controlled study of Butterbur extract Ze 339." Phytotherapy research: PTR, 19(6): 530-537.

School, H. M. (2010). "Stress and the sensitive gut." Retrieved Nov 25, 2017, from health.harvard.edu/newsletters/Harvard_Mental_Health_Letter/2010/August/stress-and-the-sensitive-gut?utm_source=mental&utm_medium=pressrelease&utm_campaign=mental0810.

School, H. M. (2013). "Blueberries, strawberries protect the heart, from the Harvard Heart Letter." Retrieved Nov 23, 2017, from health.harvard.edu/press_releases/blueberries-strawberries-protect-the-heart.

Shahar, E., et al. (2004). "Effect of vitamin E supplementation on the regular treatment of seasonal allergic rhinitis." Annals of Allergy, Asthma & Immunology, 92(6): 654-658.

Shamliyan, T. A., et al. (2013). "Preventive pharmacologic treatments for episodic migraine in adults." Journal of general internal medicine, 28(9): 1225-1237.

Simmons, A. L., et al. (2014). "What are we putting in our food that is making us fat? Food additives, contaminants, and other putative contributors to obesity." Current obesity reports, 3(2): 273-285.

Society, N. A. M. (2017). "The 2017 hormone therapy position statement of the North American Menopause Society." Menopause (New York, NY), 24(7): 728-753.

Somer, E. (1999). Food and Mood:: The Complete Guide To Eating Well and Feeling Your Best, Macmillan.

Spain, E. (2014). "Scientists Find Heart Disease Can Be Reversed by Adopting Healthy Habits." Retrieved Nov 22, 2017, from feinberg.northwestern.edu/news/2014/06/reverse_heart_disease.html.

Staff, M. C. (2014). "Diseases and Conditions: Diabetes Risk Factors." Retrieved Nov 23, 2017, from http://www.mayoclinic.org/diseases-conditions/diabetes/basics/risk-factors/con-20033091.

Staff, M. C. (2015, June 12, 2015). "Cholesterol: Top foods to improve your numbers." Retrieved Nov 22, 2017, from mayoclinic.org/diseases-conditions/high-blood-cholesterol/in-depth/cholesterol- levels/art-20048245.

Stojanovska, L., et al. (2014). "To exercise, or, not to exercise, during menopause and beyond." Maturitas, **77**(4): 318-323.

Suarez, K., et al. (2010). "Psychological stress and self-reported functional gastrointestinal disorders." The Journal of nervous and mental disease, **198**(3): 226-229.

Sullivan, P. S., et al. (2012). "Successes and challenges of HIV prevention in men who have sex with men." The Lancet, **380**(9839): 388-399.

Thorne Research, I. (2000). "Berberine." Altern Med Rev, **5**(2): 175-177.

UChospitals (2017). "Light Therapy for Skin." Retrieved Nov 24, 2017, from uchospitals.edu/specialties/dermatology/light-therapy/.

UCL (2014). "Diabetes treatments 'do more harm than good' for many people." Retrieved Nov 24, 2017, from ucl.ac.uk/news/news-articles/0714/010714-Diabetes-treatments-do-more-harm- than-good.

UMMC (2015). "Feverfew." Retrieved Nov 24, 2017, from http://www.umm.edu/health/medical/altmed/herb/feverfew.

UMMC (2015, Aug 6, 2015). "Vitamin B1 (Thiamine)." Retrieved Nov 24, 2017, from http://www.umm.edu/health/medical/altmed/supplement/vitamin-b1-thiamine.

UMMC (2016). "Elderberry." Retrieved Nov 26, 2017, from http://www.umm.edu/health/medical/altmed/herb/elderberry.

UMMC (2016). "osteoarthritis." Retrieved Nov 22, 2017, from http://www.umm.edu/health/medical/altmed/condition/osteoarthritis.

UMMC (2016). "Sinusitis." Retrieved Nov 26, 2017, from umm.edu/health/medical/altmed/condition/sinusitis.

van Dam, R. M., et al. (2002). "Dietary patterns and risk for type 2 diabetes mellitus in US men." Annals of internal medicine, 136(3): 201-209.

Van Dam, R. M., et al. (2006). "Coffee, caffeine, and risk of type 2 diabetes." Diabetes care, 29(2): 398-403.

Vanuytsel, T., et al. (2014). "Treatment of abdominal pain in irritable bowel syndrome." Journal of gastroenterology, 49(8): 1193-1205.

Vitacost (2017). "Nature's Way Chamomile Standardized -- 60 Capsules." Retrieved Nov 24, 2017, from vitacost.com/natures-way-chamomile-standardized.

Watch, H. M. s. H. (2015). "Adding folate to blood pressure medication reduces stroke." Retrieved Nov 23, 2017, from https://www.health.harvard.edu/diseases-and-conditions/adding-folate-to-blood-pressure-medication-reduces-stroke.

Wells, R. E., et al. (2014). "Meditation for migraines: a pilot randomized controlled trial." Headache: The Journal of Head and Face Pain, 54(9): 1484-1495.

Wepner, F., et al. (2014). "Effects of vitamin D on patients with fibromyalgia syndrome: a randomized placebo-controlled trial." PAIN®, 155(2): 261-268.

WHFoods (2017). "The best ways to prepare and store garlic." Retrieved Nov 23, 2017, from whfoods.com/genpage.php?tname=george&dbid=136.

Witt, C. M., et al. (2006). "Acupuncture in patients with osteoarthritis of the knee or hip: a randomized, controlled trial with an additional nonrandomized arm." Arthritis & Rheumatology, 54(11): 3485-3493.

Witte, A. V., et al. (2014). "Effects of resveratrol on memory performance, hippocampal functional connectivity, and glucose metabolism in healthy older adults." Journal of Neuroscience, 34(23): 7862-7870.

Wu, L., et al. (2014). "Walnut-enriched diet reduces fasting non-HDL-cholesterol and apolipoprotein B in healthy Caucasian subjects: a randomized controlled cross-over clinical trial." Metabolism, 63(3): 382-391.

Xiong, X., et al. (2015). "Massage therapy for essential hypertension: a systematic review." Journal of human hypertension, 29(3): 143-151.

Yina, J., et al. (2008). "Efficacy of berberine in patients with type 2 diabetes." Metabolism, **57**(5): 712-717.

Ying, X., et al. (2013). "Piperine inhibits IL-β induced expression of inflammatory mediators in human osteoarthritis chondrocyte." International Immunopharmacology, **17**(2): 293-299.

Younge, J. O., et al. (2015). "Mind–body practices for patients with cardiac disease: a systematic review and meta-analysis." European journal of preventive cardiology, **22**(11): 1385-1398.

Yudkin, J. S. and V. M. Montori (2014). "Too Much Medicine: The epidemic of pre-diabetes: the medicine and the politics." The BMJ, **349**.

Zhang, S., et al. (2014). "Sinupret activates CFTR and TMEM16A-dependent transepithelial chloride transport and improves indicators of mucociliary clearance." PloS one, **9**(8): e104090.

PART III NOTES

Allergies, K. w. f. (2017). "Frequently Asked Questions About the Food Allergen Labeling Consumer Protection Act (FALCPA)." Retrieved Nov 27, 2017, from http://www.kidswithfoodallergies.org/page/label-law-food-allergen-labeling-consumer-protection-act.aspx.

Altshul, S. (2013). "Body fat is the deadliest organ." Retrieved Nov 27, 2017, from https://www.prevention.com/health/diabetes/avoid-belly-fat.

Arab, L., et al. (2009). "Green and black tea consumption and risk of stroke." Stroke, **40**(5): 1786-1792.

Bamia, C., et al. (2015). "Coffee, tea and decaffeinated coffee in relation to hepatocellular carcinoma in a European population: multicentre, prospective cohort study." International journal of cancer, **136**(8): 1899-1908.

Barlow, R. (2013). "A drink a day raises cancer risk, study says." Retrieved Nov 27, 2017, from http://www.bu.edu/today/2013/a-drink-a-day-raises-cancer-risk-study-says/.

Bazzano, L. A., et al. (2014). "Effects of Low-Carbohydrate and Low-Fat DietsA Randomized TrialEffects of Low-Carbohydrate and Low-Fat Diets." Annals of internal medicine, **161**(5): 309-318.

Becker, R. and G. Selden (1998). The body electric: Electromagnetism and the foundation of life, Harper Collins.

Bidel, S., et al. (2006). "Coffee consumption and risk of total and cardiovascular mortality among patients with type 2 diabetes." Diabetologia, **49**(11): 2618-2626.

Brehm, B. J. and D. A. D'alessio (2008). "Benefits of high-protein weight loss diets: enough evidence for practice?" Current Opinion in Endocrinology, Diabetes and Obesity, **15**(5): 416-421.

Brown, A. C. (2012). "Gluten sensitivity: problems of an emerging condition separate from celiac disease." Expert review of gastroenterology & hepatology, **6**(1): 43-55.

CDC (2017). "Chronic Disease Overview." from https://www.cdc.gov/chronicdisease/overview/index.htm.

centre, T. b. (nd). " the buddhistcentre: buddhism for today." Retrieved Nov 28, 2017, from https://thebuddhistcentre.com/text/loving-kindness-meditation.

Cheung, L. (nd). "Definition of Mindful eating." Retrieved Nov 27, 2017, from https://www.lexiconoffood.com/definition/definition-mindful-eating.

Chödrön, P. (2016). How to meditate: A practical guide to making friends with your mind, Jaico Publishing House.

Church, D. (2009). The genie in your genes: Epigenetic medicine and the new biology of intention, Elite Books.

Ciardi, C., et al. (2012). "Food additives such as sodium sulphite, sodium benzoate and curcumin inhibit leptin release in lipopolysaccharide-treated murine adipocytes in vitro." British journal of nutrition, **107**(6): 826-833.

Cohen, S., et al. (2012). "Chronic stress, glucocorticoid receptor resistance, inflammation, and disease risk." Proceedings of the National Academy of Sciences, **109**(16): 5995-5999.

Cohen, S., et al. (1991). "Psychological stress and susceptibility to the common cold." New England journal of medicine, **325**(9): 606-612.

Conley, C. C., et al. (2016). Emotions and Emotion Regulation in Breast Cancer Survivorship. Healthcare, Multidisciplinary Digital Publishing Institute.

Davis, W. (2014). Wheat belly: lose the wheat, lose the weight, and find your path back to health, Rodale.

Di Raimondo, D., et al. (2013). "Metabolic and anti-inflammatory effects of a home-based programme of aerobic physical exercise." International journal of clinical practice, 67(12): 1247-1253.

Drweil (2017). "Three breathing exercise and techniques." Retrieved Nov 28, 2017, from https://www.drweil.com/health-wellness/body-mind-spirit/stress-anxiety/breathing-three-exercises/.

EFT (nd). "Emotional Freedom Techniques: The birth of EFT." Retrieved Nov 28, 2017, from http://eft-help.com/intro/EFThistory.htm.

Elsawy, B. and K. E. Higgins (2010). "Physical activity guidelines for older adults." American family physician, 81(1): 55-59.

Floegel, A., et al. (2012). "Coffee consumption and risk of chronic disease in the European Prospective Investigation into Cancer and Nutrition (EPIC)–Germany study." The American journal of clinical nutrition 95(4): 901-908.

Fowler, S. P., et al. (2008). "Fueling the obesity epidemic? Artificially sweetened beverage use and long-term weight gain." Obesity, 16(8): 1894-1900.

Goleman, D. (1996). "Emotional Intelligence. Why It Can Matter More than IQ." Learning, 24(6): 49-50.

Guest, A. and M. Apgar (2002). "Promoting and prescribing exercise for the elderly." American family physician, 65: 3.

Gunnars, K. (2017). "23 Studies on Low-Carb and Low-Fat Diets — Time to Retire The Fad." Retrieved Nov 26, 2017, from https://www.healthline.com/nutrition/23-studies-on-low-carb-and-low-fat-diets.

HSPH (2017). "Healthy Drinks." Retrieved Nov 27, 2017, from https://www.hsph.harvard.edu/nutritionsource/healthy-drinks/.

HSPH (2017). "Omega-3 Fatty Acids: An Essential Contribution." Retrieved Nov 26, 2017, from hsph.harvard.edu/nutritionsource/omega-3/.

IFT (2017). "9 fats to include in a healthy diet." Retrieved Nov 26, 2017, from ift.org/newsroom/news-releases/2014/september/17/9-fats-to-include-in-a-healthy-diet.aspx.

Institute, H. (2017). "Our purpose." Retrieved Nov 28, 2017, from heartmath.org.

Institute, R. (2017). "Homepage." Retrieved Nov 25, 2017, from rodaleinstitute.org.

Kabat-Zinn, J. (2005). Guided Mindfulness Meditation (Guided Mindfulness)[UNABRIDGED](Audio CD), Sounds True.

Kahleova, H., et al. (2014). "Eating two larger meals a day (breakfast and lunch) is more effective than six smaller meals in a reduced-energy regimen for patients with type 2 diabetes: a randomised crossover study." Diabetologia, 57(8): 1552-1560.

Kalish, N. (2011). "10 Best Healing Herbs." Retrieved Nov 26, 2017, from https://www.prevention.com/mind-body/natural-remedies/best-healing-herbs-top-10.

Kornfield, J. (2005). Meditation for beginners: Six guided meditations for insight, inner clarity, and cultivating a compassionate heart, Random House.

Kruk, J. (2007). "Physical activity in the prevention of the most frequent chronic diseases: an analysis of the recent evidence." Asian Pacific Journal of Cancer Prevention, 8(3): 325.

Lian, X.-Q., et al. (2014). "The influence of regular walking at different times of day on blood lipids and inflammatory markers in sedentary patients with coronary artery disease." Preventive medicine, 58: 64-69.

Lipton, B. H. (2015). The Biology of Belief 10th Anniversary Edition: Unleashing the Power of Consciousness, Matter & Miracles, Hay House, Inc.

Mangin, M., et al. (2014). "Inflammation and vitamin D: the infection connection." Inflammation Research, 63(10): 803-819.

MedlinePlus (2017). "Black Tea." Retrieved Nov 27, 2017, from https://medlineplus.gov/druginfo/natural/997.html.

Michaëlsson, K., et al. (2014). "Milk intake and risk of mortality and fractures in women and men: cohort studies." BMJ, 349: g6015.

Mons, U., et al. (2014). "A reverse J-shaped association of leisure time physical activity with prognosis in patients with stable coronary heart disease: evidence from a large cohort with repeated measurements." Heart: heartjnl-2013-305242.

Moore, C. (2014). The resilience breakthrough: 27 tools for turning adversity into action, Greenleaf Book Group.

Naparstek, B. (2016). Guided imagery: A portable, scalable, user-friendly 24/7 self administered audio intervention for hospital patients and their families. Keck Medicine, USC.

nccaom (nd). "Home." Retrieved Nov 24, 2017, from nccaom.org.

Nestle, M. (2006). "What to eat: An aisle-by-aisle guide to savvy food choices and good eating." The Free Library.

NIDDK (2014). "Lactose Intolerance." Retrieved Nov 27, 2017, from https://www.niddk.nih.gov/health-information/digestive-diseases/lactose-intolerance.

Ortner, N. (2013). The Tapping Solution: A Revolutionary System for Stress-free Living, Hay House, Inc.

Paddock, C. (2012). "Stress may cause illness by changing genes." Retrieved Nov 28, 2017, from https://www.medicalnewstoday.com/articles/249215.php.

PCRM (nd). "Health Concerns about Dairy Products." Retrieved Nov 28, 2017, from http://www.pcrm.org/health/diets/vegdiets/health-concerns-about-dairy-products.

Perlmutter, D. (2014). Grain Brain: The Surprising Truth about Wheat, Carbs, and Sugar-Your Brain's Silent Killers, Hachette UK.

Pert, C. (1999). Molecules of emotion: the science behind mind–body medicine. New York: Touchstone, Simon and Schuster.

Prevention (nd). "The Smoothie Cure For Gas And Bloating." Retrieved Nov 27, 2017, from https://www.prevention.com/mind-body/natural-remedies/natural-remedy-gas-and-bloating.

Prevention (nd). "Spices can alleviate common health problems." Retrieved Nov 26, 2017, from prevention .com/food/food-remedies/spices-can-alleviate-common-health- problems.

Rabkin, J. G. and E. L. Struening (1976). "Life events, stress, and illness." Science, **194**(4269): 1013-1020.

Reports, C. (2017). Taking antibiotics off your fast food menu, Consumer Reports.

Rossy, L. (2016). The Mindfulness-Based Eating Solution: Proven Strategies to End Overeating, Satisfy Your Hunger, and Savor Your Life, New Harbinger Publications.

Samaha, F. F., et al. (2003). "A low-carbohydrate as compared with a low-fat diet in severe obesity." N Engl J Med, 2003 (348): 2074-2081.

School, H. M. (2011, March 18, 2016). "Understanding the stress response: Chronic activation of this survival mechanism impairs health." Retrieved Nov 26, 2017, from https://www.health.harvard.edu/staying-healthy/understanding-the-stress-response.

SEHN (nd). "Precautionary principle-FAQs." Retrieved Nov 26, 2017.

Seligman, M. E. (2012). Flourish: A visionary new understanding of happiness and well-being, Simon and Schuster.

Shamard, C. (2017). " Adult food allergies on the rise, report finds, but cause still unclear." Retrieved Nov 27, 2017, from https://www.nbcnews.com/health/health-news/adult-food-allergies-rise-report-finds-cause-still-unclear-n805316.

Shiraev, T. and G. Barclay (2012). "Evidence based exercise: Clinical benefits of high intensity interval training." Australian family physician, 41(12): 960.

Simmons, A. L., et al. (2014). "What are we putting in our food that is making us fat? Food additives, contaminants, and other putative contributors to obesity." Current obesity reports 3(2): 273-285.

Sirois, F. M., et al. (2015). "Self-compassion, affect, and health-promoting behaviors." Health Psychology, 34(6): 661.

Smith, J., et al. (2017). Badditives!: The 13 Most Harmful Food Additives in Your Diet - And How to Avoid Them, Skyhorse Publishing Company, Incorporated.

Suez, J., et al. (2014). "Artificial sweeteners induce glucose intolerance by altering the gut microbiota." Nature, 514(7521): 181-186.
Sullivan, P. S., et al. (2012). "Successes and challenges of HIV prevention in men who have sex with men." The Lancet, 380(9839): 388-399.

Sydney, T. U. o. (2017, May 2017). "Search for glycemic index." Retrieved Nov 26, 2017, from glycemicindex.com.

UMMC (2015). "Green Tea." Retrieved Nov 27, 2017, from http://www.umm.edu/health/medical/altmed/herb/green-tea.

universe, E. (nd). "6 successful sessions with a war veteran." Retrieved Nov 28, 2017, from http://www.eftuniverse.com/trauma-and-abuse/6-successful-sessions-with-a-war-veteran.

USDA (2017). "Organic agriculture." Retrieved Nov 25, 2017, from usda.gov/wps/portal/usda/usdahome?contentidonly=true&contentid=organic-agriculture.html.

USGS (2016). "The water in you." Retrieved Nov 26, 2017, from https://water.usgs.gov/edu/propertyyou.html.

Veerman, J. L., et al. (2011). "Television viewing time and reduced life expectancy: a life table analysis." British journal of sports medicine: bjsports085662.

Volek, J. S., et al. (2009). "Carbohydrate restriction has a more favorable impact on the metabolic syndrome than a low fat diet." Lipids, **44**(4): 297-309.

Watch, H. M. s. H. (2009). "Walking your steps to health." Retrieved Nov 23, 2017, from https://www.health.harvard.edu/newsletter_article/walking-your-steps-to-health.

Weber, B. (2013). "High-fiber diet linked to lower risk of heart disease." Retrieved Nov 26, 2017, from medicalnewstoday.com/articles/270378.php.

WebMD (2011). "Moderate alcohol drinking may cut A lzheimers risk." Retrieved Nov 27, 2017, from webmd.com/alzheimers/news/20110817/moderate-alcoholdrinking-may-cut-alzheimers-risk.

WebMD (2017). "Alcohol and Heart Disease." Retrieved Nov 27, 2017, from https://www.webmd.com/heart-disease/guide/heart-disease-alcohol-your-heart.

WHFoods (nd). "Are colored potatoes healthier than white potatoes?". Retrieved Nov 26, 2017, from whfoods.org/genpage.php?tname=dailytip&dbid=122.

WHfoods (nd). "Beef, grass-fed." Retrieved Nov 27, 2017, from http://whfoods.com/genpage.php?tname=foodspice&dbid=141.

WHFoods (nd). "Omega-3 fatty acids." Retrieved Nov 27, 2017, from http://whfoods.com/genpage.php?tname=nutrient&dbid=84.

Winter, R. (2009). A consumer's dictionary of food additives: Descriptions in plain English of more than 12,000 ingredients both harmful and desirable found in foods, Crown Archetype.

Endnotes

1. Whittaker, B., *Ex-DEA agent: Opioid crisis fueled by drug industry and Congress*. 2017, CBS News: CBS News 60 Minutes Politics.

2. Sarpatwari, A., M. Sinha, and A. Kesselheim, *The Opioid Epidemic: Fixing a Broken Pharmaceutical Market"*. Harvard Law and Policy Review, 2017. **11**: p. 463-484.

3. Cha, A. *Researchers: Medical errors now third leading cause of death in the United States*. Washington Post 2016 [cited 2017 Nov 18]; Available from: https://www.washingtonpost.com/news/to-your-health/wp/2016/05/03/researchers-medical-errors-now-third-leading-cause-of-death-in-united-states/?utm_term=.1e0c1c1bc6ea.

4. Makary, M. and M. Daniel, *Medical Errors—The Third Leading Cause of Death in the US*. BMJ, 2016. **353**.

5. Will, M. *The 16 countries with the world's best healthcare systems*. 2017 Jan13, 2017 [cited 2017 Nov 18]; Available from: http://nordic.businessinsider.com/the-16-countries-with-the-worlds-best-healthcare-systems-2017-1/.

6. Buttorff, C., T. Ruder, and M. Bauman, *Multiple Chronic Conditions in the United States*. 2017, RAND Corporation: Santa Monica, CA.

7. McLean, B., *Everything You Know About Martin Shkreli Is Wrong—Or Is It?"*, in *Vanity Fair*. 2015.

8. Spain, E. *Scientists Find Heart Disease Can Be Reversed by Adopting Healthy Habits*. 2014 [cited 2017 Nov 22]; Available from: feinberg.northwestern.edu/news/2014/06/reverse_heart_disease.html.

9. eDrugSearch. *New Chart Exposes the Inhumanity of US Drug Prices Compared to Other Countries*. 2017 [cited 2017 Nov 20]; Available from: https://edrugsearch.com/chart-inhumanity-us-drug-prices/.

10. Jones, C.M., et al., *Alcohol involvement in opioid pain reliever and benzodiazepine drug abuse-related emergency department visits and drug-related deaths-United States, 2010*. MMWR Morb Mortal Wkly Rep, 2014. **63**(40): p. 881-5.

11. Meier, B., *Narcotics Maker Guilty of Deceit Over Marketing*, in *The New York Times/Business Day*. 2007: The New York Times/Business Day.

12. NIDA. *Overdose Death Rates*. 2017 Sept 2017 [cited 2017 Nov 20]; Available from: https://www.drugabuse.gov/related-topics/trends-statistics/overdose-death-rates.

13. CDC. *Opioid Overdose*. 2017 [cited 2017 Nov 20]; Available from: https://www.cdc.gov/drugoverdose/.

14. Kearns, C., L. Schmidt, and S. Glantz, *Sugar Industry and Coronary Heart Disease Research: A Historical Analysis of Internal Industry Documents*. JAMA, 2016. **176**(11): p. 1680-1685.

15.   Moss, M., *Salt Sugar Fat: How the Food Giants Hooked Us. , 2013*. 2013, New York City, NY: Random House Publishing Group.

16.   **Huen, K.**, et al., *Organophosphate pesticide levels in blood and urine of women and newborns living in an agricultural community*. Environ Res, 2012. **117**: p. 8-16.

17.   ewg. *Nation's Pediatricians, EWG Urge EPA to Ban Pesticide that Harms Kids' Brains*. 2017 [cited 2017 Nov 23]; Available from: https://www.ewg.org/testimony-official-correspondence/nation-s-pediatricians-ewg-urge-epa-ban-pesticide-harms-kids#.Wf8QZ2hSyyK.

18.   Hedlund, B. *Homepage*. 2017 [cited 2017 Nov 23]; Available from: www.baumhedlundlaw.com.

19.   CDC. *Infographic: Antibiotic Resistance The Global Threat*. 2017 [cited 2017 Nov 20]; Available from: https://www.cdc.gov/globalhealth/infographics/antibiotic-resistance/antibiotic_resistance_global_threat.htm

20.   Davis, K., et al. *Mirror, Mirror on the Wall, 2014 Update: How the U.S. Health Care System Compares Internationally, The Commonwealth Fund, June 2014*. 2014 [cited 2017 Nov 20]; Available from: http://www.commonwealthfund.org/publications/fund-reports/2014/jun/mirror-mirror.

21.   Walker, E.R. and B.G. Druss, *Cumulative burden of comorbid mental disorders, substance use disorders, chronic medical conditions, and poverty on health among adults in the USA*. Psychology, health & medicine, 2017. **22**(6): p. 727-735.

22.   Zhong, W., et al. *Age and sex patterns of drug prescribing in a defined American population*. in *Mayo Clinic Proceedings*. 2013. Elsevier.

23.   Kantor, E.D., et al., *Trends in prescription drug use among adults in the United States from 1999-2012*. Jama, 2015. **314**(17): p. 1818-1830.

24.   Edney, A. *Drug Quality in China Still Poses Risks for U.S. Market*. 2014 [cited 2017 Nov 19]; Available from: www.bloomberg.com/news/print2014-04-03/drug-quality-in-china-still-poses-risks-for-u-s-market.html.

25.   Center, J.D. *Oral Diabetes Medications Summary Chart*. 2017 [cited 2017 Vov 18]; Available from: joslin.org/info/oral_diabetes_medications_summary_chart.html.

26.   NIH. *Understand your risk for high blood pressure*. 2017 [cited 2017 Nov 20]; Available from: nhlbi.nih.gov/health-topics/topics/hbp/printall-index.html; heart.org/HEARTORG/Conditions/HighBloodPressure/UnderstandYourRiskForHighBloodPressure/Understand-Your-Risk-For-High-Blood-Pressure_UCM_002052_Article.jsp;.

27.   Johnson, D.A. and E.C. Oldfield, *Reported side effects and complications of long-term proton pump inhibitor use: dissecting the evidence*. Clinical gastroenterology and hepatology, 2013. **11**(5): p. 458-464.

28.   Brown, T. *100 Best-Selling, Most Prescribed Branded Drugs Through March.* 2015 [cited 2017 Nov 21]; Available from: https://www.medscape.com/viewarticle/844317.

29.   Fluoridation. *Fluoridation status of some countries.* nd [cited 2017 Nov 21]; Available from: http://www.fluoridation.com/c-country.htm.

30.   Network, F.A. *National Research Council.* 2017 [cited 2017 Nov 21]; Available from: fluoridealert.org/researchers/nrc/findings/.

31.   Network, F.A. *Statements from European Health, Water & Environment Authorities on Water Fluoridation.* 2007 2007 [cited 2017 Nov 21].

32.   Sugiyama, T., et al., *Different time trends of caloric and fat intake between statin users and nonusers among US adults: gluttony in the time of statins?* JAMA internal medicine, 2014. **174**(7): p. 1038-1045.

33.   Dueñas-Laita , A., F. Pineda , and A. Armentia *Hypersensitivity to Generic Drugs with Soybean Oil.* New England Journal of Medicine, 2009. **361**(13): p. 1317-1318.

34.   Reeve, E., et al., *A systematic review of the emerging definition of 'deprescribing' with network analysis: implications for future research and clinical practice.* British journal of clinical pharmacology, 2015. **80**(6): p. 1254-1268.

35.   Potter, K., et al., *Deprescribing in frail older people: a randomised controlled trial.* PLoS one, 2016. **11**(3): p. e0149984.

36.   Pongdee, T. *Colds, Allergies and Sinusitis—How to Tell the Difference.* 2012 [cited 2017 Nov 21]; Available from: aaaai.org/Aaaai/media/MediaLibrary/PDF%20Documents/Libraries/EL-allergies-colds-allergies-sinusitis-patient.pdf.

37.   Chatzi, L., et al., *Protective effect of fruits, vegetables and the Mediterranean diet on asthma and allergies among children in Crete.* Thorax, 2007. **62**(8): p. 677-683.

38.   Schapowal, A., *Treating intermittent allergic rhinitis: a prospective, randomized, placebo and antihistamine-controlled study of Butterbur extract Ze 339.* Phytotherapy research: PTR, 2005. **19**(6): p. 530-537.

39.   Health, N.L. *Conditions we treat.* 2017 [cited 2017 Nov 21]; Available from: med.nyu.edu/content?ChunkIID=21574.

40.   Shahar, E., G. Hassoun, and S. Pollack, *Effect of vitamin E supplementation on the regular treatment of seasonal allergic rhinitis.* Annals of Allergy, Asthma & Immunology, 2004. **92**(6): p. 654-658.

41.   Medicinenet. *fexofenadine - oral, Allegra.* 2017 [cited 2017 Nov 21]; Available from: medicinenet.com/fexofenadine-oral/page2.htm.

42.   Gray, S.L., et al., *Cumulative use of strong anticholinergics and incident dementia: a prospective cohort study.* JAMA internal medicine, 2015. **175**(3): p. 401-407.

43.   aafa. *Allergies.* 2017 [cited 2017 Nov 21]; Available from: aafa.org/display.cfm?id=9&sub=24&cont=34.

44. Salo, P.M., et al., *Prevalence of allergic sensitization in the United States: results from the National Health and Nutrition Examination Survey (NHANES) 2005-2006.* Journal of Allergy and Clinical Immunology, 2014. **134**(2): p. 350-359.

45. NIH. *Prevalence of allergies the same, regardless of where you live.* 2014 March 4, 2014 [cited 2017 Nov 21]; Available from: nih.gov/news/health/mar2014/niehs-04.htm.

46. Bredesen, D.E., *Reversal of cognitive decline: A novel therapeutic program.* Aging (Albany NY), 2014. **6**(9): p. 707.

47. Foundation, A. *Osteoarthritis.* nd [cited 2017 Nov 21]; Available from: arthritis.org/arthritis-facts/disease-center/osteoarthritis.php.

48. Foundation, A. *Snow conference.* 2012 2012 [cited 2017 Nov 21]; Available from: arthritistoday.org/about-arthritis/types-of-arthritis/osteoarthritis/treatment- plan/snow-conference-2012.php.

49. Foundation, A. *Cause of Osteoarthritis.* 2012 [cited 2017 Nov 21]; Available from: arthritistoday.org/about-arthritis/types-of-arthritis/osteoarthritis/who-gets-oa- and-why/cause-of-osteoarthritis.php.

50. Lv, H. and G. She, *Naturally occurring diarylheptanoids.* Natural product communications, 2010. **5**(10): p. 1687-1708.

51. Abas, F., et al., *Biological evaluation of curcumin and related diarylheptanoids.* Zeitschrift für Naturforschung C, 2006. **61**(9-10): p. 625-631.

52. Ying, X., et al., *Piperine inhibits IL-β induced expression of inflammatory mediators in human osteoarthritis chondrocyte.* International immunopharmacology, 2013. **17**(2): p. 293-299.

53. Witt, C.M., et al., *Acupuncture in patients with osteoarthritis of the knee or hip: a randomized, controlled trial with an additional nonrandomized arm.* Arthritis & Rheumatology, 2006. **54**(11): p. 3485-3493.

54. UMMC. *osteoarthritis.* 2016 [cited 2017 Nov 22]; Available from: http://www.umm.edu/health/medical/altmed/condition/osteoarthritis.

55. consumerlab.com. *Product Review: Acetyl-L-Carnitine Supplements Review.* 2012 Apr 5, 2016 [cited 2017 Nov 23]; Available from: consumerlab.com/reviews/Acetyl-L-Carnitine-Supplements-Review/Acetyl-L- Carnitine/.

56. Kim, J., et al., *Comparative clinical trial of S-adenosylmethionine versus nabumetone for the treatment of knee osteoarthritis: an 8-week, multicenter, randomized, double-blind, double-dummy, Phase IV study in Korean patients.* Clinical therapeutics, 2009. **31**(12): p. 2860-2872.

57. AHA. *Atherosclerosis and Stroke.* 2014 Oct 24, 2016 [cited 2017 Nov 22]; Available from: strokeassociation.org/STROKEORG/LifeAfterStroke/HealthyLivingAfterStroke/ UnderstandingRiskyConditions/Atherosclerosis-and-Stroke_UCM_310426_ Article.jsp.

58.   AHA. *What is cardiovascular disease?* 2017 [cited 2017 Nov 22];
        Available from:
        heart.org/HEARTORG/Caregiver/Resources/WhatisCardiovascularDisease
        / What-is-Cardiovascular-Disease_UCM_301852_Article.jsp.

59.   NIH. *High Blood Cholesterol: What You Need To Know.* 2005 June 2005
        [cited 2017 Nov 22]; Available from:
        nhlbi.nih.gov/health/resources/heart/heart-cholesterol-hbc-what-
        html.htm.

60.   HSPH. *Fats and Cholesterol.* 2017 [cited 2017 Nov 22]; Available from:
        hsph.harvard.edu/nutritionsource/fats-full-story/.

61.   Abramson, J. and R. Redberg. *Don't Give More Patients Statins.* 2013
        [cited 2017 Nov 22]; Available from:
        http://www.nytimes.com/2013/11/14/opinion/dont-give-more-patients-
        statins.html.

62.   Novella, S. *Statins – The Cochrane Review.* 2011 [cited 2017 Nov 19];
        Available from: sciencebasedmedicine.org/statins-the-cochrane-.

63.   Naci, H. and J.P. Ioannidis, *Comparative effectiveness of exercise and drug
        interventions on mortality outcomes: metaepidemiological study.* Bmj,
        2013. **347**: p. f5577.

64.   Sullivan, P.S., et al., *Successes and challenges of HIV prevention in men
        who have sex with men.* The Lancet, 2012. **380**(9839): p. 388-399.

65.   MedlinePlus. *Triglyceride level.* 2017 [cited 2017 Nov 21]; Available from:
        nlm.nih.gov/medlineplus/ency/article/003493.htm.

66.   Staff, M.C. *Cholesterol: Top foods to improve your numbers.* 2015 June 12,
        2015 [cited 2017 Nov 22]; Available from: mayoclinic.org/diseases-
        conditions/high-blood-cholesterol/in-depth/cholesterol- levels/art-
        20048245.

67.   Hastings, D. *The 25 Best Foods For Your Heart.* 2013 Jan 23, 2013 [cited
        2017 Nov 22]; Available from:
        https://www.prevention.com/health/health-concerns/best-foods-for-
        heart-health?s=25.

68.   Watch, H.M.s.H. *Adding folate to blood pressure medication reduces
        stroke.* 2015 [cited 2017 Nov 23]; Available from:
        https://www.health.harvard.edu/diseases-and-conditions/adding-folate-
        to-blood-pressure-medication-reduces-stroke.

69.   WHFoods. *The best ways to prepare and store garlic.* 2017 [cited 2017
        Nov 23]; Available from:
        whfoods.com/genpage.php?tname=george&dbid=136.

70.   eatright. *Understanding the New Nutrition Facts Label.* 2017 [cited 2017
        Nov 23]; Available from:
        eatright.org/Public/content.aspx?id=6442472548.

71.   School, H.M. *Blueberries, strawberries protect the heart, from the Harvard
        Heart Letter.* 2013 [cited 2017 Nov 23]; Available from:

health.harvard.edu/press_releases/blueberries-strawberries-protect-the-heart.

72. AHA. *The American Heart Association's Diet and Lifestyle Recommendations*. 2017 [cited 2017 Nov 25]; Available from: http://www.heart.org/HEARTORG/ GettingHealthy/NutritionCenter/HealthyEating/Trans-Fats_UCM_301120_ Article.jsp.

73. Altshul, S. *Docs gone wild*. 2014 [cited 2017 Nov 23].

74. Wu, L., et al., *Walnut-enriched diet reduces fasting non-HDL-cholesterol and apolipoprotein B in healthy Caucasian subjects: a randomized controlled cross-over clinical trial.* Metabolism, 2014. **63**(3): p. 382-391.

75. Hypertension-cholesterol. *Hypertension*. nd [cited 2017 Nov 23]; Available from: http://hypertension-cholesterol.com/hypertension-cholesterol/hypertension-1-2557.%20html.

76. Lian, X.-Q., et al., *The influence of regular walking at different times of day on blood lipids and inflammatory markers in sedentary patients with coronary artery disease.* Preventive medicine, 2014. **58**: p. 64-69.

77. Castano, G., et al., *Effects of policosanol 20 versus 40 mg/day in the treatment of patients with type II hypercholesterolemia: a 6-month double-blind study.* International journal of clinical pharmacology research, 2001. **21**(1): p. 43-57.

78. Lee, T. *Ask the doctor: Is no-flush niacin as effective as other types of niacin?* 2010 [cited 2017 Nov 23]; Available from: https://www.health.harvard.edu/newsletter_article/is-no-flush-niacin-as-effective-as-other-kinds-of-niacin.

79. AHA. *High stress, hostility, depression linked with increased stroke risk*. 2014 [cited 2017 Nov 23]; Available from: http://newsroom.heart.org/news/high-stress-hostility-depression-linked-with-increased-stroke-risk.

80. Rognmo, Ø., et al., *High intensity aerobic interval exercise is superior to moderate intensity exercise for increasing aerobic capacity in patients with coronary artery disease.* European Journal of Cardiovascular Prevention & Rehabilitation, 2004. **11**(3): p. 216-222.

81. CDC. *Leading causes of death*. 2017 March 17, 2017 [cited 2017 Nov 23]; Available from: cdc.gov/nchs/fastats/leading-causes-of-death.htm.

82. NHLBI. *Description of High Blood Pressure*`. 2015 Sept 10, 2015 [cited 2017 Nov 23]; Available from: nhlbi.nih.gov/health/health-topics/topics/hbp/#.

83. Younge, J.O., et al., *Mind–body practices for patients with cardiac disease: a systematic review and meta-analysis.* European journal of preventive cardiology, 2015. **22**(11): p. 1385-1398.

84. Xiong, X., S. Li, and Y. Zhang, *Massage therapy for essential hypertension: a systematic review.* Journal of human hypertension, 2015. **29**(3): p. 143-151.

85. Givi, M., *Durability of effect of massage therapy on blood pressure.* International journal of preventive medicine, 2013. **4**(5): p. 511.

86. Anglia, U.o.E. *Eating blueberries can guard against high blood pressure, according to new research.* 2011 Jan 15, 2011 [cited 2017 Nov 23]; Available from: sciencedaily.com/releases/2011/01/110114155241.htm.

87. AHA. *Eating probiotics regularly may improve your blood pressure.* nd [cited 2017 Nov 25]; Available from: http://newsroom.heart.org/news/eating-probiotics-regularly-may-improve-your-blood-%20pressure.

88. MedlinePlus. *High blood pressure - medicine-related.* 2017 Nov 6, 2017 [cited 2017 Nov 23]; Available from: https://medlineplus.gov/ency/article/000155.htm.

89. Ried, K., et al., *Does chocolate reduce blood pressure? A meta-analysis.* BMC medicine, 2010. **8**(1): p. 39.

90. CDC. *Myalgic Encephalomyelitis/Chronic Fatigue Syndrome.* 2017 Nov 7, 2017 [cited 2017 Nov 23]; Available from: cdc.gov/cfs/symptoms/.

91. Rockett, D. *'Unrest' puts spotlight on disease that affects millions, including Riverside girl, 12.* 2017 [cited 2017 Nov 23]; Available from: http://www.chicagotribune.com/lifestyles/health/ct-life-me-cfs-unrest-film-20170928-story.html.

92. Kaplan, M. *Worn Out At the Finish Line.* 2014 [cited 2017 Nov 22]; Available from: http://anapsid.org/cnd/coping/hillenbrand.html.

93. Huth, T., et al., *Pilot study of natural killer cells in chronic fatigue syndrome/myalgic encephalomyelitis and multiple sclerosis.* Scandinavian journal of immunology, 2016. **83**(1): p. 44-51.

94. Marshall-Gradisnik, S.M., et al., *Examination of single nucleotide polymorphisms (SNPs) in transient receptor potential (TRP) ion channels in chronic fatigue syndrome patients.* Immunology and Immunogenetics Insights, 2015. **7**: p. 1.

95. Clinic, M. *Chronic fatigue syndrome.* 2017 Oct 5, 2017 [cited 2017 Nov 23]; Available from: mayoclinic.org/diseases-conditions/chronic-fatigue-syndrome/basics/treatment/ con-20022009.

96. Castro-Marrero, J., et al., *Does oral coenzyme Q10 plus NADH supplementation improve fatigue and biochemical parameters in chronic fatigue syndrome?* 2015, Mary Ann Liebert, Inc. 140 Huguenot Street, 3rd Floor New Rochelle, NY 10801 USA.

97. Crosta, P. *What is Lyrica (pregabalin)?: Uses, dosage, and side effects.* 2017 [cited 2017 Nov 23]; Available from: medicalnewstoday.com/articles/151139.php.

98. Roundtable, T.M. *Fibromyalgia: New Clinical Concepts.* 2012 [cited 2017 Nov 23]; Available from: themedicalroundtable.com/article/fibromyalgia-new-clinical-concepts.

99. fmswaws. *Treatments-Medications.* 2014 [cited 2017 Nov 23]; Available from: fmswaws.org/medications.html.

100. Wepner, F., et al., *Effects of vitamin D on patients with fibromyalgia syndrome: a randomized placebo-controlled trial.* PAIN®, 2014. **155**(2): p. 261-268.

101. Cordero, M.D., et al., *Can coenzyme q10 improve clinical and molecular parameters in fibromyalgia?* 2013, Mary Ann Liebert, Inc. 140 Huguenot Street, 3rd Floor New Rochelle, NY 10801 USA.

102. Milner, J. *New Insights into the Mechanism of Action of Antioxidants.* nd nd [cited 2017 Nov 23].

103. Häuser, W., et al., *Efficacy of different types of aerobic exercise in fibromyalgia syndrome: a systematic review and meta-analysis of randomised controlled trials.* Arthritis research & therapy, 2010. **12**(3): p. R79.

104. Bernardy, K., et al., *Cognitive behavioural therapies for fibromyalgia syndrome.* The Cochrane database of systematic reviews, 2012. **9**.

105. NIMH. *Anxiety Disorders.* 2016 [cited 2017 Nov 23]; Available from: https://www.nimh.nih.gov/health/topics/anxiety-disorders/index.shtml.

106. NIMH. *Depression.* 2016 [cited 2017 Nov 23]; Available from: nimh.nih.gov/health/topics/depression/index.shtml.

107. Cohen, H. *Depression versus Anxiety.* 2016 July 17, 2016 [cited 2017 Nov 23]; Available from: https://www.nimh.nih.gov/health/topics/depression/index.shtml.

108. Lewis, J.E., et al., *The effect of methylated vitamin B complex on depressive and anxiety symptoms and quality of life in adults with depression.* ISRN psychiatry, 2013. **2013**.

109. ADAA. *Generalized Anxiety Disorder (GAD.* Understanding the facts 2016 [cited 2017 Nov 23]; Available from: adaa.org/understanding-anxiety/generalized-anxiety-disorder-gad.

110. ADAA. *Symptoms.* 2016 [cited 2017 Nov 23]; Available from: https://adaa.org/understanding-anxiety/generalized-anxiety-disorder-gad/symptoms.

111. NIMH. *Post-Traumatic Stress Disorder.* 2016 [cited 2017 Nov 23]; Available from: https://www.nimh.nih.gov/health/topics/anxiety-disorders/index.shtml.

112. Drugs.com. *U.S. Pharmaceutical Sales - Q4 2013.* 2014 [cited 2017 Nov 23]; Available from: https://www.drugs.com/stats/top100/sales.

113. Medicinenet. *Aripiprazole (Abilify, Abilify Maintena, Aristrada).* 2017 [cited 2017 Nov 23]; Available from: medicinenet.com/aripiprazole/article.htm.

114. Friedman, R. *A Call for Caution on Antipsychotic Drugs.* 2012 [cited 2017 Nov 23]; Available from: http://www.nytimes.com/2012/09/25/health/a-call-for-caution-in-the-use-of-antipsychotic-drugs.html.

115. Maslej, M.M., et al., *The Mortality and Myocardial Effects of Antidepressants Are Moderated by Preexisting Cardiovascular Disease: A*

Meta-Analysis. Psychotherapy and Psychosomatics, 2017. **86**(5): p. 268-282.

116.	Brooks, M. *Antidepressants Tied to a Significantly Increased Risk for Death.* 2017 [cited 2017 Nov 23]; Available from: https://www.medscape.com/viewarticle/886015.

117.	ADAA. *Medication.* 2016 [cited 2017 Nov 23]; Available from: adaa.org/finding-help/treatment/medication.

118.	MedlinePlus. *Venlafaxine.* 2014 [cited 2017 Nov 23]; Available from: nlm.nih.gov/medlineplus/druginfo/meds/a694020.html.

119.	MedlinePlus. *Duloxetine.* 2016 [cited 2017 Nov 23]; Available from: https://medlineplus.gov/druginfo/meds/a604030.html.

120.	Osher, Y. and R. Belmaker, *Omega-3 fatty acids in depression: A review of three studies.* CNS neuroscience & therapeutics, 2009. **15**(2): p. 128-133.

121.	Somer, E., *Food and Mood:: The Complete Guide To Eating Well and Feeling Your Best.* 1999: Macmillan.

122.	Beck. *What is Cognitive Behavior Therapy (CBT)?* 2016 [cited 2017 Nov 25]; Available from: https://beckinstitute.org/get-informed/what-is-cognitive-therapy/.

123.	Institute, S.A. *DSM-5 Definition of Social Anxiety Disorder.* nd [cited 2017 Nov 24]; Available from: socialanxietyinstitute.org/dsm-definition-social-anxiety-disorder.

124.	Blumenthal, J.A., P.J. Smith, and B.M. Hoffman, *Is exercise a viable treatment for depression?* ACSM's health & fitness journal, 2012. **16**(4): p. 14.

125.	Babyak, M., et al., *Exercise treatment for major depression: maintenance of therapeutic benefit at 10 months.* Psychosomatic medicine, 2000. **62**(5): p. 633-638.

126.	Blumenthal, J.A., et al., *Effects of exercise training on older patients with major depression.* Archives of internal medicine, 1999. **159**(19): p. 2349-2356.

127.	Blumenthal, J.A., et al., *Depression as a risk factor for mortality after coronary artery bypass surgery.* The Lancet, 2003. **362**(9384): p. 604-609.

128.	Blumenthal, J.A., et al., *Exercise and pharmacotherapy in the treatment of major depressive disorder.* Psychosomatic medicine, 2007. **69**(7): p. 587.

129.	nccaom. *Home.* nd [cited 2017 Nov 24]; Available from: nccaom.org.

130.	Ritsner, M.S., et al., *L-theanine relieves positive, activation, and anxiety symptoms in patients with schizophrenia and schizoaffective disorder: an 8-week, randomized, double-blind, placebo-controlled, 2-center study.* Journal of Clinical Psychiatry, 2011. **72**(1): p. 34.

131.	UMMC. *Vitamin B1 (Thiamine).* 2015 Aug 6, 2015 [cited 2017 Nov 24]; Available from: http://www.umm.edu/health/medical/altmed/supplement/vitamin-b1-thiamine.

132. McVeigh, G. *Mood Booster: B12*. 2011 [cited 2017 Nov 24]; Available from: prevention.com/mind-body/natural-remedies/vitamin-b12-and-depression.

133. Altshul, S. *21 Healing Herbs And Supplements Doctors Prescribe*. 2014 [cited 2017 Nov 24]; Available from: https://www.prevention.com/mind-body/herbs-and-supplements-natural-remedies-doctors-prescribe.

134. Lopresti, A.L., et al., *Curcumin for the treatment of major depression: a randomised, double-blind, placebo controlled study*. Journal of affective disorders, 2014. **167**: p. 368-375.

135. consumerlab.com. *Turmeric curcumin supplements spice review*. nd [cited 2017 Nov 25]; Available from: https://www.consumerlab.com/reviews/turmeric-curcumin-supplements-spice-review/%20turmeric/.

136. Vitacost. *Nature's Way Chamomile Standardized -- 60 Capsules*. 2017 [cited 2017 Nov 24]; Available from: vitacost.com/natures-way-chamomile-standardized.

137. Amsterdam, J.D., et al., *Chamomile (matricaria recutita) may have antidepressant activity in anxious depressed humans-an exploratory study*. Alternative therapies in health and medicine, 2012. **18**(5): p. 44.

138. NIDDK. *Diabetes Prevention Program*. nd [cited 2017 Nov 24]; Available from: diabetes.niddk.nih.gov/dm/pubs/preventionprogram.

139. CDC. *Pennsylvania*. nd [cited 2017 Nov 25]; Available from: https://www.cdc.gov/diabetes/prevention/recognition/states/Pennsylvania.%20htm?choice=states%2FPennsylvania.htm.

140. Altshul, S., *Get a leg up on diabetes*. 2013, Prevention.

141. Staff, M.C. *Diseases and Conditions: Diabetes Risk Factors*. 2014 [cited 2017 Nov 23]; Available from: http://www.mayoclinic.org/diseases-conditions/diabetes/basics/risk-factors/con-20033091.

142. van Dam, R.M., et al., *Dietary patterns and risk for type 2 diabetes mellitus in US men*. Annals of internal medicine, 2002. **136**(3): p. 201-209.

143. Akbaraly, T., et al., *Does overall diet in midlife predict future aging phenotypes? A cohort study*. The American journal of medicine, 2013. **126**(5): p. 411-419. e3.

144. UCL. *Diabetes treatments 'do more harm than good' for many people*. 2014 [cited 2017 Nov 24]; Available from: ucl.ac.uk/news/news-articles/0714/010714-Diabetes-treatments-do-more-harm- than-good.

145. Yudkin, J.S. and V.M. Montori, *Too Much Medicine: The epidemic of pre-diabetes: the medicine and the politics*. The BMJ, 2014. **349**.

146. Moore, E.M., et al., *Increased risk of cognitive impairment in patients with diabetes is associated with metformin*. Diabetes care, 2013. **36**(10): p. 2981-2987.

147. Rhee, M.K., et al., *Many Americans have pre-diabetes and should be considered for metformin therapy*. Diabetes Care, 2010. **33**(1): p. 49-54.

148.   Feinman, R.D., et al., *Dietary carbohydrate restriction as the first approach in diabetes management: critical review and evidence base.* Nutrition, 2015. **31**(1): p. 1-13.

149.   Mitrou, P., et al., *Vinegar consumption increases insulin-stimulated glucose uptake by the forearm muscle in humans with type 2 diabetes.* Journal of diabetes research, 2015. **2015**.

150.   Van Dam, R.M., et al., *Coffee, caffeine, and risk of type 2 diabetes.* Diabetes care, 2006. **29**(2): p. 398-403.

151.   Gulati, S., et al., *Effects of pistachio nuts on body composition, metabolic, inflammatory and oxidative stress parameters in Asian Indians with metabolic syndrome: a 24-wk, randomized control trial.* Nutrition, 2014. **30**(2): p. 192-197.

152.   Altshul, S., *Outsmart diabetes.* 2013, Prevention.

153.   Yina, J., H. Xing, and J. Yeb, *Efficacy of berberine in patients with type 2 diabetes.* Metabolism, 2008. **57**(5): p. 712-717.

154.   Gunn, J., C. Che, and N. Farnsworth, *Diabetes and Natural Products.* Bioactive Food as Dietary Interventions for Diabetes, ed. R. Watson and P. Preedy. 2013, San Diego, CA: Academic Press   381-394.

155.   Witte, A.V., et al., *Effects of resveratrol on memory performance, hippocampal functional connectivity, and glucose metabolism in healthy older adults.* Journal of Neuroscience, 2014. **34**(23): p. 7862-7870.

156.   Bhatt, J.K., S. Thomas, and M.J. Nanjan, *Resveratrol supplementation improves glycemic control in type 2 diabetes mellitus.* Nutrition research, 2012. **32**(7): p. 537-541.

157.   McIntosh, J. *What's to know about eczema?* 2017 [cited 2017 Nov 24]; Available from: https://www.medicalnewstoday.com/articles/14417.php.

158.   Habashy, J., D. Robles, and W. James. *Psoriasis.* 2017 [cited 2017 Nov 24]; Available from: https://emedicine.medscape.com/article/1943419-overview.

159.   Katta, R. and S.P. Desai, *Diet and dermatology: the role of dietary intervention in skin disease.* The Journal of clinical and aesthetic dermatology, 2014. **7**(7): p. 46.

160.   Gulliver, W.P. and H.J. Donsky, *A report on three recent clinical trials using Mahonia aquifolium 10% topical cream and a review of the worldwide clinical experience with Mahonia aquifolium for the treatment of plaque psoriasis.* American journal of therapeutics, 2005. **12**(5): p. 398-406.

161.   Thorne Research, I., *Berberine.* Altern Med Rev, 2000. **5**(2): p. 175-7.

162.   Millsop, J.W., et al., *Diet and psoriasis, part III: role of nutritional supplements.* Journal of the American Academy of Dermatology, 2014. **71**(3): p. 561-569.

163.   UChospitals. *Light Therapy for Skin.* 2017 [cited 2017 Nov 24]; Available from: uchospitals.edu/specialties/dermatology/light-therapy/.

164.   ewg. *Homepage.* 2016 [cited 2016 Nov 25]; Available from: https://www.ewg.org/.

165. NLM. *Migraine*. nd [cited 2017 Nov 25]; Available from: https://www.ncbi.nlm.nih.gov/pubmedhealth/PMHT0024778/.

166. Ramsden, C.E., et al., *Targeted alteration of dietary n-3 and n-6 fatty acids for the treatment of chronic headaches: a randomized trial*. PAIN®, 2013. **154**(11): p. 2441-2451.

167. Harrar, S. and S.A. O'Donnell, *The Woman's Book of Healing Herbs: healing teas, tonics, supplements, and formulas*. 1999: Rodale Press.

168. NHF. *Headache Sufferers' Diet*. 2012 [cited 2017 Nov 13]; Available from: http://www.headaches.org/2012/01/13/headache-sufferers-diet/.

169. Chawla, J. *Migraine Headache Treatment & Management*. 2017 [cited 2017 Nov 24]; Available from: emedicine.medscape.com/article/1142556-treatment.

170. Lawler, S.P. and L.D. Cameron, *A randomized, controlled trial of massage therapy as a treatment for migraine*. Annals of Behavioral Medicine, 2006. **32**(1): p. 50-59.

171. Arnadottir, T.S. and A.K. Sigurdardottir, *Is craniosacral therapy effective for migraine? Tested with HIT-6 Questionnaire*. Complementary therapies in clinical practice, 2013. **19**(1): p. 11-14.

172. Wells, R.E., et al., *Meditation for migraines: a pilot randomized controlled trial*. Headache: The Journal of Head and Face Pain, 2014. **54**(9): p. 1484-1495.

173. Mauskop, A. and B. Fox, *What Your Doctor May Not Tell You About (TM): Migraines: The Breakthrough Program That Can Help End Your Pain*. 2007: Grand Central Publishing.

174. Pareek, A., et al., *Feverfew (Tanacetum parthenium L.): A systematic review*. Pharmacognosy reviews, 2011. **5**(9): p. 103.

175. UMMC. *Feverfew*. 2015 [cited 2017 Nov 24]; Available from: http://www.umm.edu/health/medical/altmed/herb/feverfew.

176. Maghbooli, M., et al., *Comparison between the efficacy of ginger and sumatriptan in the ablative treatment of the common migraine*. Phytotherapy research, 2014. **28**(3): p. 412-415.

177. Shamliyan, T.A., et al., *Preventive pharmacologic treatments for episodic migraine in adults*. Journal of general internal medicine, 2013. **28**(9): p. 1225-1237.

178. NIDDK. *Irritable Bowel Syndrome (IBS)*. nd [cited 2017 Nov 23]; Available from: digestive.niddk.nih.gov/ddiseases/pubs/ibs/.

179. Newman, A.M., *The Essential IBS Book: Understanding and Managing Irritable Bowel Syndrome & Functional Dyspepsia*. Robert Rose. Inc. Toronto, Canada, 2011.

180. Lashner, B. *Best and Worst Foods for IBS*. 2014 [cited 2017 Nov 23]; Available from: health.clevelandclinic.org/2014/02/take-control-of-ibs-with-low-fodmap-diet/.

181. Sambrook, J. *IBS Diet Sheet*. nd [cited 2017 Nov 23]; Available from: patient.co.uk/health/irritable-bowel-syndrome-diet-sheet.

182. Fujimura, K.E., et al., *Role of the gut microbiota in defining human health.* Expert review of anti-infective therapy, 2010. **8**(4): p. 435-454.

183. Khanna, S. and P.K. Tosh. *A clinician's primer on the role of the microbiome in human health and disease.* in *Mayo Clinic Proceedings.* 2014. Elsevier.

184. AMA. *Human Microbiome.* nd [cited 2017 Nov 26]; Available from: academy.asm.org/images/stories/documents/FAQ_Human_Microbiome. pdf.

185. Suarez, K., et al., *Psychological stress and self-reported functional gastrointestinal disorders.* The Journal of nervous and mental disease, 2010. **198**(3): p. 226-229.

186. School, H.M. *Stress and the sensitive gut.* 2010 [cited 2017 Nov 25]; Available from: health.harvard.edu/newsletters/Harvard_Mental_Health_Letter/2010/ August/stress-and-the-sensitive-gut?utm_source=mental&utm_ medium=pressrelease&utm_campaign=mental0810.

187. Javed, Y. and A. Zagham, *Role of Omega-3 Fatty Acids in Irritable Bowel Syndrome (IBS).* International Journal of Pharmacological Research, 2016. **6**(8): p. 1-6.

188. Vanuytsel, T., J.F. Tack, and G.E. Boeckxstaens, *Treatment of abdominal pain in irritable bowel syndrome.* Journal of gastroenterology, 2014. **49**(8): p. 1193-1205.

189. drweil. *Irritable Bowel Syndrome.* nd [cited 2017 Nov 26]; Available from: https://www.drweil.com/.

190. NIDDK. *Acid Reflux (GER & GERD) in Adults.* nd [cited 2017 Nov 25].

191. Paddock, C. *Stress may cause illness by changing genes.* 2012 [cited 2017 Nov 28]; Available from: https://www.medicalnewstoday.com/articles/249215.php.

192. Masters, P.A., *Insomnia.* Annals of internal medicine, 2014. **161**(7): p. ITC1-ITC1.

193. *Prevention,* E.o., *The Belly Melt Diet.* 2012, Emmaus, PA: Rodale.

194. NINDS. *Brain Basics: Understanding Sleep.* nd [cited 2017 Nov 23]; Available from: https://www.ninds.nih.gov/Disorders/Patient-Caregiver-Education/Understanding-Sleep.

195. McIntosh, J. *Serotonin: Facts, What Does Serotonin Do?* 2016 [cited 2017 Nov 25]; Available from: medicalnewstoday.com/articles/232248.php.

196. Grisanti, R. *Insomnia Solution.* nd [cited 2017 Nov 26]; Available from: functionalmedicineuniversity.com/public/906.cfm.

197. Breus, M.J. *Kiwi: Super Food for Sleep?* 2013 [cited 2017 Nov 26]; Available from: psychologytoday.com/blog/sleep-newzzz/201311/kiwi-super-food-sleep.

198. Lin, H.-H., et al., *Effect of kiwifruit consumption on sleep quality in adults with sleep problems.* Asia Pacific journal of clinical nutrition, 2011. **20**(2): p. 169-174.

199. MedlinePlus. *Zolpidem.* 2017 May 15, 2017 [cited 2017 Nov 26]; Available from: nlm.nih.gov/medlineplus/druginfo/meds/a693025.html.

200. MIRECC/CoE. *Benzodiazepines.* nd [cited 2017 Nov 26]; Available from: https://www.mirecc.va.gov/visn4/bhl/docs/benzodiazepines.pdf.

201. Passos, G.S., et al., *Exercise improves immune function, antidepressive response, and sleep quality in patients with chronic primary insomnia.* BioMed research international, 2014. **2014.**

202. Khalsa, S.B.S., *Treatment of chronic insomnia with yoga: a preliminary study with sleep–wake diaries.* Applied psychophysiology and biofeedback, 2004. **29**(4): p. 269-278.

203. Abbasi, B., et al., *The effect of magnesium supplementation on primary insomnia in elderly: A double-blind placebo-controlled clinical trial.* Journal of research in medical sciences: the official journal of Isfahan University of Medical Sciences, 2012. **17**(12): p. 1161.

204. Kling, J., *he Strange Case of Premarin.* Modern Drug Discovery, 2000. **3**(8): p. 46-52.

205. Society, N.A.M., *The 2017 hormone therapy position statement of the North American Menopause Society.* Menopause (New York, NY), 2017. **24**(7): p. 728-753.

206. Herber-Gast, G.-C.M. and G.D. Mishra, *Fruit, Mediterranean-style, and high-fat and-sugar diets are associated with the risk of night sweats and hot flushes in midlife: results from a prospective cohort study.* The American journal of clinical nutrition, 2013. **97**(5): p. 1092-1099.

207. Ross, S.M., *Menopause: a standardized isopropanolic black cohosh extract (remifemin) is found to be safe and effective for menopausal symptoms.* Holistic nursing practice, 2012. **26**(1): p. 58-61.

208. Stojanovska, L., et al., *To exercise, or, not to exercise, during menopause and beyond.* Maturitas, 2014. **77**(4): p. 318-323.

209. Markham, H. *4 Ways To Fight Your Night Sweats.* 2013 [cited 2017 Nov 26]; Available from: prevention.com/health/health-concerns/activity-linked-fewer-night-sweats- menopause.

210. Dog, T.L. *3 Ways To Cool Hot Flashes.* 2013 [cited 2017 Nov 26]; Available from: https://www.prevention.com/health/health-concerns/natural-remedies-hot-flashes.

211. Clinic, C. *Menopause & Osteoporosis.* 2015 [cited 2017 Nov 26]; Available from: my.clevelandclinic.org/health/diseases_conditions/hic-what-is-perimenopause- menopause-postmenopause/hic_Menopause_and_Osteoporosis.

212. Chiu, H.-Y., et al., *Effects of acupuncture on menopause-related symptoms and quality of life in women in natural menopause: a meta-analysis of randomized controlled trials.* Menopause, 2015. **22**(2): p. 234-244.

213. Ladabaum, U., et al., *Obesity, abdominal obesity, physical activity, and caloric intake in US adults: 1988 to 2010.* The American journal of medicine, 2014. **127**(8): p. 717-727. e12.

214. Simmons, A.L., J.J. Schlezinger, and B.E. Corkey, *What are we putting in our food that is making us fat? Food additives, contaminants, and other putative contributors to obesity.* Current obesity reports, 2014. **3**(2): p. 273-285.

215. Kemps, E., M. Tiggemann, and S. Hollitt, *Exposure to television food advertising primes food-related cognitions and triggers motivation to eat.* Psychology & health, 2014. **29**(10): p. 1192-1205.

216. Prevention. *Eating pepper helps you eat fewer calories.* nd [cited 2017 Nov 26]; Available from: prevention .com/food/healthy-eating-tips/eating-pepper-helps-you-eat-fewer-calories.

217. Prevention. *Natural remedies: Safety herbal supplements.* nd [cited 2017 Nov 24]; Available from: prevention.com/mind-body/natural-remedies/safety-herbal-supplements?page=3&cm_BULbczB8WctNB879b%24ADD8jS47h=1412283273&cm_BUPYW3B8WctNB879b%24ADD8jS3oh=1413319480.

218. MedlinePlus. *Sinusitis.* 2016 [cited 2017 Nov 26]; Available from: nlm.nih.gov/medlineplus/sinusitis.html.

219. PCOM. *Improve Your Sinuses Today: What to Eat to Avoid Inflammation.* 2017 [cited 2017 Nov 26]; Available from: pacificcollege.edu/acupuncture-massage-news/articles/1126-improve-your- sinuses-today-what-to-eat-to-avoid-inflammation.html.

220. Connect, N. *Sinusitis: Dietary and Lifestyle Recommendations to improve symptoms.* nd [cited 2017 Nov 26]; Available from: naturopathconnect.com/articles/sinusitis-dietary/.

221. UMMC. *Elderberry.* 2016 [cited 2017 Nov 26]; Available from: http://www.umm.edu/health/medical/altmed/herb/elderberry.

222. UMMC. *Sinusitis.* 2016 [cited 2017 Nov 26]; Available from: umm.edu/health/medical/altmed/condition/sinusitis.

223. Glatthaar-Saalmüller, B., et al., *Antiviral activity in vitro of two preparations of the herbal medicinal product Sinupret® against viruses causing respiratory infections.* Phytomedicine, 2011. **19**(1): p. 1-7.

224. Zhang, S., et al., *Sinupret activates CFTR and TMEM16A-dependent transepithelial chloride transport and improves indicators of mucociliary clearance.* PloS one, 2014. **9**(8): p. e104090.

225. Gunnars, K. *23 Studies on Low-Carb and Low-Fat Diets — Time to Retire The Fad.* 2017 [cited 2017 Nov 26]; Available from: https://www.healthline.com/nutrition/23-studies-on-low-carb-and-low-fat-diets.

226. Samaha, F.F., et al., *A low-carbohydrate as compared with a low-fat diet in severe obesity.* N Engl J Med, 2003. **2003**(348): p. 2074-2081.

227. Volek, J.S., et al., *Carbohydrate restriction has a more favorable impact on the metabolic syndrome than a low fat diet.* Lipids, 2009. **44**(4): p. 297-309.

228. Brehm, B.J. and D.A. D'alessio, *Benefits of high-protein weight loss diets: enough evidence for practice?* Current Opinion in Endocrinology, Diabetes and Obesity, 2008. **15**(5): p. 416-421.

229. Sydney, T.U.o. *Search for glycemic index.* 2017 May 2017 [cited 2017 Nov 26]; Available from: glycemicindex.com.

230. Bazzano, L.A., et al., *Effects of Low-Carbohydrate and Low-Fat DietsA Randomized TrialEffects of Low-Carbohydrate and Low-Fat Diets.* Annals of internal medicine, 2014. **161**(5): p. 309-318.

231. Weber, B. *High-fiber diet linked to lower risk of heart disease.* 2013 [cited 2017 Nov 26]; Available from: medicalnewstoday.com/articles/270378.php.

232. HSPH. *Omega-3 Fatty Acids: An Essential Contribution.* 2017 [cited 2017 Nov 26]; Available from: hsph.harvard.edu/nutritionsource/omega-3/.

233. IFT. *9 fats to include in a healthy diet.* 2017 [cited 2017 Nov 26]; Available from: ift.org/newsroom/news-releases/2014/september/17/9-fats-to-include-in-a- healthy-diet.aspx.

234. WHFoods. *Are colored potatoes healthier than white potatoes?* nd [cited 2017 Nov 26]; Available from: whfoods.org/genpage.php?tname=dailytip&dbid=122.

235. Prevention. *Spices can alleviate common health problems.* nd [cited 2017 Nov 26]; Available from: prevention .com/food/food-remedies/spices-can-alleviate-common-health- problems.

236. Kalish, N. *10 Best Healing Herbs.* 2011 [cited 2017 Nov 26]; Available from: https://www.prevention.com/mind-body/natural-remedies/best-healing-herbs-top-10.

237. SEHN. *Precautionary principle-FAQs.* nd [cited 2017 Nov 26].

238. WHfoods. *Beef, grass-fed.* nd [cited 2017 Nov 27]; Available from: http://whfoods.com/genpage.php?tname=foodspice&dbid=141.

239. WHFoods. *Omega-3 fatty acids.* nd [cited 2017 Nov 27]; Available from: http://whfoods.com/genpage.php?tname=nutrient&dbid=84.

240. allergies, K.w.f. *Frequently Asked Questions About the Food Allergen Labeling Consumer Protection Act (FALCPA).* 2017 [cited 2017 Nov 27]; Available from: http://www.kidswithfoodallergies.org/page/label-law-food-allergen-labeling-consumer-protection-act.aspx.

241. Smith, J., et al., *Badditives!: The 13 Most Harmful Food Additives in Your Diet - And How to Avoid Them.* 2017: Skyhorse Publishing Company, Incorporated.

242. Fowler, S.P., et al., *Fueling the obesity epidemic? Artificially sweetened beverage use and long-term weight gain.* Obesity, 2008. **16**(8): p. 1894-1900.

243. Winter, R., *A consumer's dictionary of food additives: Descriptions in plain English of more than 12,000 ingredients both harmful and desirable found in foods*. 2009: Crown Archetype.

244. Institute, R. *Homepage*. 2017 [cited 2017 Nov 25]; Available from: rodaleinstitute.org.

245. USDA. *Organic agriculture*. 2017 [cited 2017 Nov 25]; Available from: usda.gov/wps/portal/usda/usdahome?contentidonly=true&contentid=organic-agriculture.html.

246. Ciardi, C., et al., *Food additives such as sodium sulphite, sodium benzoate and curcumin inhibit leptin release in lipopolysaccharide-treated murine adipocytes in vitro*. British journal of nutrition, 2012. **107**(6): p. 826-833.

247. Shamard, C. *Adult food allergies on the rise, report finds, but cause still unclear*. 2017 [cited 2017 Nov 27]; Available from: https://www.nbcnews.com/health/health-news/adult-food-allergies-rise-report-finds-cause-still-unclear-n805316.

248. Davis, W., *Wheat belly: lose the wheat, lose the weight, and find your path back to health*. 2014: Rodale.

249. Perlmutter, D., *Grain Brain: The Surprising Truth about Wheat, Carbs, and Sugar-Your Brain's Silent Killers*. 2014: Hachette UK.

250. Brown, A.C., *Gluten sensitivity: problems of an emerging condition separate from celiac disease*. Expert review of gastroenterology & hepatology, 2012. **6**(1): p. 43-55.

251. Michaëlsson, K., et al., *Milk intake and risk of mortality and fractures in women and men: cohort studies*. Bmj, 2014. **349**: p. g6015.

252. PCRM. *Health Concerns about Dairy Products*. nd [cited 2017 Nov 28]; Available from: http://www.pcrm.org/health/diets/vegdiets/health-concerns-about-dairy-products.

253. NIDDK. *Lactose Intolerance*. 2014 [cited 2017 Nov 27]; Available from: https://www.niddk.nih.gov/health-information/digestive-diseases/lactose-intolerance.

254. Reports, C., *Taking antibiotics off your fast food menu*. 2017, Consumer Reports.

255. USGS. *The water in you*. 2016 [cited 2017 Nov 26]; Available from: https://water.usgs.gov/edu/propertyyou.html.

256. HSPH. *Healthy Drinks*. 2017 [cited 2017 Nov 27]; Available from: https://www.hsph.harvard.edu/nutritionsource/healthy-drinks/.

257. UMMC. *Green Tea*. 2015 [cited 2017 Nov 27]; Available from: http://www.umm.edu/health/medical/altmed/herb/green-tea.

258. Arab, L., W. Liu, and D. Elashoff, *Green and black tea consumption and risk of stroke*. Stroke, 2009. **40**(5): p. 1786-1792.

259. MedlinePlus. *Black Tea*. 2017 [cited 2017 Nov 27]; Available from: https://medlineplus.gov/druginfo/natural/997.html.

260. Prevention. *The Smoothie Cure For Gas And Bloating.* nd [cited 2017 Nov 27]; Available from: https://www.prevention.com/mind-body/natural-remedies/natural-remedy-gas-and-bloating.

261. Floegel, A., et al., *Coffee consumption and risk of chronic disease in the European Prospective Investigation into Cancer and Nutrition (EPIC)–Germany study.* The American journal of clinical nutrition, 2012. **95**(4): p. 901-908.

262. Bidel, S., et al., *Coffee consumption and risk of total and cardiovascular mortality among patients with type 2 diabetes.* Diabetologia, 2006. **49**(11): p. 2618-2626.

263. Bamia, C., et al., *Coffee, tea and decaffeinated coffee in relation to hepatocellular carcinoma in a European population: multicentre, prospective cohort study.* International journal of cancer, 2015. **136**(8): p. 1899-1908.

264. Nestle, M., *What to eat: An aisle-by-aisle guide to savvy food choices and good eating.* The Free Library, 2006.

265. Suez, J., et al., *Artificial sweeteners induce glucose intolerance by altering the gut microbiota.* Nature, 2014. **514**(7521): p. 181-186.

266. WebMD. *Moderate alcohol drinking may cut A lzheimers risk.* 2011 [cited 2017 Nov 27]; Available from: webmd.com/alzheimers/news/20110817/moderate-alcohol-drinking-may-cut-alzheimers-risk.

267. Barlow, R. *A drink a day raises cancer risk, study says.* 2013 [cited 2017 Nov 27]; Available from: http://www.bu.edu/today/2013/a-drink-a-day-raises-cancer-risk-study-says/.

268. WebMD. *Alcohol and Heart Disease.* 2017 [cited 2017 Nov 27]; Available from: https://www.webmd.com/heart-disease/guide/heart-disease-alcohol-your-heart.

269. Mangin, M., R. Sinha, and K. Fincher, *Inflammation and vitamin D: the infection connection.* Inflammation Research, 2014. **63**(10): p. 803-819.

270. Kahleova, H., et al., *Eating two larger meals a day (breakfast and lunch) is more effective than six smaller meals in a reduced-energy regimen for patients with type 2 diabetes: a randomised crossover study.* Diabetologia, 2014. **57**(8): p. 1552-1560.

271. Cheung, L. *Definition of Mindful eating.* nd [cited 2017 Nov 27]; Available from: https://www.lexiconoffood.com/definition/definition-mindful-eating.

272. Rossy, L., *The Mindfulness-Based Eating Solution: Proven Strategies to End Overeating, Satisfy Your Hunger, and Savor Your Life.* 2016: New Harbinger Publications.

273. CDC. *Chronic Disease Overview.* 2017; Available from: https://www.cdc.gov/chronicdisease/overview/index.htm.

274. Veerman, J.L., et al., *Television viewing time and reduced life expectancy: a life table analysis.* British journal of sports medicine, 2011: p. bjsports085662.

275. Kruk, J., *Physical activity in the prevention of the most frequent chronic diseases: an analysis of the recent evidence.* Asian Pacific Journal of Cancer Prevention, 2007. **8**(3): p. 325.

276. Elsawy, B. and K.E. Higgins, *Physical activity guidelines for older adults.* American family physician, 2010. **81**(1): p. 55-9.

277. Mons, U., H. Hahmann, and H. Brenner, *A reverse J-shaped association of leisure time physical activity with prognosis in patients with stable coronary heart disease: evidence from a large cohort with repeated measurements.* Heart, 2014: p. heartjnl-2013-305242.

278. Di Raimondo, D., et al., *Metabolic and anti-inflammatory effects of a home-based programme of aerobic physical exercise.* International journal of clinical practice, 2013. **67**(12): p. 1247-1253.

279. Watch, H.M.s.H. *Walking your steps to health.* 2009 [cited 2017 Nov 23]; Available from: https://www.health.harvard.edu/newsletter_article/walking-your-steps-to-health.

280. Shiraev, T. and G. Barclay, *Evidence based exercise: Clinical benefits of high intensity interval training.* Australian family physician, 2012. **41**(12): p. 960.

281. Altshul, S. *Body fat is the deadliest organ.* 2013 [cited 2017 Nov 27]; Available from: https://www.prevention.com/health/diabetes/avoid-belly-fat.

282. Guest, A. and M. Apgar, *Promoting and prescribing exercise for the elderly.* American family physician, 2002. **65**: p. 3.

283. School, H.M. *Understanding the stress response: Chronic activation of this survival mechanism impairs health.* 2011 March 18, 2016 [cited 2017 Nov 26]; Available from: https://www.health.harvard.edu/staying-healthy/understanding-the-stress-response.

284. Rabkin, J.G. and E.L. Struening, *Life events, stress, and illness.* Science, 1976. **194**(4269): p. 1013-1020.

285. Cohen, S., et al., *Chronic stress, glucocorticoid receptor resistance, inflammation, and disease risk.* Proceedings of the National Academy of Sciences, 2012. **109**(16): p. 5995-5999.

286. Cohen, S., D.A. Tyrrell, and A.P. Smith, *Psychological stress and susceptibility to the common cold.* New England journal of medicine, 1991. **325**(9): p. 606-612.

287. Becker, R. and G. Selden, *The body electric: Electromagnetism and the foundation of life.* 1998: Harper Collins.

288. Lipton, B.H., *The Biology of Belief 10th Anniversary Edition: Unleashing the Power of Consciousness, Matter & Miracles.* 2015: Hay House, Inc.

289. Pert, C., *Molecules of emotion: the science behind mind–body medicine*. New York: Touchstone. 1999, Simon and Schuster.

290. Church, D., *The genie in your genes: Epigenetic medicine and the new biology of intention*. 2009: Elite Books.

291. Chödrön, P., *How to meditate: A practical guide to making friends with your mind*. 2016: Jaico Publishing House.

292. Kornfield, J., *Meditation for beginners: Six guided meditations for insight, inner clarity, and cultivating a compassionate heart*. 2005: Random House.

293. Kabat-Zinn, J., *Guided Mindfulness Meditation (Guided Mindfulness)[UNABRIDGED](Audio CD)*. 2005: Sounds True.

294. Naparstek, B., *Guided imagery: A portable, scalable, user-friendly 24/7 self administered audio intervention for hospital patients and their families*. 2016: Keck Medicine, USC.

295. EFT. *Emotional Freedom Techniques: The birth of EFT*. nd [cited 2017 Nov 28]; Available from: http://eft-help.com/intro/EFThistory.htm.

296. Ortner, N., *The Tapping Solution: A Revolutionary System for Stress-free Living*. 2013: Hay House, Inc.

297. universe, E. *6 successful sessions with a war veteran*. nd [cited 2017 Nov 28]; Available from: http://www.eftuniverse.com/trauma-and-abuse/6-successful-sessions-with-a-war-veteran.

298. Institute, H. *Our purpose*. 2017 [cited 2017 Nov 28]; Available from: heartmath.org.

299. Sirois, F.M., R. Kitner, and J.K. Hirsch, *Self-compassion, affect, and health-promoting behaviors*. Health Psychology, 2015. **34**(6): p. 661.

300. centre, T.b. *the buddhistcentre: buddhism for today*. nd [cited 2017 Nov 28]; Available from: https://thebuddhistcentre.com/text/loving-kindness-meditation.

301. Drweil. *Three breathing exercise and techniques*. 2017 [cited 2017 Nov 28]; Available from: https://www.drweil.com/health-wellness/body-mind-spirit/stress-anxiety/breathing-three-exercises/.

302. Goleman, D., *Emotional Intelligence. Why It Can Matter More than IQ*. Learning, 1996. **24**(6): p. 49-50.

303. Conley, C.C., B.T. Bishop, and B.L. Andersen. *Emotions and Emotion Regulation in Breast Cancer Survivorship*. in *Healthcare*. 2016. Multidisciplinary Digital Publishing Institute.

304. Seligman, M.E., *Flourish: A visionary new understanding of happiness and well-being*. 2012: Simon and Schuster.

305. Moore, C., *The resilience breakthrough: 27 tools for turning adversity into action*. 2014: Greenleaf Book Group.

Made in the USA
Columbia, SC
21 March 2018